Get Through

**Final FRCR Part A:
SBAs for the Modular Examination**

To our families, with love

Get Through

Final FRCR Part A: SBAs for the Modular Examination

Megan Bydder MB ChB MRCP FRCR
Specialist Registrar in Radiology, University Hospital of North Staffordshire,
Stoke-on-Trent, UK

Alexander Clark MA(Cantab) MB BChir FRCR
Consultant Radiologist, University Hospital of North Staffordshire, Stoke-on-Trent, UK

Nicholas Coupe BSc MB ChB MRCS
Specialist Registrar in Radiology, University Hospital of North Staffordshire,
Stoke-on-Trent, UK

John Pattison MB BS MRCS FRCR
Consultant Radiologist, Royal Shrewsbury Hospital, Shrewsbury, UK

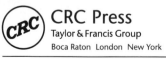

CRC Press
Taylor & Francis Group
Boca Raton London New York

CRC Press is an imprint of the
Taylor & Francis Group, an **informa** business

First published in Great Britain in 2009 by the Royal Society of Medicine Press Ltd
Reprinted in 2012 by Hodder Arnold

Published 2014 by
CRC Press
Taylor & Francis Group
6000 Broken Sound Parkway NW, Suite 300
Boca Raton, FL 33487-2742

Visit the Taylor & Francis Web site at
http://www.taylorandfrancis.com

and the CRC Press Web site at
http://www.crcpress.com

Contents

Preface

In 2008 the Royal College of Radiologists announced proposed changes to the format of the Examinations for the Fellowship in Clinical Radiology, which included the introduction of single best answer questions (SBAs) for the Final FRCR Part A examination from the Autumn 2009 sitting.

SBAs are being increasingly adopted by the Royal Colleges, because they have a number of advantages over traditional true/false multiple-choice questions. In particular they are better suited to the assessment of higher levels of knowledge such as problem-solving and decision-making, and are more relevant to everyday clinical practice.

The modular format of the Final FRCR Part A examination remains, and the following six modules are examined:

  Module 1: Cardiothoracic and Vascular
  Module 2: Musculoskeletal and Trauma
  Module 3: Gastrointestinal
  Module 4: Genitourinary, Adrenal, Obstetrics & Gynaecology, and
      Breast
  Module 5: Paediatrics
  Module 6: Central Nervous System and Head & Neck

Each module consists of a single paper of two hours in duration containing 75 questions. Radiological anatomy and techniques continue to be part of the Final FRCR Part A examination, but physics is now examined entirely in the First FRCR examination. Negative marking has been discontinued. Further detailed guidance is available from the College website (www.rcr.ac.uk).

This book contains six chapters mirroring the six modules of the Final FRCR Part A examination, each of which contains 100 single best answer format questions. The questions have been written using the commonly used radiology textbooks, together with specialist textbooks and radiology journals. All questions are accompanied by detailed explanations, and are comprehensively referenced for further reading. Many of the journal references are available in free full-text version on the internet. To provide additional feedback, each question is assigned a difficulty level, ranging from * (easiest) to ***** (most difficult).

This book aims to give radiology trainees a valuable insight into the new Final FRCR Part A examination format, while providing a comprehensive collection of practice questions to aid thorough preparation for the examination.

Single best answer question (SBA) format

SBAs are composed of a stem, often in the form of a clinical scenario, followed by a question to which the candidate must select a single response from a list of possible options. The options consist of one correct answer and a number of incorrect options or distractors, which are not necessarily completely wrong, merely less correct in the given scenario.

When attempting SBAs, it is advisable to read the question carefully and attempt to formulate the answer initially without looking at the options. If you are unsure of the answer, it is usually possible to eliminate several of the distractors, improving your chances of guessing the answer correctly. If you are unable to answer the question straight away, return to it at a later stage. Ensure that you give yourself time to attempt all the questions, and do not leave any out, as incorrect answers are no longer penalised.

In our experience, attempting practice questions is essential for optimal exam preparation, as a means of identifying gaps in knowledge and, when performed under examination conditions, as a valuable self-assessment technique. In addition, increasing familiarity with the examination format is likely to enhance performance.

Further information about single best answer format questions and guidance on attempting them can be obtained from these sources:

Case SM, Swanson DB. *Constructing Written Test Questions for the Basic and Clinical Sciences*, 3rd edn. Philadelphia: National Board of Medical Examiners. Available at: www.nbme.org/publications/item-writing-manual.html.

McCoubrie P, McKnight L. Single best answer MCQs: a new format for the FRCR part 2a exam. *Clin Radiol* 2008; 63: 506–10.

Abbreviations

2D	two-dimensional
ADC	apparent diffusion coefficient
AFP	alfa-fetoprotein
AIDS	acquired immune deficiency syndrome
AP	anteroposterior
β-hCG	beta-human chorionic gonadotrophin
CA-15-3	cancer antigen 15-3
CA-125	cancer antigen 125
CA-19-9	carbohydrate antigen 19-9
CEA	carcinoembryonic antigen
CMV	cytomegalovirus
CNS	central nervous system
CSF	cerebrospinal fluid
CT	computed tomography
CT KUB	computed tomography of the kidneys, ureters and bladder
DMSA	dimercaptosuccinic acid
DNA	deoxyribonucleic acid
DTPA	diethylene triamine pentaacetic acid
DWI	diffusion-weighted imaging
ECD	ethyl cysteine dimer
ECG	electrocardiogram
ERCP	endoscopic retrograde cholangiopancreatography
^{18}FDG	[^{18}F]-fluorodeoxyglucose
FLAIR	fluid-attenuated inversion recovery
FNA	fine-needle aspiration
FOV	field of view
GCS	Glasgow Coma Scale
Gd	gadolinium
GI	gastrointestinal
HIV	human immunodeficiency virus
HMPAO	hexamethylpropylene amine oxime
HMSO	Her Majesty's Stationery Office
HU	Hounsfield units
IDA	iminodiacetic acid
^{111}In	indium-111
IQ	intelligence quotient
IVC	inferior vena cava
IVU	intravenous urogram
MAA	macroaggregated albumin
MAG3	mercaptoacetyltriglycine
MIBG	metaiodobenzylguanidine
MR	magnetic resonance
MRCP	magnetic resonance cholangiopancreatography
MRI	magnetic resonance imaging
Na$^+$/K$^+$ ATPase	sodium–potassium adenosine triphosphatase
PA	posteroanterior
pANCA	perinuclear anti-neutrophil cytoplasmic antibody

PET	positron emission tomography
PET/CT	combined positron emission and computed tomography
PSA	prostate-specific antigen
SPECT	single photon emission computed tomography
STIR	short TI inversion recovery
SVC	superior vena cava
T1W	T1-weighted
T2W	T2-weighted
T2*W	T2*-weighted
^{99m}Tc	technetium-99m
TNM	TNM Classification of Malignant Tumours
$\dot{V}/\dot{Q}$	ventilation–perfusion
WHO	World Health Organization

MODULE I
CARDIOTHORACIC AND VASCULAR

Module 1: Cardiothoracic and Vascular: Questions

1) A 40-year-old male presents with shortness of breath. He also has lower back pain and stiffness of the spine. A chest radiograph shows bilateral upper-zone fibrosis with elevation of the hila. Spinal ligamentous ossification is also noted. High-resolution CT shows peripheral interstitial changes with traction bronchiectasis and paraseptal emphysematous changes in the upper zones. What is the most likely diagnosis?

   a. ankylosing spondylitis
   b. Reiter's syndrome
   c. tuberculosis
   d. sarcoidosis
   e. chronic extrinsic allergic alveolitis

2) In acute respiratory distress syndrome what is the first change usually seen on the chest radiograph?

   a. confluent consolidation
   b. pleural effusions
   c. increased heart size with globular shape
   d. volume loss with atelectasis
   e. patchy ill-defined opacities

3) A 32-year-old female presents with shortness of breath and haemoptysis. There is no leg swelling and an ECG is normal. A chest radiograph shows a triangular, pleurally based opacity in the right mid-zone with an ipsilateral effusion. Which investigation would be most helpful in making the diagnosis?

   a. $\dot{V}/\dot{Q}$ scan
   b. CT pulmonary angiogram
   c. conventional pulmonary angiogram
   d. high-resolution CT
   e. staging CT of chest

4) A 56-year-old female patient presents with shortness of breath. A chest radiograph is unremarkable. A high-resolution CT scan is performed which shows mosaic perfusion with no air trapping on expiratory scan. What is the most likely diagnosis?

   a. bronchiolitis obliterans
   b. cystic fibrosis
   c. hypersensitivity pneumonitis
   d. chronic thromboembolic disease
   e. asthma

5) A 28-year-old male with known Marfan's syndrome presents with chest pain and shortness of breath. An echocardiogram is performed. What are the most likely findings?

a. aortic regurgitation and dilatation
b. pulmonary stenosis
c. aortic stenosis and post-stenotic dilatation
d. global myocardial wall thickening
e. ventricular septal defect

6) Into which structure does the thoracic duct normally drain?

a. left brachiocephalic vein
b. left internal jugular vein
c. left subclavian vein
d. superior vena cava
e. junction of left subclavian and internal jugular veins

7) A 43-year-old man with a previous history of polytrauma requiring a long period in intensive care for acute respiratory distress syndrome presents with shortness of breath. An abnormal chest radiograph prompts a high-resolution CT scan. What are the most likely findings?

a. bronchiectasis in the lower lobes
b. pleural effusions
c. fibrosis with volume loss in the upper lobes
d. reticular changes in the anterior aspects of the lungs
e. reticular changes in the posterior aspects of the lungs

8) In systemic sclerosis, what is the most common pulmonary finding on CT?

a. consolidation secondary to aspiration pneumonia
b. pulmonary hypertension
c. pleural effusions
d. interstitial lung disease
e. pulmonary emboli

9) A 28-year-old female presents with menorrhagia and dysmenorrhoea. An ultrasound scan shows a large fibroid in the uterus measuring 7 cm. An MR scan confirms an intramural fibroid which enhances vividly. The patient undergoes uterine artery embolization. What is the commonest complication occurring in the first 12 months following this procedure?

a. premature ovarian failure
b. failure of therapy with need for re-embolization or hysterectomy
c. hysterectomy for uterine infection or pain
d. persistent non-offensive vaginal discharge
e. post-embolization syndrome

10) A 55 year old presents with chest pain. His blood tests show a mild troponin rise, but an ECG is normal. A chest radiograph shows bilateral, symmetrical, hilar adenopathy but no other abnormality. Which feature on cardiac MRI would make cardiac sarcoid a more likely diagnosis than ischaemia secondary to coronary artery disease?

   a. delayed hyperenhancement of lateral wall
   b. full-thickness, abnormal, high T2 signal in lateral wall
   c. reduced inferior wall motility
   d. partial-thickness, abnormal, high T2 signal with subendocardial sparing at base of septum
   e. segmental area of reduced enhancement in lateral wall on early phase study

11) Which of the following best describes the radiographic changes seen in acute rejection of a lung transplant?

   a. mosaic perfusion and air trapping
   b. pleural effusion and septal thickening with no left ventricular dysfunction
   c. bilateral consolidation at the bases
   d. increased lung volumes
   e. globular heart and bat-wing perihilar consolidation

12) An 87-year-old male presents with fever and cough. A chest radiograph shows dense consolidation in the right mid-zone, which is seen to be in the apical segment of the lower lobe on a lateral view. The oblique fissure is seen to be bulging away from the consolidation. There is an associated effusion. What is the most likely diagnosis?

   a. *Haemophilus influenzae* pneumonia
   b. *Staphylococcus aureus* pneumonia
   c. *Streptococcus pneumoniae* pneumonia
   d. Klebsiella pneumonia
   e. Legionnaires' disease

13) A 76-year-old female presents with haemoptysis and cough. A chest radiograph shows a mass in the right upper lobe that contains a crescent of air. Which feature on CT would make a cavitating malignancy more likely than aspergilloma?

   a. thin cavity wall
   b. high-density central mass
   c. enhancing central mass
   d. calcification
   e. adjacent bronchiectasis

14) A 42-year-old male presents with stridor and persistent cough. He previously has had several nosebleeds. Bloods show mild renal impairment. A chest radiograph shows multiple cavitary lesions with irregular lining, predominantly in the lower lobes. What is the most likely diagnosis?

a. metastatic disease from nasopharyngeal carcinoma
b. Wegener's granulomatosis
c. sarcoidosis
d. pyogenic abscesses
e. systemic lupus erythematosus

15) A 32-year-old male presents with increasing shortness of breath following a road traffic accident, in which he sustained multiple long bone fractures. At 48 hours post-injury, his chest radiograph is normal. The next day a $\dot{V}/\dot{Q}$ scan shows patchy, mottled, peripheral perfusion defects. The following day a chest radiograph shows patchy, bilateral, alveolar infiltrates. What is the most likely diagnosis?

a. fat embolism
b. thrombotic embolism
c. atypical infection
d. pulmonary contusions
e. pulmonary oedema

16) A 50-year-old male with known chronic asthma is seen in an outpatient clinic. He has no current symptoms. A 'routine' chest radiograph is performed. Which feature is most likely to be seen?

a. hyperexpansion
b. peribronchial cuffing
c. bronchiectasis
d. parenchymal scars
e. normal chest radiograph

17) A 65-year-old man presents with painful wrists and ankles. There is no digital clubbing. A chest radiograph shows a well-defined pleural mass, forming an obtuse angle with the chest wall. CT confirms an ovoid, pleurally based, enhancing mass with no bone destruction, effusion or volume loss. Radiographs of the wrists and ankles show symmetrical periosteal reaction. What is the most likely diagnosis?

a. hypertrophic osteoarthropathy with bronchogenic carcinoma
b. hypertrophic osteoarthropathy with malignant mesothelioma
c. hypertrophic osteoarthropathy with pleural fibroma
d. rheumatoid arthritis
e. tuberculosis

18) A right-sided aortic arch with mirror-image branching is most frequently associated with which congenital cardiac abnormality?

a. pulmonary atresia and ventricular septal defect
b. truncus arteriosus
c. uncomplicated ventricular septal defect
d. Fallot's tetralogy
e. corrected transposition of the great vessels

19) A 68-year-old man presents with increasing dyspnoea. He has a history of asbestos exposure. CT of the chest demonstrates bilateral pleural thickening with calcification, and a 3 cm, rounded, lower lobe mass. This is related to an area of pleural thickening, with bronchovascular markings coursing from it towards the hilum in a curved path. What is the most likely diagnosis?

a. rounded atelectasis
b. bronchogenic carcinoma
c. tuberculosis
d. silicosis
e. round pneumonia

20) A 43-year-old female with Churg–Strauss syndrome has a high-resolution CT. What is the most likely finding?

a. small centrilobular nodules
b. bullous disease
c. bilateral, symmetrical, hilar lymphadenopathy
d. tumour-like mass
e. pleural effusion

21) A 32-year-old male presents with headaches and bilateral lower limb claudication. He is noted to have weak pulses in the lower limbs. A chest radiograph shows a 'figure-3' indentation of the aorta and inferior rib notching. The cardiac apex is elevated. There is no previous medical history. What is the most likely diagnosis?

a. superior vena caval obstruction
b. aortic dissection
c. coarctation of the aorta
d. aortic thrombosis
e. transposition of the great vessels

22) A 25-year-old male presents with recurrent epistaxis, which is progressively worsening. On examination he is noted to have multiple, red, vascular skin blemishes. A chest radiograph shows several opacities in the lung measuring up to 3 cm with bands of opacification extending to the hila. No calcification is seen. What is the most likely diagnosis?

a. hereditary haemorrhagic telangiectasia
b. neurofibromatosis
c. tuberous sclerosis
d. Wegener's granulomatosis
e. sarcoidosis

23) A 40-year-old female presents with a stroke, which is confirmed on CT of brain. She gives a history of worsening claudication of the limbs and a long history of fever and myalgia. CT of the neck and thorax shows thickening of the arterial walls of the aorta and major vessels with irregular stenotic lesions throughout the aorta, with focal areas of dilatation and stenosis in the brachiocephalic arteries and carotid arteries. What is the most likely diagnosis?

a. fibromuscular dysplasia
b. syphilis
c. atherosclerosis
d. Marfan's syndrome
e. Takayasu's arteritis

24) The bronchial tree receives blood from one right and two left bronchial arteries. From which vessel does the single right artery usually arise?

a. aorta
b. joint origin with left bronchial arteries
c. second posterior right intercostal artery
d. third posterior right intercostal artery
e. fourth posterior right intercostal artery

25) A patient with known polyarteritis nodosa presents with acute left loin pain. Which of the following is most likely to be seen on ultrasound scan?

a. hydronephrosis
b. a solid mass with a perinephric collection
c. multiple renal artery aneurysms and perinephric collection
d. crossed fused ectopia
e. small kidneys with increased echogenicity

26) A 5-year-old female presents with intermittent, colicky, epigastric discomfort with no specific features. A CT shows transverse colon protruding through a small defect anteriorly in the diaphragm in a parasternal position. What is the most likely diagnosis?

a. Bochdalek's hernia
b. Morgagni's hernia
c. rolling hiatus hernia
d. eventration
e. septum transversum defect

27) A 45-year-old female presents with malaise and cough. She has a history of multiple allergies. Her blood results show an eosinophilia, and the chest radiograph reveals two areas of peripheral consolidation. A further chest radiograph 2 days later shows these to be resolving. Which of the following is the most likely diagnosis?

a. histiocytosis
b. pseudomonas pneumonia
c. Klebsiella pneumonia
d. Loeffler's syndrome
e. lipoid pneumonia

28) A 26-year-old intravenous drug user presents with reduced conscious level, associated pyrexia and malaise. Clinically, there is a systolic murmur, mild hypotension and an elevated white cell count. A chest radiograph shows multiple opacities in the mid and lower zones, some of which are cavitating. What is the most appropriate next investigation?

a. CT of the thorax
b. transthoracic echocardiogram
c. white cell scan
d. MRI of the heart
e. transoesophageal echocardiogram

29) A 64-year-old man presents with pain in the left arm when exercising, associated with a headache. The clinical team suspect subclavian steal syndrome. Ultrasound scan, however, shows normal flow in the carotid and vertebral arteries bilaterally. What is most likely to happen to the flow in the vessels during patient exercise to reproduce the pain?

a. reversal of flow in the right carotid artery
b. reversal of flow in the left carotid artery
c. reversal of flow in the right vertebral artery
d. reversal of flow in the left vertebral artery
e. no change

30) A 19-year-old male presents following blunt chest trauma, with dyspnoea, chest pain and haemoptysis. A chest radiograph shows bilateral pneumothoraces, subcutaneous emphysema and bilateral fractures of multiple upper ribs. The pneumothoraces fail to resolve despite chest drains and he needs intubation and ventilation. Which finding at CT would be most suggestive of the diagnosis of tracheal injury?

a. pneumomediastinum
b. bilateral pneumothorax
c. mediastinal haematoma
d. focal overdistension of endotracheal tube cuff
e. chylothorax

31) An 80-year-old man presents with haemoptysis and a mass on chest radiograph. A biopsy shows non-small-cell lung cancer. CT of chest shows a 4 cm, right middle lobe mass with pleural tethering but no chest wall invasion. Lymph nodes are seen at the right hilum (17 mm short axis), in the subcarinal space (20 mm short axis) and in the aortopulmonary space (8 mm short axis). No other abnormalities are seen. What is the TNM stage?

a. T2 N1 M0
b. T2 N2 M0
c. T2 N3 M0
d. T3 N1 M0
e. T3 N2 M0

32) A 48-year-old female with known lung cancer undergoes an ^{18}FDG PET/CT scan. The tumour is highly FDG avid. Several areas of moderate uptake are noted on the study. Which of the following findings is of concern with regard to metastatic disease?

a. diffuse thyroid uptake
b. symmetrical nasopharyngeal tonsil uptake
c. diffuse uptake in caecal wall
d. focal paravertebral muscle uptake
e. focal uterine cavity uptake

33) A 42-year-old female with tuberous sclerosis presents with flank pain. Ultrasound scan and CT demonstrate a 7 cm renal angiomyo-lipoma, with multiple similar smaller lesions in both kidneys. No evidence of acute haemorrhage is seen. She undergoes embolization with polyvinyl alcohol particles. After 48 hours, she presents again with flank pain and is found to have a large perinephric haematoma on the side of the embolization. What is the most likely cause?

a. vascular trauma during embolization
b. spontaneous haemorrhage from non-embolized lesion
c. post-embolization rupture
d. revascularization of embolized lesion
e. inadequate embolization material used

34) In ventilation–perfusion scintigraphy, which of the following is suggestive of an intermediate probability of pulmonary embolism?

   a. matched non-segmental defects with a normal chest radiograph
   b. multiple unmatched small perfusion defects with normal ventilation
   c. large, segmental, matched defect with similar-sized opacity on chest radiograph
   d. reverse mismatch
   e. two large, unmatched, segmental, perfusion defects

35) A 78-year-old man presents with superior vena caval syndrome. A CT scan shows an irregular mass in the superior mediastinum causing near-total occlusion of the superior vena cava. There is no sign of respiratory compromise or raised intracranial pressure. Which of the following would be the most appropriate next step in the patient's management?

   a. obtain tissue diagnosis
   b. chemotherapy
   c. radiotherapy
   d. stenting of superior vena cava
   e. surgical bypass

36) A 68-year-old patient presents with cough and dyspnoea. A chest radiograph is performed. Which feature would suggest sarcoidosis as a more likely diagnosis than tuberculosis?

   a. pleural effusion
   b. cavitating upper lobe lesion
   c. calcified lung lesion
   d. symmetrical hilar lymphadenopathy
   e. consolidation

37) A 57-year-old man presents with chest pain and fever after an episode of vomiting. A chest radiograph shows a small left pleural effusion and pneumomediastinum. Which investigation will best establish the diagnosis?

   a. CT of the chest
   b. barium swallow
   c. water-soluble contrast swallow
   d. MRI
   e. transoesophageal echocardiogram

38) A 65-year-old male presents with a 2-month history of cough and dyspnoea and has had swelling of the face, neck and arms for 1 week. He has had tuberculosis in the past. CT shows an irregular right paratracheal mass with calcification that is compressing the superior vena cava and right main bronchus, with patchy consolidation in the right lung. What is the most likely diagnosis?

a. small-cell carcinoma
b. lymphoma
c. malignant teratoma
d. fibrosing mediastinitis
e. bronchogenic cyst

39) A 48-year-old female patient presents with mild dyspnoea on exertion. A chest radiograph shows fine calcification overlying the cardiac silhouette adjacent to the left sternal edge at the level of the fourth intercostal space. What is the most likely cause?

a. rheumatic heart disease
b. bicuspid valve
c. syphilis
d. ankylosing spondylitis
e. normal ageing

40) A 37-year-old male presents to accident and emergency following smoke inhalation in a fire. He feels well and a chest radiograph is normal. The following day he re-presents feeling short of breath and unwell. What are the most likely findings on the chest radiograph now?

a. pulmonary oedema
b. pleural effusions
c. upper-zone consolidation
d. diffuse reticular change
e. pneumothorax

41) A 40-year-old female with known history of seizures and low IQ presents with severe shortness of breath, progressively worsening over a number of years. A chest radiograph shows extensive honey-combing throughout both lungs, which are of normal volume. A small pneumothorax is also seen on the right side. What is the most likely diagnosis?

a. sarcoidosis
b. cystic fibrosis
c. tuberous sclerosis
d. lymphangiomyomatosis
e. idiopathic pulmonary fibrosis

42) A 28-year-old male is involved in a road traffic accident and sustains chest trauma. He has chest pain and bruising over the chest with reduced blood pressure. A chest radiograph shows a shift of the trachea to the right at T3–4 level with depression of the left main bronchus and loss of clarity of the aortic knuckle. Which diagnosis should be considered?

a. aortic rupture
b. bronchial rupture
c. superior vena caval laceration
d. azygos vein injury
e. internal mammary artery injury

43) A 35 year old with asthma presents with malaise, flu-like illness and cough. Previous similar episodes have occurred. A chest radiograph shows patchy airspace opacification in the mid and upper zones. Which feature on high-resolution CT would make allergic bronchopulmonary aspergillosis a more likely diagnosis than extrinsic allergic alveolitis?

a. widespread centrilobular micronodules <3 mm
b. tubular finger-like opacities
c. bronchiectasis
d. upper-zone fibrosis
e. pleural effusion

44) A 38-year-old pregnant female presents with haemoptysis and shortness of breath. A chest radiograph shows a large effusion, which is drained and found to be chylous. What is the most likely diagnosis?

a. histiocytosis
b. tuberous sclerosis
c. neurofibromatosis
d. lymphangiomyomatosis
e. idiopathic pulmonary fibrosis

45) A 42-year-old female patient presents with a swollen calf, and deep venous thrombosis is suspected clinically. The D-dimer is elevated. Doppler ultrasound scan shows no thrombus in the thigh or calf veins. Spectral Doppler shows continuous signal with no respiratory variation. Which further investigation may be of value?

a. no further investigation – normal findings
b. pelvic ultrasound
c. CT pulmonary angiogram
d. chest radiograph
e. echocardiogram

46) A 27-year-old female with known sickle cell disease has an out-patient appointment. She is feeling unwell and bloods show an anaemia. A chest radiograph shows a right-sided, lobulated, para-mediastinal mass in the lower thorax with widening of the rib spaces. CT shows no calcification or bone erosion. What is the most likely diagnosis?

a. neurogenic tumour
b. bronchogenic cyst
c. Bochdalek's hernia
d. tuberculous abscess
e. extramedullary haematopoiesis

47) A 52-year-old male presents with dyspnoea and cough. A chest radiograph shows an ill-defined opacity in the right mid-zone, obscuring the heart border. A lateral view shows a thin wedge-shaped opacity with base in contact with the pleura anteroin-feriorly, and pointing posterosuperiorly. What is the most likely diagnosis?

a. right middle lobe collapse
b. right middle lobe consolidation
c. right lower lobe collapse
d. right lower lobe consolidation
e. encysted pleural fluid

48) A 42-year-old female patient presents with dyspnoea and pleuritic chest pain. She has previously had pulmonary emboli diagnosed. A CT pulmonary angiogram is performed. Which feature would indicate chronic rather than acute thrombus on the CT?

a. complete occlusion of segmental vessel
b. filling defects centrally with peripheral contrast enhancement
c. peripheral mural filling defect forming acute angle with wall
d. peripheral mural filling defect forming obtuse angle with wall
e. linear atelectasis

49) A 50-year-old male presents with gradual onset dyspnoea and cough. There is no preceding history. A chest radiograph shows bilateral 'bat-wing' consolidation, with normal heart size and no effusion. High-resolution CT shows diffuse ground-glass change with intralobular and interlobular septal thickening ('crazy-paving' appearance). What is the most likely diagnosis?

a. pulmonary oedema
b. atypical pneumonia
c. pulmonary alveolar proteinosis
d. acute respiratory distress syndrome
e. hypersensitivity pneumonitis

50) A 56-year-old male presents with wheezing, cough and recurrent chest infections. A chest radiograph shows right middle lobe consolidation. CT of the chest shows a 3 cm mass arising within the right middle lobe bronchus with distal collapse and consolidation. Which feature of the mass would make hamartoma more likely than carcinoid?

   a. central location
   b. presence of calcification
   c. cavitation
   d. presence of fat
   e. prominent enhancement

51) A 52-year-old female presents with cough. She is on dialysis, but, apart from abnormal urea and creatinine, her bloods are normal. A chest radiograph is abnormal and high-resolution CT is performed. This demonstrates fluffy, nodular, 5–10 mm opacities of airspace-type appearance with foci of calcification, in an upper lobe distribution with subpleural sparing. Calcification of chest wall vessels is noted. What is the most likely cause of the appearances?

   a. varicella
   b. chronic renal failure
   c. tuberculosis
   d. histoplasmosis
   e. talcosis

52) A 75-year-old man presents with worsening shortness of breath. He was a mine worker. A chest radiograph shows multiple nodules in the upper zones with a large upper-zone mass on the left. CT confirms multiple small nodules up to 5 mm with a sausage-shaped mass paralleling the mediastinum. What is the most likely diagnosis?

   a. coal worker's pneumoconiosis with bronchogenic carcinoma
   b. coal worker's pneumoconiosis with progressive massive fibrosis
   c. tuberculosis
   d. primary lung carcinoma with metastases
   e. chronic extrinsic allergic alveolitis

53) A 25-year-old male presents with dyspnoea on exertion, cough and haemoptysis. He has a history of recurrent chest infections as a child. A chest radiograph shows a hyperlucent left lung. A pulmonary embolus is suspected and a V/Q scan is arranged. This shows reduced perfusion and ventilation of the left lung, with delayed washout on ventilation. What is the most likely diagnosis?

a. acute pulmonary embolus
b. Macleod's syndrome
c. congenital lobar emphysema
d. Poland's syndrome
e. hypogenetic lung syndrome

54) Which of the following is the most typical description of a myxoma?

a. left atrial mass, no atrial enlargement, pulmonary oedema
b. right atrial mass, enlarged right atrium, clear lungs
c. left atrial mass, enlarged left atrium, calcified lung nodules, pulmonary oedema
d. right atrial mass, enlarged right atrium, pulmonary oedema
e. left atrial mass, dilated superior vena cava, inferior vena cava and azygos vein

55) A 58-year-old male presents with malaise and left chest discomfort. A chest radiograph shows a well-defined mass in the left paravertebral region. CT shows that this is fatty but has soft-tissue stranding within it. Some enhancement of soft-tissue elements is seen along with foci of calcification. What is the most likely diagnosis?

a. lipoma
b. liposarcoma
c. hamartoma
d. neurofibroma
e. thymolipoma

56) In patients with rheumatoid arthritis, what is the commonest pulmonary finding seen on the chest radiograph?

a. pleural effusion
b. fibrosis
c. pulmonary nodules
d. bronchiectasis
e. heart failure

57) A 35-year-old man presents following a chest injury. A chest radiograph shows a smooth, curvilinear, tubular opacity adjacent to the right heart border. No other abnormality is seen. The accident and emergency team are requesting a CT of the chest. What is the most likely diagnosis?

a. pulmonary contusion
b. pneumothorax
c. pericardial injury
d. extralobar sequestration
e. partial anomalous pulmonary venous return

58) In multidetector CT angiography of the lower limbs, the effects of calcification on the images can be reduced by the use of which post-processing technique?

a. curved planar reformat
b. maximum-intensity projection
c. minimum-intensity projection
d. volume rendering
e. digital subtraction of pre- and post-contrast studies

59) A 52-year-old male presents with mild dyspnoea. A chest radiograph shows a raised left hemidiaphragm which demonstrates paradoxical movement on fluoroscopy. Which of the following would be the most likely cause?

a. Pancoast's tumour
b. left lower lobe tumour
c. mediastinal small cell carcinoma
d. eventration
e. cerebrovascular accident

60) A 74-year-old male presents with low back pain. MRI shows some degenerative changes but no disc protrusion or neural compromise. A 6 cm, abdominal aortic aneurysm is seen, which has an irregular wall, with patchy high signal within mural thrombus and in the wall on T1W images. No perianeurysmal fluid to suggest leak is seen. What advice should be given regarding the aneurysm?

a. follow-up with ultrasound scan
b. follow-up with CT
c. follow-up with MRI
d. routine referral to vascular surgeon
e. emergency assessment by vascular surgeon

61) A 44-year-old male presents with a solitary pulmonary nodule on a chest radiograph performed for a suspected chest infection. CT shows this to be 20 mm in diameter with a central cavity and smooth internal walls. No additional findings are seen. Which investigation should be arranged?

a. none; findings are entirely benign
b. CT enhancement study
c. interval volumetric CT
d. contrast MRI
e. ^{18}FDG PET/CT scan

62) In coronary artery anatomy, the vessel supplying the sinoatrial node most commonly arises from which structure?

a. left anterior descending/anterior interventricular artery
b. circumflex artery
c. right coronary artery
d. right coronary sinus at aortic root
e. left coronary artery main stem

63) In MRI of the heart in the assessment of hypertrophic cardiomyopathy, muscle mass is best assessed by using a steady-state free-precession sequence in which plane?

a. left ventricular vertical long axis
b. left ventricular horizontal long axis
c. left ventricular short axis
d. left ventricular short axis oblique
e. four-chamber plane

64) A 33-year-old female with renal failure has an indwelling right internal jugular venous catheter. She presents with swelling of the right arm. Ultrasound Doppler scan of the neck and arm veins is performed. Which feature would suggest occlusion of the right brachiocephalic vein?

a. collapse of right internal jugular vein on sniffing
b. variation of flow with respiration in right subclavian vein
c. variation with cardiac cycle in right subclavian vein
d. continuous monophasic flow in the right subclavian vein
e. collapse of the left internal jugular vein on sniffing

65) A 43-year-old female presents with stridor. A chest radiograph shows a superior mediastinal mass with narrowing of the trachea and displacement to the right. Foci of calcification are seen within it. What is the most likely diagnosis?

    a. thymoma
    b. teratoma
    c. aneurysm of the aortic arch
    d. thyroid goitre
    e. lymph node mass

66) A 56-year-old male has a cough. A chest radiograph and CT chest show a 2 cm rounded mass in the apex of the left lung not amenable to biopsy. An ^{18}FDG PET/CT scan is arranged for further assessment. Which technique may help to improve characterization of the lesion as benign or malignant using the standardized uptake value (SUV)?

    a. maximum SUV corrected for lean body mass
    b. maximum SUV corrected for body weight
    c. metabolic tumour burden (volume × average SUV)
    d. dual time point assessment of SUV
    e. assessment of SUV centrally and peripherally in the lesion

67) A 20 year old presents with shortness of breath and cough. A chest radiograph shows a well-defined right hilar mass. CT shows a 4 cm, rounded, soft-tissue mass arising from the mediastinum adjacent to the right side of the carina. The attenuation value of the lesion is 10 HU. No other abnormal findings are seen. What is the most likely diagnosis?

    a. bronchogenic cyst
    b. pericardial cyst
    c. carcinoid tumour
    d. lymphoma
    e. bronchogenic carcinoma

68) A 16-year-old male presents with sudden shortness of breath. A chest radiograph shows multiple, bilateral nodules measuring up to 3 cm, some of which are calcified. There is a moderate left pneumothorax. The patient has been undergoing treatment for a malignant tumour. What is the most likely diagnosis?

    a. metastases secondary to Wilms' tumour
    b. metastases secondary to osteosarcoma
    c. metastases secondary to testicular tumour
    d. abscesses secondary to immunosuppression
    e. varicella pneumonia secondary to immunosuppression

69) A 64-year-old male presents with worsening shortness of breath and haemoptysis. A chest radiograph shows a right hilar mass with extensive reticulation in the ipsilateral lung, with Kerley A and B lines and reduced lung volumes. The left lung is clear. CT of the chest demonstrates the right hilar mass, and a thickened parenchymal polygonal network within the mid and lower zones of the ipsilateral lung. Beaded thickening of the interlobular septa is also noted. What is the most likely diagnosis?

a. lymphangitis carcinomatosis
b. idiopathic pulmonary fibrosis
c. extrinsic allergic alveolitis
d. histiocytosis
e. sarcoidosis

70) A 38-year-old male presents with a cough, not responding to antibiotics. A chest radiograph shows reticular change in both lungs with normal volumes. High-resolution CT confirms multiple thin-walled cysts with centrilobular nodules of 3–10 mm throughout the lungs. The intervening lung is normal. No pleural effusion is present. What is the most likely diagnosis?

a. neurofibromatosis
b. tuberous sclerosis
c. lymphangiomyomatosis
d. histocytosis
e. usual interstitial pneumonitis

71) In patients undergoing lung resection for malignancy, which imaging investigation is the best predictor of postoperative lung function?

a. perfusion scintigraphy
b. ventilation scintigraphy
c. ventilation and perfusion scintigraphy
d. helical CT of the lungs
e. dynamic MRI of the lungs

72) A 42-year-old male suffers a chest injury in a road traffic accident. The presenting chest radiograph shows fractures of the fifth and sixth ribs on the right side with patchy airspace changes. He is admitted and has supportive care. A repeat chest radiograph shows the consolidation to have largely resolved, but a rounded opacity is now present with an air–fluid level. He is otherwise well. What is the most likely diagnosis?

a. abscess
b. bronchopleural fistula
c. bronchogenic cyst
d. pulmonary infarct
e. pulmonary laceration

73) A 52-year-old man presents 1 year post-heart transplantation and has a routine follow-up chest radiograph. This shows multiple nodules of varying sizes, with enlarged hilar lymph nodes. What is the most likely diagnosis?

a. graft-versus-host disease
b. aspergillosis
c. cytomegalovirus infection
d. post-transplantation lymphoproliferative disorder
e. Epstein–Barr virus infection

74) A 48-year-old female patient presents with right upper quadrant discomfort. She has previously had a liver biopsy for deranged liver function tests, which was normal. Ultrasound scan shows a rounded, 2 cm, low-echogenicity lesion related to a branch of the hepatic artery. This shows arterial-type flow throughout on Doppler. Which minimally invasive treatment option should be offered?

a. injection of thrombin
b. transcatheter coil embolization
c. transcatheter placement of covered stent
d. embolization of hepatic artery
e. no endovascular treatment

75) Which lung segments are separated by the superior accessory fissure?

a. apical segment of lower lobes from other lower lobe segments
b. apical segment of right upper lobe from other upper lobe segments
c. superior segment of lingula from inferior segment of lingula
d. lingular segment of upper lobe from remainder of left upper lobe
e. right middle lobe from right lower lobe

76) In normal anatomy, which vascular structure lies most anteriorly at the level of the thoracic inlet, posterior to the manubrium?

a. left common carotid artery
b. brachiocephalic artery
c. superior vena cava
d. left brachiocephalic vein
e. right brachiocephalic vein

77) Which of the following descriptions would be most suggestive of a pulmonary hamartoma on imaging?

   a. round, 2 cm, soft-tissue mass with no calcification or fat, in a central location
   b. irregular, 8 cm mass with cavitation and associated effusion
   c. multiple lesions of 1–3 cm with calcification, throughout lungs
   d. lobulated, 3 cm mass with calcification and fat, in a peripheral location
   e. peripheral, 5 cm lesion with no calcification, and band-like opacity connecting it to the hilum

78) In persistent left-sided superior vena cava, drainage usually occurs into which structure?

   a. left atrium
   b. right atrium
   c. normal right superior vena cava
   d. hemiazygos vein
   e. coronary sinus

79) An 18-year-old male presents with a chest radiograph performed for immigration purposes. He is noted to have dextrocardia. Further investigation reveals nasal polyposis and bronchiectasis. Which further investigation should be considered?

   a. renal function
   b. CT of brain
   c. fertility assessment
   d. renal angiogram
   e. thyroid function test

80) A CT scan performed on a patient shows a soft-tissue mass in the medial aspect of the left lung, invading the mediastinum between the aortic arch and pulmonary artery. Neither vessel is compromised. Which symptom may the patient have presented with?

   a. stridor
   b. dysphagia
   c. pain
   d. swelling of face and neck
   e. hoarse voice

81) A 65-year-old male presents with chest pain and is referred for myocardial perfusion imaging, as he is unable to exercise due to osteoarthritis of the hips. He is known to have asthma requiring regular inhalers and often has a wheeze. Which pharmacological stress agent should be used?

a. adenosine
b. dipyridamole
c. dobutamine
d. glyceryl trinitrate
e. arbutamine

82) A 78-year-old patient who had an endovascular aortic aneurysm repair undergoes a routine 6-month follow-up scan. This shows that the aneurysm sac has increased in size compared with the 1-month follow-up scan. On the delayed-phase part of the scan, there is contrast seen in the periphery of the aneurysm sac, not in contact with the stent. What is the most likely diagnosis?

a. type I endoleak
b. type II endoleak
c. type III endoleak
d. type IV endoleak
e. type V endoleak

83) In thoracic lymphoma, which feature would favour non-Hodgkin's lymphoma over Hodgkin's disease?

a. predominantly anterior mediastinal lymph nodal involvement
b. predominantly middle mediastinal lymph nodal involvement
c. predominantly posterior mediastinal lymph nodal involvement
d. nodal calcification
e. mass larger than 5 cm

84) In normal anatomy, which structure lies immediately anterior to the left main bronchus at the left hilum?

a. left pulmonary artery
b. left inferior pulmonary vein
c. left superior pulmonary vein
d. left phrenic nerve
e. left vagus nerve

85) A 62-year-old male presents with increasing shortness of breath. Clinically, he has oedematous ankles, raised central venous pressure, ascites and hepatomegaly. Blood tests show mildly raised inflammatory markers. Which feature on CT would make restrictive cardiomyopathy a more likely diagnosis than constrictive pericarditis?

a. dilated inferior vena cava
b. pleural effusions
c. normal pericardial thickness
d. pericardial calcification
e. previous coronary artery surgery

86) In an adult patient, which structure, along with the right atrium and superior vena cava, forms the right mediastinal border?

a. right brachiocephalic vein
b. inferior vena cava
c. right ventricle
d. trachea
e. brachiocephalic artery

87) In bronchopulmonary sequestration, which of the following features would be more suggestive of intralobar than extralobar type?

a. enclosed in visceral pleura
b. no connection to bronchial tree
c. systemic venous drainage
d. presentation in infancy
e. systemic arterial supply

88) In anatomy of the aortic arch, after the normal configuration of vessels (brachiocephalic, left common carotid and left subclavian arteries), what is the next most common configuration seen?

a. left vertebral artery arising from the arch between left common carotid and subclavian arteries
b. common origin of the brachiocephalic artery and left common carotid artery
c. right subclavian arising distal to the left subclavian artery
d. common origin of left common carotid and left subclavian arteries
e. double arch with common carotid and subclavian arteries arising from each side

89) A 20-year-old male has a chest radiograph following a slow-to-resolve chest infection. There is a mass arising from the mediastinum on the right side. Teratoma is suspected. Which feature on CT would suggest that the lesion is more likely to be benign?

a. lobulated margin
b. calcification
c. pleural effusion
d. pericardial effusion
e. mass projecting from both sides of the mediastinum

90) An 82-year-old man has known renal cell carcinoma, which is inoperable due to co-morbidity. He presents with haematuria that necessitates embolization. He has prophylactic antibiotics during and after the procedure. Twenty-four hours later he presents with loin pain and fever. Blood tests show raised inflammatory markers. A CT scan shows an area of lack of enhancement involving the tumour and adjacent renal parenchyma, with locules of gas within this area. What is the most likely diagnosis?

a. urinary tract infection
b. pyelonephritis
c. abscess
d. post-embolization syndrome
e. unintentional embolization of non-target organ

91) A 60-year-old female presents with increasing shortness of breath. She is known to have rheumatoid arthritis. A chest radiograph shows reticulonodular changes, and high-resolution CT is performed. Which feature would suggest underlying sarcoidosis as a more likely diagnosis than rheumatoid lung?

a. lower-zone predominance of reticulation
b. mid-zone predominance of reticulation
c. pleural effusion
d. multiple nodules larger than 20 mm
e. cardiomegaly

92) A 23-year-old female who is 23 weeks' pregnant presents with pleuritic chest pain, and pulmonary embolus is suspected. She asks about the relative radiation doses for CT pulmonary angiogram and ventilation–perfusion ($\dot{V}/\dot{Q}$) scintigraphy. What is the dose for a CT pulmonary angiogram relative to a $\dot{V}/\dot{Q}$ scan?

   a. CT pulmonary angiogram has a higher total body dose but a lower uterine dose
   b. CT pulmonary angiogram has the same total body dose but a lower uterine dose
   c. CT pulmonary angiogram has a higher total body dose and uterine dose
   d. CT pulmonary angiogram has a lower total body dose and uterine dose
   e. CT pulmonary angiogram has a higher total body dose but the same uterine dose

93) Which of the following would be most in keeping with the appearance of pulmonary hydatid disease?

   a. multiple subcentimetre nodules throughout both lungs with no cavitation
   b. unilateral patchy alveolar changes with unilateral hilar lymphadenopathy
   c. solitary ovoid mass with air–fluid level and floating debris
   d. bilateral basal reticular change
   e. 3 cm, rounded mass with central calcification

94) A 56-year-old female has arthralgia. A chest radiograph shows erosion of the lateral ends of the clavicles, superior notching of the third to fifth ribs, and narrowing of the humeral–acromial space. What is the most likely diagnosis?

   a. hyperparathyroidism
   b. rheumatoid arthritis
   c. osteoarthritis
   d. cleidocranial dysostosis
   e. neurofibromatosis

95) In the left lower lobe of the lung, the bronchi to which segments share a common origin?

   a. posterior basal and lateral basal
   b. lateral basal and anterior basal
   c. anterior basal and medial basal
   d. medial basal and posterior basal
   e. apical and posterior basal

96) A 35-year-old female who smokes presents with hypertension and renal impairment. Ultrasound scan shows normal appearance of the kidneys. Doppler of the renal arteries demonstrates a peak velocity of 180 cm/s and no diastolic flow. Angiography shows multiple stenoses of the renal arteries bilaterally with a normal aorta. Which therapeutic option should be offered?

a. angiotensin-converting enzyme inhibitors
b. other antihypertensives
c. angioplasty
d. surgical correction
e. no definitive therapy is of value

97) On high-resolution CT of the chest, how can mosaic perfusion be distinguished from ground-glass opacification?

a. the opaque areas have abnormally small vessels
b. the lucent areas have abnormally small vessels
c. mosaic perfusion is restricted to lower zones
d. mosaic perfusion is restricted to subpleural regions
e. cannot be reliably distinguished

98) A 59 year old with a history of ventricular arrhythmia presents with dyspnoea on exertion. A chest radiograph shows alveolar and interstitial opacification with frank consolidation at the right lung base, which is of high density. There is no peripheral oedema or cyanosis, and the heart size is normal. What is the most likely diagnosis?

a. congestive heart failure
b. sarcoidosis
c. extrinsic allergic alveolitis
d. allergic bronchopulmonary aspergillosis
e. amiodarone pulmonary disease

99) A 67 year old presents with shortness of breath. A chest radiograph shows a reticulonodular pattern with hilar adenopathy. Which feature on high-resolution CT would make silicosis a more likely diagnosis than sarcoidosis?

a. nodules >10 mm
b. calcified hilar lymph nodes
c. traction bronchiectasis
d. honeycombing
e. progressive massive fibrosis

100) A 25-year-old male presents with haemoptysis. A chest radiograph shows symmetrical, bilateral, perihilar consolidation, extending to the bases but with sparing of the apices. There is mild hilar enlargement. The patient is also found to be in renal failure. Appearances on the chest radiograph subsequently progress to an interstitial pattern. What is the most likely diagnosis?

a. primary pulmonary haemosiderosis
b. secondary pulmonary haemosiderosis
c. Goodpasture's syndrome
d. hereditary haemorrhagic telangiectasia
e. histoplasmosis

Module 1: Cardiothoracic and Vascular: Answers

1) a. *
Pulmonary changes occur in ankylosing spondylitis in 1% of patients, with reticulonodular abnormality in the upper zones progressing to confluent opacification and fibrosis. There may be apical bullous formation and cavitation mimicking tuberculosis. No granulomatous disease is seen. Ossification of spinal ligaments is typical in ankylosing spondylitis. Upper-zone fibrosis is seen with tuberculosis, sarcoidosis and chronic extrinsic allergic alveolitis, but spinal ossification is not a feature of these conditions. The reciprocal is true of Reiter's syndrome.

Chapman & Nakielny (2003), 534–5; Dähnert (2007), 46–7.

2) e. ***
Acute respiratory distress syndrome (ARDS) commences with interstitial oedema, progressing to congestion and extensive alveolar, and interstitial oedema and haemorrhage. The chest radiograph is often normal for the first 24 hours, before patchy opacities appear in both lungs. These progress to massive airspace consolidation over the following 24–48 hours. True volume loss, atelectasis, cardiomegaly and effusions are not seen in ARDS.

Desai (2002).

3) b. ***
The differential diagnosis is between pulmonary embolus or pneumonia with effusion, with investigation directed accordingly. High-resolution CT would be unhelpful with lack of contrast. A staging chest CT is performed in the aortic phase of contrast so pulmonary arteries will be suboptimally seen. CT pulmonary angiogram is the best investigation in this case, because, when there is consolidation/opacification present on a chest radiograph, a $\dot{V}/\dot{Q}$ scan has a high likelihood of being non-diagnostic. Conventional pulmonary angiography is a high-risk procedure and is rarely performed in modern practice.

Sutton (2002), 237–9; Dähnert (2007), 523–6.

4) d. *
Mosaic perfusion is caused by abnormalities of ventilation, or vascular obstruction. Expiratory scans help to distinguish causes by establishing whether there is air trapping. With no air trapping present, pulmonary emboli of any cause are most likely. Air trapping would suggest airway

disease such as bronchiolitis obliterans, or other causes of small airway obstruction such as bronchiectasis or cystic fibrosis.

Chapman & Nakielny (2003), 173; Dähnert (2007), 525.

5) a. ***
Marfan's syndrome is an autosomal dominant connective tissue disorder. It predominantly affects the musculoskeletal system but 60–98% of patients have cardiovascular manifestations. There is myxomatous degeneration of the aortic wall, leading to dilatation of the aortic root and aortic regurgitation. There is an association with congenital heart disease, incomplete coarctation and atrial septal defects.

Dähnert (2007), 115–16.

6) e. ***
The thoracic duct starts at the cisterna chyli at the level of T12. It passes behind the right diaphragmatic crus and crosses right to left in the thorax behind the oesophagus. It terminates by draining into the junction between the left subclavian and internal jugular veins, usually as two or three branches.

Butler et al (1999), 141.

7) d. ****
In most patients who survive acute respiratory distress syndrome (ARDS), there is no functional deficit. Where investigated, however, the most common abnormality detected is a reticular pattern in the ventral non-dependent lung. The extent of this is negatively related to the extent of opacification in the acute phase and strongly related to the duration of mechanical ventilation. Bronchiectasis is seen in both acute and chronic phases but is less common than reticular change. Upper-lobe fibrosis is not associated with ARDS.

Desai (2002).

8) d. ****
All of these features can occur, but 65% of patients have fibrosis on CT, although only 30% of patients with systemic sclerosis have clinically significant lung disease. The commonest interstitial lung disease is non-specific interstitial pneumonitis, seen in two-thirds of cases. This is less coarse and extensive than usual interstitial pneumonitis, the other type seen, and is almost always associated with ground-glass opacification. Other respiratory features seen in systemic sclerosis are organizing pneumonia, pulmonary haemorrhage, pleural thickening and malignancy.

Madani et al (2008).

9) e. ***

Post-embolization syndrome occurs in up to 52% of patients and is characterized by a flu-like illness with malaise and fever. This is self-limiting and lasts for up to 10 days. Failure of therapy with the need for re-embolization or hysterectomy occurs in 10% within the first 12 months, but increases to 20–25% at 5 years. A persistent non-offensive discharge per vaginum, which is negative on bacterial culture, occurs in 7–14% of patients and appears to be more common with submucosal fibroids. Hysterectomy for uterine sepsis or intractable pain is required in 2.9% in the first year. Premature ovarian failure is seen in approximately 1–2% of patients, but this increases with age, rising to 25% in the over-45 age group.

Watkinson & Nicholson (2007).

10) d. *****

Acute cardiac sarcoid is seen on MRI as high T2 signal in the myocardium, which may be associated with wall thickening secondary to oedema. Early enhancement may also be seen with sarcoid on post-contrast scans. Delayed hyperenhancement can occur in acute sarcoid, but is also seen in non-viable myocardium secondary to ischaemia. However, in non-ischaemic conditions, it is often seen only involving the central section of the wall with subendocardial sparing. Acute sarcoid may also cause nodular high-signal areas of high T2 signal. It usually involves the base of the septum and left ventricle, but rarely the papillary muscle or right ventricle. Distribution rarely conforms to vascular territories.

Vignaux (2005).

11) b. *****

Acute rejection usually develops 7–10 days post-surgery. Most patients experience at least one episode during their life. Clinically, there are reduced arterial oxygen levels without infection, associated with fatigue and reduced exercise tolerance. Chest imaging findings include ground-glass opacity, heterogeneous perihilar opacification and new enlarging pleural effusion with septal thickening, with no signs of left ventricular failure. Pleural oedema, peribronchial cuffing and airspace shadowing may also occur.

Dähnert (2007), 506–8.

12) d. ****

Klebsiella pneumonia is typically seen in elderly, debilitated men and produces dense, lobar consolidation, with bulging of the fissure sometimes seen. This may also be seen with pneumococcal pneumonia, but less commonly. *Klebsiella* may also cause empyema (the commonest cause) and patchy bronchopneumonia. Cavitation occurs in 50%. *Staphylococcus aureus* pneumonia has a bronchopneumonic pattern which may coalesce, and cavitation is common. Multiple abscesses tend to occur in intravenous drug addicts. Effusions and empyema are common. Streptococcal pneumonia occurs in all ages, especially young adults, and often produces a lobar consolidation in the basal region. *Haemophilus influenzae* pneumonia has no characteristic appearance. Legionnaires' disease causes a spreading consolidation of bronchopneumonic type.

Dähnert (2007), 504.

13) c. ***

Aspergilloma appears as a solid mass in a thin-walled cavity, which lies in a dependent position and is mobile. A crescent-shaped airspace is typical. It may calcify and be associated with pleural thickening. In contrast, cavitating malignancy often has irregular thick-walled margins with a central mass that often enhances, and is fixed and non-mobile. Calcification may occur in relation to malignancy but is usually adjacent to, rather than in, the lesion and is usually seen with a scar carcinoma. Neither causes high-density lesions. Adjacent bronchiectasis is more often seen when there has been previous infection such as tuberculosis, producing a cavity in which an aspergilloma develops.

Park et al (2007).

14) b. ***

The combination of nosebleeds and cavitatory nodules is very suggestive of Wegener's granulomatosis, especially with renal impairment. In the lungs there is often patchy alveolar infiltration, pleural effusions and cavitatory nodules. Systemic lupus erythematosus produces similar appearances by the same mechanism of vasculitis. Sarcoidosis produces many lung changes but cavitatory nodules are rare. Metastatic nasopharyngeal carcinomas are usually squamous cell tumours and can produce cavitatory metastases, but primary tumours usually present with nasal obstruction, although they may cause epistaxis. Renal impairment is not a feature. Multiple abscesses are not usually associated with epistaxis and present acutely, typically in intravenous drug users.

Sutton (2002), 201; Dähnert (2007), 541–2.

15) a. ***

In a patient who has sustained multiple fractures, fat embolism should always be considered when a patient is short of breath in the presence of a normal chest radiograph. This manifests on a $\dot{V}/\dot{Q}$ scan as mottled peripheral perfusion defects. Chest radiograph remains normal for up to 72 hours, when discoid atelectasis, diffuse alveolar infiltrates and consolidation may develop. Fat embolism may precede the development of acute respiratory distress syndrome. Pulmonary contusions usually manifest earlier, within the first 24 hours.

Dähnert (2007), 495.

16) e. *

In chronic asthma, the majority of patients (73%) have normal appearances on chest radiographs between acute episodes. Features such as bronchiectasis or parenchymal scarring may be seen, especially with episodes of repeated infection. Hyperexpansion and peribronchial cuffing are features seen during acute exacerbations of asthma.

Dähnert (2007), 467–8.

17) c. ***

The periosteal reaction is typical of hypertrophic osteoarthropathy (HOA), which has many causes, both intra- and extrathoracic. It is associated with bronchogenic carcinoma and malignant mesothelioma, but features of the described lesion are not typical of either of these, and are more in keeping with pleural fibroma. These are associated with HOA in 20–35% of cases and rarely with clubbing. They may arise in pleura adjacent to the chest wall or in a fissure, and can vary in size from 2 cm to 30cm in diameter. Tuberculosis is a rare cause of HOA. Rheumatoid arthritis is associated with bilateral periosteal reactions, but not HOA.

Sutton (2002), 102, 1231; Dähnert (2007), 106, 513.

18) d. *****

There is a 98% incidence of associated congenital heart disease with a right-sided aortic arch with mirror-image branching. Nearly all of these cases will be tetralogy of Fallot. All of the given options are associated with right-sided aortic arch, as well as dextrocardia with situs inversus and double-outlet right ventricle. Right-sided aortic arch with left subclavian artery is associated with only a 12% incidence of congenital heart disease, again with Fallot's tetralogy being the most commonly associated abnormality.

Chapman & Nakielny (2003), 205.

19) a. **

Rounded atelectasis is an infolding of pleura associated with atelectasis, which occurs in the posterior lower lobes and abuts an area of pleural thickening. Often a 'comet's tail' of bronchovascular markings is seen curving towards the hilum. Bronchogenic carcinoma may occur with asbestos exposure, but is usually of bronchioalveolar cell type and has a latent period of 25–35 years. Round pneumonia produces spherical consolidation with air bronchograms. Silicosis may cause conglomerate masses, usually in the mid or upper zones, or progressive massive fibrosis, but reticulonodular changes predominate.

Sutton (2002), 179.

20) a. ****

Churg—Strauss syndrome is rare, though pulmonary abnormalities are a common feature of the condition. Typically airspace and airway patterns are seen with the following features — centrilobular nodules, ground-glass opacities, bronchial wall thickening, bronchiectasis, consolidation and septal thickening. Lymphadenopathy may be seen in the mediastinum and at the hila but is not a common feature. Large nodules may occur but a tumour-like mass is not a feature. Pleural effusions and bullae are not seen.

Kim et al (2007b).

21) c. **

Adults presenting with coarctation usually have headaches (due to hypertension) and claudication (due to hypoperfusion). The chest radiograph shows an indentation on the lateral margin of the aorta ('figure-3' sign) and elevation of the cardiac apex due to left ventricular hypertrophy. Rib notching is seen in adults, usually over 20 years, and affects the third to eighth ribs. Superior vena caval obstruction may cause rib notching but also causes a 'nipple' on the side of the aorta due to dilated collaterals (accessory hemiazygos). Aortic thrombosis may present similarly to coarctation, but the 'figure-3' sign is not seen. Transposition presents in the first 2 weeks of life.

Dähnert (2007), 630–1.

22) a. **

Hereditary haemorrhagic telangiectasia (HHT), or Rendu—Osler—Weber syndrome, is a disorder that produces telangiectasia, arteriovenous malformations (AVMs) and aneurysms, affecting multiple organ systems. Recurrent epistaxis is seen in up to 85% of cases. Up to 15% of patients with HHT have multiple pulmonary AVMs, and 60% of patients with pulmonary AVMs have HHT. Wegener's granulomatosis is also associated with epistaxis, due to granulomas of the nasal septum, but pulmonary findings are of multiple granulomas.

Dähnert (2007), 497.

23) e. ****

Takayasu's arteritis is a granulomatous inflammatory condition of unknown cause. It is the only aortitis to cause stenosis/occlusion of the aorta. It produces irregular short or long stenotic lesions within the aorta. Involvement of the great vessels usually produces multisegmental dilatation with segmental septation. Atherosclerosis tends to occur in older patients. Syphilis produces aneurysms of the ascending aorta with extensive calcification. Marfan's syndrome produces aneurysms and occasionally is associated with aortic coarctation.

Dähnert (2007), 655–6.

24) d. ***

The bronchial tree derives its arterial supply via bronchial arteries. The two left-sided vessels arise direct from the aorta. The solitary right artery usually arises from the right third posterior intercostal artery. These vessels supply the bronchi from the carina to the respiratory bronchioles.

Butler et al (1999), 138–40.

25) c. ****

Polyarteritis nodosa is a systemic necrotizing inflammation of medium-sized and small muscular arteries. No glomerulonephritis (small, echogenic kidneys) is present. The condition most commonly affects the kidneys (85%) and is usually seen as multiple small intrarenal aneurysms, which may disappear due to thrombosis. Recognized complications are perinephric or subcapsular haemorrhage due to aneurysm rupture. Crossed fused ectopia and hydronephrosis are not recognized features of polyarteritis nodosa.

Dähnert (2007), 649–50.

26) b. ***

A Morgagni hernia is due to a developmental defect anteromedially in the diaphragm between the septum transversum and left (10%) or right (90%) costal margins. They are usually asymptomatic but can produce pain. They are usually small and present in older children or adults. A Bochdalek hernia is a posterolateral developmental defect. It tends to be large, is more common on the left and presents in infancy. Rolling hiatus hernia is herniation of the stomach through the oesophageal hiatus alongside the oesophagus. A septum transversum defect is a defect in the central tendon.

Dähnert (2007), 489–91.

27) d. ***

Loeffler's syndrome is of unknown aetiology and is characterized by areas of non-segmental consolidation, which are peripherally situated and transient. Histiocytosis produces ill-defined nodules which cavitate, first producing thick-walled and then thin-walled cysts. Klebsiella pneumonia usually affects the upper lobes, producing dense, lobar consolidation, sometimes with bulging fissure and empyema. Pseudomonas pneumonia is patchy but extensive and usually in the lower lobes. Lipoid pneumonia is segmental and homogeneously dense, and changes only slowly.

Dähnert (2007), 506.

28) e. **

In this clinical scenario the patient is most likely to have multiple septic emboli secondary to intravenous drug usage. Given the multiple pulmonary abscesses and pneumonia, tricuspid endocarditis should be considered and an echocardiogram should be performed. Transoesophageal echocardiogram is more sensitive to valvular vegetations and should be the investigation of choice. MRI of the heart may have some value in endocarditis, but as yet its value as a routine investigation has not been proven.

Sutton (2002), 276, 279; Dähnert (2007), 531–2, 626.

29) d. ****

In subclavian steal syndrome (SSS), there is a stenosis in the subclavian artery proximal to the vertebral artery origin. This causes reversal of flow in the ipsilateral vertebral artery to maintain blood supply to the upper limb. If the stenosis is not severe, there is normal flow at rest, but exercise aggravates this by increasing the blood supply to the limb. As the stenosis is unable to accommodate the increased flow, the flow in the ipsilateral vertebral artery is reversed. This is termed 'occult SSS'.

Dähnert (2007), 654–5.

30) d. ***

Tracheobronchial injury secondary to blunt trauma presents with non-specific symptoms and signs. Persistent pneumomediastinum, pneumothorax or subcutaneous emphysema despite treatment is suggestive. Associated findings are fractures of the upper three ribs and posterior dislocation of the sternoclavicular joints. The diagnosis is confirmed by bronchoscopy. In intubated patients, focal overdistension of the cuff of the endotracheal tube is seen when the balloon bulges into the defect. Mediastinal haematoma is more suggestive of vascular injury and chylothorax is more suggestive of thoracic duct injury. These may occur in association with tracheobronchial injury.

Euathrongchit et al (2006).

31) b. ****

The T stage is T2, as the lesion is over 3 cm but there is no chest wall or mediastinal invasion or other associated feature. The nodes at the right hilum (N1) and in the subcarinal space (N2) are significantly enlarged, whereas the node in the aortopulmonary space (N3) is not (<10mm short axis), hence the N stage is N2.

Sutton (2002), 115–17.

32) d. ***

FDG uptake occurs at many sites due to physiological uptake. Muscle uptake is variable, but usually occurs throughout a muscle when physiological. Focal muscle uptake is of concern, although benign causes are not uncommon. Diffuse thyroid uptake is usually physiological, but may indicate thyroiditis, whereas focal thyroid uptake may be malignant in 20–50% of cases. Tonsillar uptake if diffuse and symmetrical is likely to be benign, but asymmetrical or focal uptake requires further assessment. Caecal uptake, if diffuse, is probably due to lymphoid uptake, but, again, focal uptake must be assessed further. FDG uptake in the uterine cavity is usually due to menstruation.

Weissleder et al (2007), 955–6.

33) c. *****
Following embolization of an angiomyolipoma, there is propensity to rupture, which appears to be more common if particulate embolization material is used alone without coiling of the feeding vessels. This latter procedure is therefore recommended by some practitioners. Vascular trauma from the original procedure may have a delayed presentation, but this is rarely seen. Spontaneous rupture of another lesion would remain a possibility, but, given the recent embolization, the cause of the haematoma would be more likely to be related to this.

Lenton et al (2008).

34) c. **
With ventilation–perfusion scintigraphy, matched segmental defects are considered low probability. When there is a similar-sized area of opacification on the chest radiograph, which indicates 'triple match', this becomes intermediate probability. Matched non-segmental defects, reverse mismatch and multiple small perfusion defects are all indicators of low probability. Two large segmental perfusion defects that are not matched are considered high probability.

Dähnert (2007), 1101–3.

35) a. ****
Wherever possible, definitive diagnosis should be obtained, as it will enable the best possible treatment. Dependent upon the cause of the obstruction, the correct therapeutic option can then be employed. Radiotherapy often gives a good response, but, in small-cell lung cancer, chemotherapy often gives good results. Stenting should be used when radiotherapy or chemotherapy has failed. Surgical therapy is usually reserved for benign causes where conservative options have failed.

Yim et al (2000), 409–24.

36) d. **
Differentiation of tuberculosis and sarcoidosis can be difficult clinically and radiologically. The presence of symmetrical hilar lymphadenopathy is seen more often with sarcoidosis than with tuberculosis. Pleural

effusions, and cavitating and calcified lesions are much more common with tuberculosis. Consolidation can be seen in both conditions, though it is again more commonly seen in tuberculosis.

Dähnert (2007), 529–31, 539–41.

37) c. ***
Oesophageal rupture is the most likely diagnosis. CT may be able to elicit suspicious signs, such as mediastinal gas, oesophageal thickening and pleural effusion, but cannot make a definitive diagnosis. A contrast swallow is best in confirming the diagnosis, but barium should not be used due to its potential to cause a severe inflammatory reaction and worsening mediastinitis.

Jeudy et al (2006).

38) d. ***
Fibrosing mediastinitis is a rare condition which has two forms: focal (usually secondary to tuberculosis or histoplasmosis) or diffuse (often idiopathic). When associated with tuberculosis, it is thought to be secondary to rupture of lymph nodes in the neck or mediastinum. Calcification is seen in 63% of cases, but the mass may be difficult to differentiate from malignant conditions when calcification is not present. Symptoms and signs are due to compression/obstruction of mediastinal structures. Small-cell carcinoma and lymphoma can produce middle mediastinal masses, but calcification is rare, unless in treated lymphoma when progressive symptoms would be unlikely. Malignant teratomas are typically anterior mediastinal masses which have well-defined lobulated margins, and usually do not calcify.

Akman et al (2004).

39) a. *
The appearances are suggestive of mitral valve calcification, which is virtually always due to rheumatic heart disease, but occasionally may occur secondary to mitral valve prolapse. The differential diagnosis of this appearance includes calcification of the right coronary artery or left circumflex artery. Bicuspid valve, syphilis, ankylosing spondylitis and normal ageing are all causes of aortic valve calcification.

Dähnert (2007), 595.

40) a. ***
Inhalation of noxious gases, including smoke, produces focal or diffuse pulmonary oedema. With smoke this may be delayed by 1–2 days. Bronchiolitis obliterans may then ensue after 1–3 weeks, especially with chemical inhalation.

Sutton (2002), 195.

41) c. **

The lung is involved in 5% of patients with tuberous sclerosis, with symptoms usually occurring in adult life, and it is predominantly women who are affected. There is interstitial fibrosis in the lower lungs with miliary nodular changes, which progress to honeycomb lung. Recurrent pneumothoraces occur in 50% of cases. Chylothorax may also be seen. Preservation of the lung volumes with honeycombing is seen in histiocytosis, neurofibromatosis and lymphangiomyomatosis, as well as tuberous sclerosis.

Chapman & Nakielny (2003), 620–1; Dähnert (2007), 331–3.

42) a. ***

Aortic injury is usually fatal, though some patients survive to reach hospital. A chest radiograph may show a variety of features including deviation of the trachea and oesophagus (position of nasogastric tube) to the right, depression of the left main bronchus, apical pleural cap and left pleural effusion. The presence of a mediastinal haematoma following trauma is more likely due to azygos or hemiazygos vein injury or possibly internal mammary or intercostal artery injury. Superior vena caval injury tends to cause right-sided mediastinal and lung changes. Bronchial rupture may be accompanied by vascular injury but would tend to present with pneumomediastinum and pneumothorax with or without collapsed lung.

Chapman & Nakielny (2003),162–4.

43) b. ***

Allergic bronchopulmonary aspergillosis (ABPA) is hypersensitivity to aspergillus in people with asthma. Typical features are of a migratory pneumonitis, predominantly in the upper lobes. It may cause bronchiectasis and upper-zone fibrosis, which are features also seen in extrinsic allergic alveolitis (EAA). Tubular opacities, indicating mucus plugging, are seen in ABPA, but not in EAA. Centrilobular nodules are seen in EAA, along with mosaic perfusion and patchy ground-glass change. Pleural effusions are rarely seen in EAA and not in ABPA.

Dähnert (2007), 416–17, 466, 494–5.

44) d. ***

Lymphangiomyomatosis is exclusively seen in women of child-bearing age and is worsened in pregnancy. Classically, it causes coarse reticular/reticulonodular interstitial changes, and patients develop recurrent chylous effusions and pneumothoraces. Lung volumes are preserved or may be increased (the only interstitial lung disease with increased lung volumes). It may progress to honeycombing. Histiocytosis usually affects men, and causes cystic change in the upper lobes, small nodules and septal thickening. Tuberous sclerosis has similar features to histiocytosis but is associated with skin changes, reduced IQ and epilepsy. Neurofibromatosis tends to cause progressive fibrosis, but effusions and pneumothoraces are uncommon. Idiopathic pulmonary fibrosis tends to affect the older age group with a reticulonodular pattern.

Dähnert (2007), 508–9.

45) b. **

Even with no clot seen, the loss of respiratory variation with continuous flow suggests a more proximal occlusion. As the limb swelling is unilateral, the most likely site of occlusion would be in the pelvic veins.

Dähnert (2007), 633–4.

46) e. ***

Extramedullary haematopoiesis occurs in conditions where there is prolonged anaemia. This can occur in the spleen, liver, lymph nodes, adrenals and many other sites. In the mediastinum it produces a rounded/lobulated, paraspinal soft-tissue mass, usually between T8 and T12. Unlike other causes of paraspinal masses, there is usually no pain or bone erosion. Bronchogenic cysts are of fluid density. Bochdalek's hernia can present in adults as a paravertebral mass, which is usually asymptomatic and contains fat as well as abdominal organs (bowel, kidney or spleen). It is usually left sided. Tuberculous abscesses are usually associated with bone destruction. Neurogenic tumours are rounded/ovoid and may extend through the intervertebral foramen into the spinal canal and/or produce bone erosion.

Sutton (2002), 1323–4; Dähnert (2007), 76.

47) a. ***

In right middle lobe collapse, the horizontal fissure and lower half of the oblique fissure converge. This creates a wedge-shaped opacity on the lateral chest radiograph. On the frontal chest radiograph, there is an ill-defined mid-zone opacity. With right middle lobe consolidation, there is a mid-zone opacity with a well-defined superior margin, as the horizontal fissure remains in a normal position and is tangential to the radiograph beam. Both obscure the right heart border. Lower lobe collapse and consolidation cause basal opacity with loss of clarity of the right hemidiaphragm. The lateral view shows a triangular opacity at the right base posteriorly, larger in consolidation than collapse.

Sutton (2002), 177–8.

48) d. ***

The differentiation of acute from chronic thromboembolic disease can be difficult. Secondary changes may be present, such as hypertrophy of the right atrium and ventricle with cardiomegaly as well as pulmonary hypertension. Chronic emboli usually form peripheral flattened defects, forming obtuse angles with the arterial wall. Complete vessel occlusion may be seen in both acute and chronic emboli. The presence of recanalization or collateral formation is also suggestive of chronicity. In addition, calcification of the clot may occur, which also indicates chronicity. Parenchymal abnormalities such as atelectasis and wedge-shaped opacities may be seen in both acute and chronic pulmonary emboli.

Dähnert (2007), 523–6.

49) c. ****
Pulmonary alveolar proteinosis is due to accumulation of proteinaceous material in the alveoli, which causes hypoxia. There is a variable combination of airspace and interstitial changes, but diffuse ground-glass opacification and 'crazy-paving' are typical. A geographic distribution is also described. Lack of other features (such as cardiomegaly, lymphadenopathy and effusion) helps to distinguish it from infection and oedema. The lack of precipitating event and slow onset makes acute respiratory distress syndrome unlikely. Hypersensitivity pneumonitis often shows no abnormality on chest radiograph, but high-resolution CT shows surprisingly marked ground-glass change and centrilobular nodules with peripheral sparing.

Pipavath & Godwin (2005).

50) d. **
Hamartomas are usually seen in the periphery of the lungs (two-thirds) with 10% being endobronchial. Calcification is seen in 15%, often popcorn type. Cavitation is rare but fat is seen in 50%. Carcinoids are usually located centrally and are endobronchial. Calcification is seen in one-third and they rarely cavitate. They do not contain fat and show prominent enhancement following contrast, as they are vascular.

Dähnert (2007), 470–1, 497.

51) b. ***
The appearances are suggestive of 'metastatic' pulmonary nodular calcification secondary to chronic renal failure. The upper lobe distribution is due to the relative alkalinity of the upper lobes, caused by the higher ventilation-to-perfusion ratio. It is often associated with calcification of chest wall vessels. Varicella produces multiple calcified nodules of 1–3 mm after the acute episode has resolved. Patients with tuberculosis or histoplasmosis, where calcified nodules are seen, have 2–5 mm, well-defined nodules, and most have calcified lymphadenopathy. Talcosis characteristically produces 1 mm, very-high density nodules.

Marchiori et al (2005).

52) b. ***

The history of mining (dust exposure) with small nodules in the upper zones is typical of pneumoconiosis. The sausage-shaped mass is characteristic of progressive massive fibrosis (PMF), although malignancy cannot be excluded. PMF is often seen to have reduced nodularity surrounding it, as it incorporates the surrounding nodules and migrates towards the hilum. Tuberculosis usually produces a generalized distribution of 2–3 mm nodules in its miliary form, often with lymphadenopathy. Metastases from primary lung cancer are not uniformly small (though they can be in thyroid cancer and melanoma). Chronic extrinsic allergic alveolitis produces fibrotic changes in the mid and lower zones.

Sutton (2002), 191–2; Dähnert (2007), 520.

53) b. ****

Macleod's (Swyer–James) syndrome is a result of acute bronchiolitis in childhood causing obliterative bronchiolitis. There is usually a history of recurrent infections. Chest radiographs show hyperlucent lung with a small or normal-sized hemithorax. High-resolution CT shows reduced vascularity and attenuation of lung with air trapping. Congenital lobar emphysema presents in the first 6 months of life with respiratory distress and a hyperlucent, overexpanded lobe (usually left upper) on the chest radiograph. Poland's syndrome is an absence of part of the pectoralis major muscle, which causes apparent hyperlucent lung, though the lung is normal. Hypogenetic lung syndrome is usually asymptomatic and causes reduced volume of lung with reduced lucency.

Dähnert (2007), 533.

54) c. ***

Myxomas are more common in the left atrium (75–80%) and present with obstruction of the mitral valve. They cause pulmonary hypertension and oedema, left atrial enlargement and ossified lung nodules. They may also cause systemic emboli. Right-sided myxomas cause tricuspid obstruction, right atrial enlargement, dilatation of the SVC, IVC and azygos veins, and reduced pulmonary vascularity. They may also cause pulmonary emboli.

Dähnert (2007), 646–7.

55) b. **

Liposarcoma is an uncommon tumour in the thorax. It contains variable amounts of fat, with soft-tissue components that may enhance following intravenous contrast. Calcification may occur within these lesions. Lipomas are more common and occur anywhere within the mediastinum. Hamartomas usually present as soft-tissue nodules within the peripheral lung and classically show popcorn calcification. They may contain fat. Neurofibromas present as paravertebral masses, often extending into the intervertebral canal, and may have fatty attenuation due to the presence of myelin. Thymolipomas occur in the anterior mediastinum and are found in young adults.

Chapman & Nakielny (2003), 189; Dähnert (2007), 114.

56) a. **

Between 2% and 54% of patients with rheumatoid arthritis have pulmonary abnormalities. Pleural abnormalities are most frequent, being either an effusion (unilateral in 92% of cases) or pleural thickening (usually bilateral). Fibrosis occurs in 30% of patients with pulmonary involvement. Nodules are unusual and seen in advanced disease. They are usually peripheral and may cavitate. Bronchial abnormalities are seen in 30% of patients with rheumatoid lung, and include bronchiectasis and bronchiolitis obliterans. Other findings include pulmonary arterial hypertension and heart failure secondary to carditis/pericarditis.

Dähnert (2007), 528–9.

57) e. ***

The appearances are classic of partial anomalous pulmonary venous return, which occurs in 0.3–0.5% of cases of congenital heart disease and is associated with atrial septal defects and hypogenetic lung. Contusions are seen as ill-defined opacities on CT, often with rib fractures. Anterior pneumothorax would cause increased conspicuity of the heart border. Pericardial injury produces a thick, irregular, shaggy, soft-tissue density adjacent to the heart border. Extralobar sequestration produces a triangular-shaped opacity adjacent to the diaphragm.

Dähnert (2007), 614.

58) a. ****

The effects of vessel calcification can be difficult to remove from CT angiogram, and ultimately axial data may be the only method to assess the vessels accurately. Curved planar reformat images may be helpful to show the lumen. This can be more problematic in small vessels. Maximum-intensity projections can be severely affected by calcification, which 'hides' the lumen. Digital subtraction CT is feasible but has not yet been adequately proven to be of value. Minimum-intensity projections are of no value.

Kock et al (2007).

59) c. **

Diaphragmatic elevation with paradoxical motion is usually due to phrenic nerve paralysis. Mediastinal tumours are one of the commonest causes. Pancoast's tumours invade the brachial plexus, though they can uncommonly invade the phrenic nerve. Eventration tends not to show paradoxical motion, though it can if large. Strokes may cause diaphragmatic elevation, but due to bilateral innervation of the diaphragm, this is not usually due to phrenic nerve involvement and has other causes, such as weakness of chest wall muscles.

Chapman & Nakielny (2003), 158; Dähnert (2007), 448.

60) e. *****
The patchy high T1 signal in the mural thrombus and wall is suggestive of haemorrhage and the aneurysm is therefore unstable. Impending rupture should be considered and urgent surgical assessment should be sought.

Sakamoto et al (2007).

61) e. ***
Although the imaging features suggest a benign nodule, malignancy cannot be excluded and further investigation is warranted. CT enhancement studies may be helpful in solid nodules, but are of less value when a nodule is cavitating. An [18]FDG PET/CT scan has both high sensitivity and specificity in assessing solitary pulmonary nodules, with accuracy over 90%. In particular there is a high specificity for a lesion that shows no FDG uptake being benign. Follow-up is still recommended to ensure no growth and exclude a very low-grade tumour. Interval CT may be considered an option, but in a young patient, unless there are exceptional circumstances, aiming to characterize the lesion is considered more appropriate. MRI is of no proven value in the evaluation of lung nodules.

Hartman (2005).

62) c. ****
The artery to the sinoatrial node arises from the right coronary artery in about 60% of people. In about 40%, the artery arises from the circumflex artery. Much less commonly, it arises directly from the right coronary sinus.

Butler et al (1999), 164–6; Dähnert (2007), 604.

63) d. *****
In the assessment of hypertrophic cardiomyopathy, MRI is better than echocardiography due to the latter being limited by poor visualization. MRI can assess the distribution of disease and wall thickness, especially the anterolateral wall. This has important implications in assessing areas of myocardial thickness of >30mm, which is of prognostic value. Wall thickness is generally best assessed on short axis images, except at the apex when long axis planes are better, and should be done at end-diastole. The technique of assessing left ventricular volume, function and

mass, using the short axis oblique plane, is well described in the literature. Inclusion of papillary muscles varies between institutions.

Hansen & Merchant (2007).

64) d. ***
Ultrasound evaluation of the central veins is difficult, as the brachiocephalic veins and superior vena cava cannot be directly visualized. Secondary features to confirm patency can be seen, such as collapse of the internal jugular veins on sniffing (Valsalva manoeuvre), and variability of flow with respiration and the cardiac cycle. A continuous monophasic flow with loss of variability suggests a proximal occlusion or stenosis.

Weber et al (2007).

65) d. **
Thyroid goitres extend into the mediastinum in 3–17% of cases. Tracheal displacement may occur due to any adjacent enlarging mass, but narrowing is specific for thyroid lesions, especially goitre. Calcification is common. Teratomas tend to arise more often in the anterior mediastinum, though they may involve the superior mediastinum by extension. Thymomas may arise in the superior or anterior mediastinum. Either of these may show calcification. Lymph node masses tend to calcify only after treatment, such as radiotherapy for lymphoma.

Chapman & Nakielny (2003), 185–6.

66) d. *****
Dual time point assessment involves measuring the SUV at two time points to assess for change. In malignant lesions the SUV rises with time, whereas with benign lesions this tends to remain static. The maximum SUV corrected for lean body mass or weight is the standard measurement used for assessment of metabolic activity of lesions on PET. The metabolic tumour burden is currently not used in clinical practice. The assessment of uptake in the peripheral and central areas of a lesion is not a recognized technique.

Lan et al (2008).

67) a. ***
Bronchogenic cyst is an abnormality of the ventral diverticulum of the primitive foregut and is the most common foregut abnormality in the thorax. Typical appearances are of a thin-walled cyst containing mucus or fluid. CT shows a well-defined mass of water density in 50% (0–10 HU) or slightly higher density in the rest (10–50 HU); 86% are mediastinal and 50% pericarinal. Pericardial cysts largely occur in the cardiophrenic angle and are rarely mediastinal. Like bronchogenic cysts,

these may change shape with position and respiration. Carcinoids occur in the lungs within bronchi and are mainly central. These are solid and may calcify. Bronchogenic carcinomas are usually solid, and centrally located in 38% of cases, where they are usually small cell tumours. These occur in the older population. Lymphadenopathy secondary to lymphoma is usually solid (unless treated) and involves multiple nodes in 95% of cases. The anterior mediastinum and retrosternal lymph nodes are usually affected first.

Sutton (2002), 74–5; Dähnert (2007), 477–8.

68) b. ****
Osteosarcoma pulmonary metastases are uncommon (seen in 2% of cases) and present as multiple masses which may calcify. There is a high incidence of associated pneumothorax. Wilms' tumours may also produce multiple pulmonary masses and may be associated with pneumothorax, but are not known to calcify. Testicular tumours may produce calcified lung metastases, but are not associated with pneumothorax. Varicella pneumonia shows patchy consolidation in the acute phase, with multiple, small, calcified nodules in the chronic phase. Abscesses may present as multiple masses but rarely calcify and often cavitate.

Sutton (2002), 1261–2; Dähnert (2007), 514–15.

69) a. **
Lymphangitis carcinomatosis is tumour cell accumulation within connective tissue, causing lymphatic obstruction. This leads to interstitial oedema. The chest radiograph may be normal, but there is often reticulonodular change with Kerley A and B lines. An ipsilateral hilar or mediastinal mass may be seen. Pulmonary fibrosis has a peripheral predominance and tends to be bilateral. Extrinsic allergic alveolitis and histiocytosis tend to be bilateral. Sarcoidosis usually produces a more nodular pattern and there is predominance in the upper lobes. Polygonal structures on CT are uncommon in sarcoidosis.

Dähnert (2007), 509.

70) d. ****
Honeycombing is seen with all of these conditions, but the combination of normal volumes, cysts and peribronchial nodules is very suggestive of histiocytosis. Often the lung bases are preserved early in the disease but the whole lung is eventually involved. Lung volumes in usual interstitial pneumonitis are reduced. Neurofibromatosis causes interstitial fibrosis with little nodularity. Tuberous sclerosis causes lower-zone fibrotic change with miliary nodules that progresses to honeycombing. Lymphangiomyomatosis produces coarse reticular change due to cyst formation, but nodularity is not seen. Pneumothoraces and pleural

effusions are seen with neurofibromatosis, tuberous sclerosis and lymphangiomyomatosis.

Dähnert (2007), 504–5.

71) b. *****
It is possible to estimate postoperative lung function (FEV$_1$ (forced expiratory volume in 1 s)) with ventilation and perfusion scintigraphy, either in isolation or combination. However, ventilation scintigraphy is the best predictor of postoperative FEV$_1$. This does underestimate the value; therefore, patients with borderline lung function should not necessarily be denied surgery on the basis of the result. CT and MRI have not been shown to be helpful in assessing postoperative lung function.

Win et al (2006), 1260–5.

72) e. ****
Pulmonary lacerations occur following trauma disrupting the lung parenchyma. The typical appearance is of a rounded cavity containing blood and/or air. On plain films, consolidation due to contusion often obscures the laceration. The laceration appears as a rounded/ovoid opacity with a pseudocapsule of compressed lung (2–3 mm), and may be fully opacified, be filled with air or have an air–fluid level. Complications are uncommon and include abscess (causes fever), bronchopleural fistula (causes pneumothorax) and progression. Bronchogenic cysts could present as an incidental finding after trauma but are usually mediastinal in location. The less common intrapulmonary bronchogenic cysts may cavitate. Pulmonary infarcts may present post-trauma due to immobilization and other risk factors causing pulmonary embolus, but these do not usually cavitate.

Miller (2006).

73) d. ****
Post-transplant lymphoproliferative disorder (PTLD) occurs after bone marrow or solid organ transplantation, usually within 2 years. The type of tumour varies. This can produce single or multiple lung nodules with or without hilar and mediastinal lymphadenopathy. The nodules may be diffuse, subpleural or peribronchial and may have a surrounding halo of ground-glass opacification. The findings in graft-versus-host disease are of bronchiolitis obliterans – hyperinflation, bronchial dilatation and wall thickening, reduced vascularity/mosaic perfusion, and air trapping. In the acute phase, it often presents as non-cardiogenic pulmonary oedema. Aspergillosis presents with nodular opacities or consolidation, which may have a halo of ground-glass opacification, but occurs in the first 30 days. Cytomegalovirus infection usually occurs within the first 6 months after bone marrow transplantation, with a variety of

appearances. Epstein–Barr virus is a causative factor in PTLD but is not in itself a cause of the pulmonary changes.

Lindell & Hartman (2005).

74) b. ****
The most likely diagnosis here is pseudoaneurysm following the biopsy. Visceral artery aneurysms, in general, affect the splenic artery most commonly, followed by the hepatic artery. They are usually solitary. Intrahepatic branch aneurysms are usually a result of trauma, infection or vasculitis, or are iatrogenic (biopsy). These are usually treated by coil embolization, although some advocate injecting thrombin into small peripheral lesions. Stent insertion is not often used, as deploying stents in the smaller branch arteries is technically difficult and the stents do not allow sufficient flow and thrombose. Embolization of the hepatic artery carries a significant risk of liver ischaemia and is not advisable.

Nosher et al (2006).

75) a. ***
The superior accessory fissure can be seen on both frontal and lateral radiographs. It is seen inferior to the horizontal fissure on the frontal projection and extends to the posterior chest wall on the lateral projection, whereas the horizontal fissure extends to the anterior chest wall. Other common accessory fissures are the inferior accessory fissure (between the medial basal segment of the lower lobe and other basal segments) and the azygos fissure (invagination of pleura into the upper lobe containing the azygos vein).

Butler et al (1999), 133–8.

76) d. ***
In the superior mediastinum the venous structures lie most anteriorly. The superior vena cava does not extend up to reach the thoracic inlet but is formed inferiorly by the convergence of the brachiocephalic veins. The right has a short vertical course to the right of the midline, while the left crosses from the root of the neck on the left to the right side of the superior mediastinum behind the manubrium, where it lies anterior to all of the other vascular structures.

Butler et al (1999), 141–4.

77) d. ***
Hamartomas are seen in 0.25% of the population and are the commonest benign lung tumour. Two-thirds are found peripherally. They are rarely multiple or cavitatory. Fifteen per cent calcify (classically popcorn) and 50% contain fat. Option (a) is more typical of carcinoid, while (c) is suggestive of multiple granulomas, probably secondary to

chickenpox. Option (e) is characteristic of pulmonary arteriovenous malformation.

Dähnert (2007), 497.

78) e. ****
Persistent left-sided superior vena cava occurs in 0.3% of the general population and in 4.3–11% of patients with congenital heart disease. It is associated with atrial septal defects and azygos continuation of the inferior vena cava. It lies lateral to the aortic arch and anterior to the left hilum. It usually drains into the coronary sinus, but rarely drains into the left atrium, causing a left-to-right shunt. The normal right-sided superior vena cava is absent in 10–18% of cases of left-sided superior vena cava.

Dähnert (2007), 598.

79) c. **
The presence of dextrocardia, nasal polyposis and bronchiectasis raises the possibility of Kartagener's syndrome. This is immotile/dysmotile cilia syndrome and may also present with deafness and infertility. There is also an association with transposition of the great vessels, pyloric stenosis, post-cricoid web and epispadias. Situs inversus is seen in 50% of cases.

Dähnert (2007), 504.

80) e. **
The space between the pulmonary artery and aortic arch is the aortopulmonary window, which contains the ligamentum arteriosum and the left recurrent laryngeal nerve. Invasion here by tumours can lead to paralysis of the left vocal fold, which attains a fixed adducted position, by involvement of the recurrent laryngeal nerve. Stridor and dysphagia could result from deeper invasion into the mediastinum, as the trachea and oesophagus form the medial border of the aortopulmonary window. Swelling of the face, neck and upper limbs occurs with superior vena cava obstruction, which is a feature of right-sided mediastinal disease.

Butler et al (1999), 144–5; Dähnert (2007), 359.

81) c. ****
In myocardial perfusion imaging, adenosine is the drug of choice, but is contraindicated in people with asthma. Dobutamine is a second-line drug that is used when adenosine is contraindicated. It has more side effects than adenosine but produces comparable imaging results. Dipyridamole is rarely used due to a poor side-effect profile and is also contraindicated in people with asthma. Arbutamine is used in some

countries but is not widely used in the UK. Glyceryl trinitrate is not used as a stress agent.

Dähnert (2007), 1112–13.

82) b. *****
Endovascular aortic aneurysm repair (EVAR) procedures require lifelong follow-up imaging – 6-monthly CT scans are recommended. Complications include expansion and rupture of the sac, or endoleak. The latter has five described types: type I – leak from stent–graft attachment, which can be subdivided into subtypes a and b, corresponding to leaks at proximal and distal attachments respectively; type II (commonest) – retrograde flow through aortic branches, usually inferior mesenteric artery or lumbar arteries; type III – structural failure of stent–graft; type IV – due to porosity of the graft; type V – endotension, which is expansion of the sac without obvious cause, although it may be due to an occult type I, II or III.

Stavropoulos & Charagundla (2007).

83) c. ***
Mediastinal nodal involvement is generally more suggestive of Hodgkin's disease, but disease is usually seen in the middle and anterior mediastinum. Posterior mediastinal involvement, with little or no anterior or middle mediastinal involvement, suggests non-Hodgkin's lymphoma as a more likely diagnosis. Calcification can occur in either condition, nearly always post-therapy. The size of the lymph node masses is not discriminatory.

Dähnert (2007), 510–12.

84) c. *
The left pulmonary artery crosses over the superior aspect of the left main bronchus giving off the upper lobe artery and the inferior pulmonary artery, and then lies posterior to the left main bronchus. The left inferior pulmonary vein drains into the left atrium and does not reach the level of the left main bronchus. The vagus nerve lies posterior to the hilum adjacent to the oesophagus. The phrenic nerve lies anterior to all of the left hilar structures on the pericardium.

Butler et al (1999), 130.

85) c. ****
Both restrictive cardiomyopathy (RCM) and constrictive pericarditis (CP) present in the same way, with signs and symptoms of reduced heart filling and venous congestion. Distinguishing between these causes is important, as CP can be cured. Pericardial calcification occurs in CP and is seen in 50% of cases on chest radiograph. Pericardial thickening of >4mm is usually seen with CP. A normal pericardial thickness excludes

CP and makes RCM a likely diagnosis instead. Previous cardiac surgery is a cause of CP.

Kim et al (2007a).

86) a. ***
In an adult, the right mediastinal border normally comprises the right brachiocephalic vein, the superior vena cava and the right atrium. In young patients the thymus may produce a characteristic sail-shaped opacity over the right mediastinal border. The right tracheal wall can be seen as the paratracheal stripe through the right brachiocephalic vein and superior vena cava. The right ventricle does not form any part of the cardiac silhouette on a frontal chest radiograph. The brachiocephalic artery lies medial to the right brachiocephalic vein and does not form any part of the mediastinal border.

Butler et al (1999), 148.

87) a. ****
Bronchopulmonary sequestration is a malformation consisting of a non-functioning lung segment with no communication to the bronchial tree and a systemic arterial supply. The intralobar type accounts for 75% of cases. It is enclosed in visceral pleura and presents in adulthood with pain, repeated infection, cough and haemoptysis. The extralobar type is enclosed in its own pleura and presents in infancy with feeding difficulties, respiratory distress, cyanosis and congestive heart failure (due to shunting). Systemic venous drainage is seen in 80% of cases of extralobar type, but only in 5% of cases of intralobar type.

Dähnert (2007), 479–81.

88) b. **
The so-called normal aortic arch anatomy is seen in only 65% of people. The next most common configuration is where the left common carotid artery arises with the brachiocephalic artery in a common origin, seen in 13%, followed by the left common carotid arising from the brachiocephalic artery (bovine origin), seen in 9%. The left vertebral artery arising direct from the arch is seen in 2.5%, and the aberrant right subclavian artery (option c) occurs in 0.5%.

Butler et al (1999), 167–168; Dähnert (2007), 602.

89) b. ****
A definite diagnosis as to whether a teratoma is benign cannot be made on radiological features. Features suggestive of a benign nature are a rounded lesion, projection from one side of the mediastinum, and calcification (especially if in the form of a tooth). A fat–fluid level is characteristic of a benign lesion but is rare. Features more suggestive of malignancy are lobulated margins, invasion into adjacent structures (may

cause pleural or pericardial effusions), and projection from both sides of the mediastinum.

Dähnert (2007), 534–5.

90) d. ***
Post-embolization syndrome usually occurs within 24–48 hours after embolization and continues for 3–7 days. It presents with pain, nausea, vomiting, malaise and fever. Blood tests show raised inflammatory markers. Gas may be seen in the infarcted tissue after embolization and is not a definite sign of abscess. Abscesses may occur but usually present later, as would other infective processes that may occur.

Sutton (2002), 459–60.

91) b. **
Sarcoidosis is seen more commonly in females and affects the thorax in 90% of cases. It usually produces adenopathy with or without parenchymal disease. There is a mid-zone predominance with irregular septal thickening, perilymphatic nodules, ground-glass opacification, traction bronchiectasis and honeycombing. Rheumatoid lung is more common in males and mostly presents with pleural abnormalities, usually an effusion. It may present with an interstitial fibrotic picture with a lower-zone predominance. Multiple large nodules of up to 7 cm in diameter are seen with rheumatoid lung. Cardiomegaly may be seen with both sarcoidosis and rheumatoid, as a result of congestive cardiac failure.

Dähnert (2007), 528–31.

92) a. ***
The total body dose for CT pulmonary angiogram is approximately 2–3 times higher than for $\dot{V}/\dot{Q}$ scanning. However the uterine, and therefore fetal, dose has been found to be higher with $\dot{V}/\dot{Q}$ scanning. A low-dose $\dot{V}/\dot{Q}$ technique can reduce this, but the uterine dose still remains higher. Regardless of technique used, there remains a risk, but the risk of death from pulmonary embolus far outweighs any radiation risk to patient or fetus.

Kluetz & White (2006).

93) c. **
The lungs are the second most frequent site affected by hydatid disease in adults, being involved in up to 25% of cases. Commonly, a solitary ovoid or spherical mass is seen in the lower lobes. These can be quite large, measuring up to 20 cm in size. There is communication with the bronchial tree, producing air–fluid levels, and the wall of the cyst may be

visible, and may appear as a curvilinear opacity or floating debris. Calcification may occur within the wall of the cyst in a few cases.

Dähnert (2007), 500–1.

94) b. ***
Erosion of the lateral ends of the clavicle is seen in several conditions, including rheumatoid arthritis, hyperparathyroidism and cleidocranial dysostosis. The associated rib notching and loss of the space between the humeral head and acromion (due to wasting/rupture of supraspinatus) are typically seen with rheumatoid arthitis. Clavicle erosions are not features of neurofibromatosis or osteoarthritis.

Chapman & Nakielny (2003), 51; Dähnert (2007), 19.

95) c. **
There are five segments to the lower lobes of both lungs, but, unlike on the right, the medial basal and anterior basal segmental bronchi on the left usually have a common origin. The medial basal segment is small due to the cardiac indentation.

Dähnert (2007), 452.

96) c. ****
The appearances are suggestive of fibromuscular hyperplasia, which is the commonest cause of renovascular hypertension in young patients and causes 35% of all renal artery stenosis. It affects the aortic branches, but not the aorta itself. Complications include giant aneurysm and arteriovenous fistula. Angioplasty has a 90% success rate with a low re-stenosis rate and is the treatment of choice. Surgical correction can be performed (end-to-end anastomosis, vein grafts) but is usually reserved for refractory cases or where there is involvement of the segmental vessels rather than the main renal arteries.

Dähnert (2007), 957–8.

97) b. *
Mosaic perfusion refers to areas of altered attenuation on CT and reflects vascular obstruction or abnormal ventilation. Differentiation from ground-glass opacification can be difficult but can usually be done by assessment of the centrilobular vessels. In comparing 'lucent' and 'opaque' areas, the area in which the vessels appear larger is generally the normal area, though this may be a difficult differentiation to make in practice, as the vessels may be of the same size throughout the lung. In mosaic perfusion, the vessels appear abnormal in the 'lucent' area, whereas, in ground-glass opacification, the vessels appear abnormal in the 'opaque' area. Expiratory scans may then help to distinguish airway

causes from vascular causes, by the presence of air trapping, which is seen with airway disease.

Chapman & Nakielny (2003), 173.

98) e. ***

Amiodarone lung disease occurs after 1–12 months of treatment. Features are of alveolar and interstitial infiltrates and high-density areas of consolidation (iodine attenuation). Heart failure usually gives a 'bat-wing' distribution of consolidation with increased heart size and vascular congestion, and often cyanosis. Sarcoidosis may produce reticulonodular changes, which coalesce to form areas of consolidation. Acute extrinsic allergic alveolitis may produce a consolidative pattern, but reticular changes are seen in the chronic stage. Allergic bronchopulmonary aspergillosis occurs in people with asthma and commonly produces fleeting areas of pneumonitis, with less common features being lobar consolidation, atelectasis and cavitation.

Dähnert (2007), 406–7.

99) e. ****

Silicosis is due to inhalation of silicon dioxide particles, and radiographic changes of chronic silicosis are seen 10–20 years after exposure. The nodules are typically less than 10mm, compared with sarcoid nodules, which can be more variable in size (acinar type 6–7mm, alveolar type >10mm). Calcified hilar lymph nodes (eggshell pattern), traction bronchiectasis and honeycombing occur in both conditions and are not discriminatory. Progressive massive fibrosis is a complication of the pneumoconioses and is not seen in sarcoidosis.

Sutton (2002), 187–91; Dähnert (2007), 532–3.

100) c. ****

Goodpasture's syndrome is an autoimmune disease characterized by glomerulonephritis and pulmonary haemorrhage. Respiratory features are usually preceded by respiratory infection. Mild haemoptysis occurs associated with cough and dyspnoea. Bilateral consolidative changes and sometimes enlarged hilar nodes may occur. Pulmonary haemosiderosis presents in a similar manner, but usually occurs in patients under 10 years of age in the primary form, with adults affected in the secondary form, which is rare. Patchy airspace change occurs in the first 2 days and then resolves. Progression to fibrosis may occur. Patients with hereditary haemorrhagic telangiectasia usually have multiple arteriovenous malformations.

Dähnert (2007), 496.

MODULE 2
MUSCULOSKELETAL AND TRAUMA

Module 2: Musculoskeletal and Trauma: Questions

1) A 34-year-old woman presents with pain and swelling of the right knee over the previous 2 months. Plain films demonstrate a well-circumscribed, expansile, lytic lesion eccentrically located in the subarticular region of the right distal femur. The lesion has a narrow, non-sclerotic zone of transition. What is the most likely diagnosis?

   a. giant cell tumour
   b. enchondroma
   c. fibrous cortical defect
   d. fibrous dysplasia
   e. aneurysmal bone cyst

2) A 30-year-old women presents to her general practitioner with fatigue and painful stiff knees. She is subsequently found to be anaemic. Plain films show an Erlenmeyer flask deformity of the distal femora with cortical thinning. There are no erosions. What is the most likely underlying condition?

   a. mucopolysaccharidosis
   b. rheumatoid arthritis
   c. Gaucher's disease
   d. Langerhans' cell histiocytosis
   e. thalassaemia major

3) Plain knee radiographs performed in accident and emergency following a sports injury in a 20-year-old footballer show an effusion, a small avulsion fracture immediately proximal to the fibular head, deepening of the lateral femoral sulcus and anterior translocation of the tibia. What is the most likely underlying ligamentous injury?

   a. complete posterior cruciate ligament rupture
   b. complete anterior cruciate ligament rupture
   c. partial anterior cruciate ligament rupture
   d. tibial collateral ligament rupture
   e. fibular collateral ligament rupture

4) CT of the cervical spine is performed on an intubated emergency patient who was a restrained driver in a high-speed motor vehicle collision. This reveals bilateral C2 pedicle fractures. What is the most likely underlying mechanism of injury?

a. hyperflexion and rotation
b. hyperextension followed by hyperflexion
c. axial loading
d. hyperextension and traction
e. hyper-rotation

5) A young patient suffers a fractured femur and acetabulum in a road traffic collision and undergoes intramedullary nailing and plate-and-screw internal fixation of the acetabulum. He is well until 8 days postoperatively, when he develops acute shortness of breath and right-sided chest pain. A chest radiograph shows only a small right-sided pleural effusion. What is the most likely diagnosis?

a. fat embolism
b. bronchial pneumonia
c. pulmonary embolism
d. pneumothorax
e. hyperventilation due to pain

6) Of the lateral fibrous structures contributing to the stability of the posterolateral corner of the knee, which is the most likely to be congenitally absent and not identified on MRI, being present in only approximately two-thirds of patients?

a. lateral collateral ligament
b. popliteus tendon
c. popliteofibular ligament
d. arcuate ligament
e. fabellofibular ligament

7) A child passenger is admitted to accident and emergency following a road traffic collision. Radiographs of the spine show a horizontal fracture involving the vertebral body and pedicles of L2. Associated injury to which of the following abdominal organs is most likely?

a. duodenum
b. pancreas
c. spleen
d. liver
e. rectum

8) A middle-aged man with no significant medical history undergoes a radiograph of the pelvis for localized tenderness following a fall. Multiple longitudinally orientated, 2–10 mm rounded densities similar to cortical bone are seen throughout the cancellous bone, in a diffuse symmetrical pattern concentrated around the acetabulum. There is no fracture. What is the most likely diagnosis?

a. osteopathia striata
b. osteopetrosis
c. bone metastases
d. melorrheostosis
e. osteopoikilosis

9) A 30-year-old man undergoes shoulder MRI for chronic anterior pain. There is no history of trauma. Sagittal images reveal an absent anterior labrum with a thickened middle glenohumeral ligament. What is the most likely diagnosis?

a. anterior labral tear
b. Bankart's lesion
c. superior labrum anterior-to-posterior (SLAP) lesion
d. glenohumeral tendonitis
e. normal variant

10) A 28-year-old physically active young man undergoes a hip MR arthrogram for chronic pain that is worse during exercise. There is a history of several months of hip pain when the patient was a teenager that was not investigated. Images show a loss of the femoroacetabular sulcus superiorly with an associated acetabular labral tear. What is the underlying condition?

a. pincer femoroacetabular impingement
b. cam femoroacetabular impingement
c. combined femoroacetabular impingement
d. traumatic labral tear
e. osteochondritis dissecans

11) You receive a referral while on call from the orthopaedic consultant regarding a middle-aged woman with a long history of simple back pain. She has attended accident and emergency complaining of worsening lower lumbar pain with a several-hour history of progressive urinary retention, faecal incontinence, saddle anaesthesia and mild bilateral leg weakness. Which method of imaging would you recommend as most appropriate?

a. plain radiography
b. myelogram
c. CT
d. CT myelogram
e. MRI

12) A female adult patient with right shoulder pain is shown to have multiple markedly expansile lytic lesions within the scapula and clavicle secondary to metastatic malignant spread. Which of the following is most likely to be the primary site of malignancy?

a. renal
b. breast
c. cervical
d. colon
e. bronchus

13) A 'fallen fragment' seen within a lytic bone lesion is most commonly associated with which of the following?

a. aneurysmal bone cyst
b. unicameral (simple) bone cyst
c. giant cell tumour
d. eosinophilic granuloma
e. chondroblastoma

14) In the spectrum of perilunate ligamentous injuries and instability, volar tilt of the lunate, seen as a triangular or 'pie-shaped' lunate on the AP projection of the wrist, is most commonly a feature of which of the following?

a. scapholunate dissociation
b. perilunate dislocation
c. lunate dislocation
d. volar intercalated segmental instability
e. dorsal intercalated segmental instability

15) On plain radiographs of the hands in a middle-aged male patient complaining of bilateral joint pain and swelling, which single feature is most likely to support a diagnosis of psoriatic arthritis over rheumatoid arthritis?

a. new bone formation
b. joint space loss
c. periarticular osteoporosis
d. periarticular erosions
e. soft-tissue swelling

16) MRI of the temporomandibular joint is performed for painful clicking, with no history of trauma. Which of the following internal derangements is the most likely underlying cause?

    a. torn intra-articular disc
    b. anteriorly displaced intra-articular disc
    c. hypertrophic/misshapen intra-articular disc
    d. erosive osteoarthritis
    e. insufficiency fracture of the condylar neck

17) In imaging of focal bone lesions in the appendicular skeleton, which of the following radiographic features is most likely to indicate an aggressive or malignant process?

    a. cortical expansion
    b. lytic process
    c. periosteal reaction
    d. multiple lesions
    e. wide zone of transition

18) In a patient who presents with acute femoral nerve radiculopathy, which of the following MRI sequences is the most useful in the diagnosis of a far lateral upper lumbar vertebral disc protrusion?

    a. sagittal STIR
    b. sagittal T1
    c. sagittal T2
    d. axial STIR
    e. axial T2

19) The presence of punctate, ring-like or arcuate calcification in a lytic bone lesion on plain radiography is most commonly associated with which of the following matrix types?

    a. osteoblastic
    b. fibrous
    c. cartilaginous
    d. cellular
    e. mixed

20) As seen on radiographs of a paediatric skeleton, generalized appendicular findings of poor mineralization of the epiphyseal centres, widening of the growth plate and cupping/fraying of the metaphyses are all frequently associated with which condition?

    a. osteogenesis imperfecta
    b. scurvy
    c. fibrous dysplasia
    d. rickets
    e. mucopolysaccharidosis

21) Which of the following skeletal findings on plain radiographs is not typically associated with achondroplasia?

a. short interpedicular distance
b. small foramen magnum
c. rhizomelia
d. horizontal acetabular roof
e. atlantoaxial instability

22) A 32-year-old woman with a long history of right knee pain undergoes radiography for atraumatic swelling of the joint and is found to have an effusion and soft-tissue swelling but no other findings. MRI shows a large anterolateral lobular intra-articular mass of low signal on T1W and T2W images, and a blooming artefact is seen on gradient echo sequences. What is the most likely condition?

a. malignant fibrous histiocytoma
b. pigmented villonodular synovitis
c. synovial osteochondromatosis
d. Baker's cyst
e. intra-articular haematoma

23) Plain radiographs of the hands in a young woman are performed for unilateral deformity. These show multiple lytic lesions in the medullary cavities of the tubular bones with cortical expansion and matrix mineralization, and associated Madelung deformity. The changes are unilateral. What is the most likely diagnosis?

a. Maffucci's syndrome
b. Ollier's disease
c. Trevor's disease
d. Lichtenstein–Jaffé disease
e. Morquio's syndrome

24) Of the following types of periosteal reaction, select the one most likely to indicate a benign process?

a. soap-bubble
b. sunray
c. hair-on-end
d. laminated
e. Codman's triangle

25) Looser's zones – transverse linear lucencies representing areas of poorly mineralized osteoid – are seen with which underlying pathological process of bone?

a. fracture
b. osteomyelitis
c. osteoporosis
d. osteopetrosis
e. osteomalacia

26) On plain radiographs of the neck in a 60-year-old man, which feature is most likely to support a diagnosis of diffuse idiopathic skeletal hyperostosis rather than ankylosing spondylitis?

a. enthesopathy
b. confluent intervertebral bony bridging
c. sparing of the posterior elements
d. sparing of the sacroiliac joints
e. changes limited to the thoracic spine

27) A lumbar spinal MRI is performed on a young man of south-east Asian origin for back pain and pyrexia of unknown origin. It reveals an anterior paraspinal soft-tissue mass at levels L1 to L3 centred at the L2–3 intervertebral disc. It is located deep to and displaces the anterior longitudinal ligament, and extends into the left psoas muscle. The mass returns intermediate signal on T1W images and high signal on T2W images. There are oedematous changes in the adjacent vertebral bodies, but the intervertebral discs are spared. What is the most likely infectious organism?

a. *Mycobacterium tuberculosis*
b. *Actinomyces*
c. HIV
d. *Staphylococcus aureus*
e. *Aspergillus fumigatus*

28) Osteoporosis circumscripta – well-defined geographic lytic lesions in the skull – represents the early stages of which condition?

a. Paget's disease
b. hyperparathyroidism
c. multiple myeloma
d. senile osteoporosis
e. sickle cell disease

29) On lateral radiographs of the thoracolumbar spine, a central anterior beak of the vertebral bodies is most likely to suggest which of the following conditions?

   a. Scheuermann's disease
   b. Morquio's syndrome
   c. Hurler's syndrome
   d. Down's syndrome
   e. achondroplasia

30) MRI of the knee in an 18-year-old man, performed for pain and limited joint movement, reveals an osteochondral lesion of the medial femoral condyle. Other than displacement, which MRI finding is the most specific indication of an unstable osteochondral fragment?

   a. joint effusion
   b. subfragmental bone resorption
   c. 3 mm cyst deep to the lesion
   d. underlying linear high signal on T2W images
   e. multiple lesions

31) Plain radiographs of the spine in a 40-year-old man performed following a road traffic collision reveal a slightly expanded midthoracic vertebral body with coarse vertical trabeculations. Subsequent CT shows a 'polka-dot' appearance to the same vertebral body in the axial plane. What is the most likely disorder affecting the vertebra?

   a. aneurysmal bone cyst
   b. osteoid osteoma
   c. haemangioma
   d. compression fracture
   e. osteopoikilosis

32) A young man complains of early morning back pain and stiffness, and undergoes plain radiographs followed by MRI of the whole spine. Which single feature is most likely to suggest a diagnosis of psoriatic arthritis over ankylosing spondylitis?

   a. syndesmophytes
   b. parasyndesmophytes
   c. asymmetrical sacroiliitis
   d. ankylosis
   e. patchy bone marrow oedema

33) A 23-year-old man falls onto his outstretched right hand with his elbow flexed. AP and lateral radiographs of the mid-forearm reveal a fracture of the middle third of the radius. Which additional radiograph should be performed?

a. clavicle
b. shoulder
c. elbow
d. oblique forearm
e. wrist

34) Which of the following is the most common type of Salter–Harris fracture, accounting for over 70% of growth-plate fractures of the immature skeleton?

a. type I
b. type II
c. type III
d. type IV
e. type V

35) A 19-year-old man presents to his general practitioner with a sudden onset of painful scoliosis. His pain improves with prescribed aspirin while awaiting MRI. MRI reveals a localized area of inflammatory change in the left pedicle of L1. Subsequent CT shows marked sclerosis in the same region with a 5 mm, cortically based central lucency. What is the most likely cause?

a. plasma cell cytoma
b. osteosarcoma
c. osteoid osteoma
d. Brodie's abscess
e. lymphoma

36) A 40-year-old man falls down the stairs and remains unconscious for several hours. On admission to hospital, he is found to have bilateral upper limb weakness, patchy sensory loss, full power in the lower limbs and a normal level of consciousness. Plain radiographs of the cervical spine and CT of the brain are normal. On MRI of the cervical spine, there is a small area of oedema identified within the cord. Clinical symptoms persist for 4 days following injury. What is the most likely diagnosis?

a. central cord syndrome
b. anterior cord syndrome
c. SCIWORA (spinal cord injury without radiological abnormality)
d. spinal shock
e. Brown-Séquard syndrome

37) Vertebral sclerosis confined to the upper and lower endplates with preservation of the intervertebral disc space ('rugger jersey spine'), is seen most commonly with which underlying condition?

a. osteoporosis
b. discitis
c. mucopolysaccharidosis
d. Paget's disease
e. renal osteodystrophy

38) A 49-year-old woman presents to her general practitioner with a history of mild midfoot pain exacerbated by walking and wearing tight shoes. Ultrasound scan demonstrates a hypoechoic, 7 mm, rounded lesion lying in the third tarsal interspace. The lesion is poorly demonstrated on MRI, returning intermediate T1 and low T2 signal. Which of the following conditions best explains these findings?

a. tendon sheath ganglion
b. tendon sheath giant cell tumour
c. synovial cyst
d. Morton's neuroma
e. paraganglioma

39) A young man is assaulted and attends accident and emergency with a painful left mandible and inability to open and close his jaw without pain. Radiographs show a simple linear fracture through the left body in the parasymphyseal region. A second fracture is most likely to be seen at which of the following sites?

a. ipsilateral condylar neck
b. ipsilateral angle
c. symphysis menti
d. contralateral body
e. contralateral condylar neck

40) On plain radiographs, which of the following is the most specific indicator of prosthetic loosening following total hip replacement?

a. sclerosis at the tip of the femoral component
b. 3 mm, lucent line at the cement/prosthesis interface
c. heterotopic bone formation
d. periprosthetic fracture
e. femoral periosteal reaction

41) A 21-year-old man presents with right hip pain. He has a history of Ewing's sarcoma of the right hemi-pelvis when aged 11, which was treated with limb-sparing surgery and chemoradiotherapy. Plain radiography shows well-defined regional sclerosis, and isotope bone scan demonstrates a corresponding photopenic area. What is the most likely cause of his pain?

a. recurrent Ewing's sarcoma
b. heterotopic ossification
c. radiation necrosis
d. osteoarthritis
e. osteosarcoma

42) On MRI performed for a tender osteochondroma of the femoral metaphysis in an adult, which feature is most useful in determining the presence of malignant change?

a. thickness of the cartilage cap
b. lesion size
c. compression of local nerves
d. fracture of the stalk
e. bursa formation

43) A middle-aged male patient who has previously undergone partial discectomy for radiculopathy, has a lumbar spine MRI due to a recurrence of his symptoms. T1W images show a low-signal area of tissue contiguous with the previously operated intervertebral disc and impinging upon the adjacent exiting nerve root. Which single additional finding favours a diagnosis of postoperative fibrosis over recurrent disc protrusion?

a. high signal on STIR sequence
b. enhancement with intravenous gadolinium
c. evolution at 6-month serial imaging
d. oedema in the surrounding bone
e. low signal on T2W images

44) Following major trauma, which of the following fractures of the thoracic skeleton is most likely to indicate a significant injury to the underlying intrathoracic viscera?

a. glenoid
b. scapular blade
c. clavicle
d. first rib
e. sternum

45) A young man sustains an obvious head injury during an assault, with clinically apparent, left temporoparietal swelling and an underlying fracture on skull radiographs. The patient's GCS is initially normal but begins to deteriorate progressively after 4 hours of observation, and CT of the brain is requested. Which finding other than a skull fracture would you expect to find on CT to explain the patient's condition?

a. diffuse axonal injury
b. haemorrhagic contusions
c. subarachnoid haemorrhage
d. subdural haematoma
e. extradural haematoma

46) On plain radiographs of the hands, hyperflexion of the proximal interphalangeal joint of the index finger, with hyperextension of the distal interphalangeal joint of the same finger, describes which deformity?

a. swan-neck
b. Boutonnière
c. mallet finger
d. baseball finger
e. Z-deformity

47) The Catterall 'head at risk' signs are plain radiographic signs that indicate a poor prognosis and increased risk of femoral head collapse in Legg–Calvé–Perthes disease. Which of the following options is not such a sign?

a. Gage's sign (wedge-shaped lysis of the femoral head)
b. calcification lateral to the epiphysis
c. lateral subluxation of the epiphysis
d. metaphyseal bone resorption
e. horizontal orientation of the growth plate

48) A young male patient sustains an external rotational injury to his left ankle and is unable to bear weight. A plain radiograph of the ankle performed in accident and emergency shows no fracture but does show soft-tissue swelling over the medial malleolus and widening of the ankle joint space medially (lateral talar shift). Which of the following additional view(s) should be performed?

a. mortise view
b. calcaneus
c. foot
d. knee
e. contralateral ankle

49) Tarsal coalition is a common cause of foot pain. Which of the following joints is most commonly affected?

 a. anterior subtalar
 b. middle subtalar
 c. posterior subtalar
 d. calcaneonavicular
 e. calcaneocuboid

50) O'Donoghue's unhappy triad consists of injuries to which three internal structures of the knee that are commonly injured together?

 a. anterior cruciate and lateral collateral ligaments, medial meniscus
 b. anterior cruciate and lateral collateral ligaments, lateral meniscus
 c. anterior cruciate and medial collateral ligaments, medial meniscus
 d. anterior cruciate and medial collateral ligaments, lateral meniscus
 e. posterior cruciate ligament, medial and lateral menisci

51) At which of the following skeletal locations does avascular osteo-necrosis typically only occur in the presence of an associated fracture?

 a. medial tibial condyle
 b. second metatarsal head
 c. lunate
 d. femoral head
 e. proximal scaphoid pole

52) A young adult male sustains an acetabular fracture in a high-speed road traffic collision. Which type of acetabular fracture is most commonly associated with significant neurological injury?

 a. posterior rim/wall
 b. anterior rim/wall
 c. transverse T-shape
 d. anterior and posterior column
 e. central dislocation

53) Of the following subtypes of osteosarcoma, which is associated with the most favourable 5-year survival?

 a. multicentric
 b. periosteal
 c. paraosteal
 d. telangiectatic
 e. soft-tissue

54) A 30-year-old woman undergoes plain radiographic imaging of the hand for a palpable, painful hard lump on the dorsum. Plain radiographs show a well-defined bony mass applied closely to the diaphysis of the second metacarpal. CT shows a wide-based pedunculated lesion with a perpendicular orientation to the diaphysis, no cartilage cap and a matrix of mature trabeculated bone. What is the most likely diagnosis?

a. osteochondroma
b. multiple osteocartilaginous exostoses
c. bizarre paraosteal osteochondromatous proliferation
d. Codman's tumour
e. dysplasia epiphysealis hemimelica

55) A young adult male sustains an anterior shoulder dislocation while playing rugby. There is no associated fracture. Following apparently uncomplicated reduction in accident and emergency, he is unable to abduct the arm and complains of numbness over the upper lateral arm. What is the most likely cause?

a. supraspinatus tendon tear
b. axillary nerve palsy
c. musculocutaneous nerve palsy
d. shoulder impingement
e. deltoid muscle tear

56) Bilateral hand radiographs performed in a 70-year-old man for painful and stiff joints reveal a symmetrical periosteal reaction involving the metacarpals, increased soft tissue of the fingertips, and an increase in the longitudinal curvature of the fingernails. Which additional imaging investigation is most appropriate?

a. CT of the hands
b. MRI of the hands
c. isotope bone scan
d. radiograph of the chest
e. radiographs of the shoulders

57) Of the following eponyms associated with fractures, which relates to a fracture–dislocation?

a. Segond
b. Jones
c. Smith
d. Barton
e. Hutchinson

58) An elderly female patient has plain radiographs performed in an outpatient clinic for bilateral painful, stiff hips, which demonstrate joint space narrowing. Which additional feature is more likely to support a diagnosis of rheumatoid arthritis rather than osteoarthritis?

a. eccentric joint space loss
b. soft-tissue swelling
c. subchondral sclerosis
d. subchondral cysts
e. protrusio acetabuli

59) A middle-aged woman, known to suffer from polyostotic fibrous dysplasia, presents with a palpable, 3 cm, soft-tissue mass in the upper left thigh. MRI shows a relatively homogeneous, smooth, well-defined lesion located in an atrophic quadriceps muscle, which returns low signal on T1W images and high signal on T2W images. Following administration of intravenous gadolinium, the lesion shows moderately intense heterogeneous enhancement. What is the most likely pathological nature of the soft-tissue lesion?

a. soft-tissue myxoma
b. malignant fibrous histiocytoma
c. soft-tissue cavernous haemangioma
d. multiple lipomatosis
e. rhabdomyosarcoma

60) Which of the following locations is most often associated with post-traumatic osteolysis?

a. coronoid process of ulna
b. surgical neck of humerus
c. lateral clavicle
d. femoral neck
e. fibular head

61) A young man is admitted in cardiac arrest following electrocution. Following successful resuscitation in accident and emergency, he complains of an acutely painful right shoulder with severely decreased range of movement. What is the most likely plain film finding?

a. anterior shoulder dislocation
b. posterior shoulder dislocation
c. acromioclavicular dislocation
d. fractured surgical neck of humerus
e. subacromial impingement

62) A middle-aged woman falls on an outstretched hand, which becomes immediately painful and swollen. A lateral radiograph shows a small fracture fragment dorsal to the carpus, and the AP radiograph appears normal. Which carpal bone is most likely to be fractured?

a. scaphoid
b. lunate
c. triquetrum
d. capitate
e. hamate

63) An elderly woman falls down the stairs and suffers a Malgaigne fracture of the pelvis and a 1% degloving injury to the left forearm. Due to significant medical co-morbidity, the decision is made not to treat with surgery. The patient dies overnight on the ward. What is the most likely mechanism of death?

a. pulmonary embolism
b. fat embolism
c. septicaemia
d. myocardial infarction
e. intra-abdominal haemorrhage

64) A 20-year-old man is a restrained driver in a high-speed road traffic collision. On admission to accident and emergency he undergoes CT of the brain for a reduced consciousness level. Images show diffuse brain injury. Which of the following findings would support a diagnosis of diffuse axonal injury rather than simple contusions?

a. corticomedullary petechial haematoma
b. anterior temporal petechial haematoma
c. basofrontal petechial haematoma
d. intraventricular haemorrhage
e. brain oedema

65) A 40-year-old woman presents to the emergency department with a painful, stiff shoulder, 12 hours after undergoing arthrography of the same joint. She describes onset of symptoms 8 hours previously with progressive worsening. She feels otherwise well with a temperature of 37.3°C. There is no overt joint swelling or overlying erythema. What is the most likely cause?

a. septic arthritis
b. chemical synovitis
c. joint haemarthrosis
d. joint effusion
e. allergic contrast reaction

66) Which of the following features is not a recognized primary musculoskeletal manifestation of the CREST (calcinosis, Raynaud's phenomenon, oesophageal involvement, sclerodactyly and telangiectasia) syndrome?

a. digital oedema
b. calcinosis
c. acro-osteolysis
d. osteoporosis
e. joint erosions

67) In reviewing a fracture of the spine at the thoracolumbar junction in a major trauma case, which single indicator on CT is most sensitive for inferring instability?

a. widened facet joints
b. two-column malalignment
c. soft-tissue swelling
d. rotational abnormality
e. increased intervertebral disc space

68) Which of the following is not a recognized cause of myeloid hyperplasia (red marrow reactivation/reconversion) in a 50-year-old adult?

a. sickle cell disease
b. smoking
c. chemotherapy
d. long-distance running
e. Gaucher's disease

69) Plain radiographs of the knees are performed in a teenage girl with growth retardation and painful, deformed lower limbs. Which radiographic finding would suggest a diagnosis of scurvy rather than rickets?

a. pathological fractures
b. bowing deformity
c. widened growth plate
d. frayed metaphysis
e. sclerotic epiphyseal rim

70) Which of the following local factors is not associated with an increased risk of fracture non-union?

a. infection
b. fracture mobility
c. avascular fragments
d. impaction
e. open fracture

71) On MRI of the foot performed for non-specific pain, which single feature is most specific for a diagnosis of sinus tarsi syndrome?

a. subtalar joint effusion
b. subtalar sclerosis
c. loss of fat signal in the sinus
d. bone marrow oedema in the talus
e. flexor tendon high signal on T2W images

72) The hypoperfusion complex, seen in patients who have suffered major blunt abdominal trauma, includes all but which of the following radiological signs on contrast-enhanced CT?

a. hyperenhancement of the adrenal glands
b. hyperenhancement of the pancreas
c. hyperenhancement of the spleen
d. collapsed inferior vena cava
e. small aorta

73) A 70-year-old man has plain radiographs of the hands and knees for joint pain and swelling, which show joint space narrowing and chondrocalcinosis. Which additional finding would support a diagnosis of haemochromatosis over pseudogout?

a. periarticular calcium deposition
b. metacarpal hooked osteophytes
c. eccentric joint space narrowing
d. large subchondral cysts
e. intra-articular loose bodies

74) A middle-aged man has a history of an undiagnosed wrist injury interfering with his playing golf. He presents with clinically apparent ulnar nerve compression at the wrist. Which of the following causes is most likely to be identified following investigation with CT and MRI?

a. non-union of hook of hamate fracture
b. non-union of scaphoid wrist fracture
c. scapholunate dissociation
d. pisiform osteoarthritis
e. triangular fibrocartilage complex tear

75) A 16-year-old female gymnast sustains a twisting injury to the knee, which becomes immediately painful and swollen, and she is unable to bear weight. Initial radiographs show an effusion but are otherwise normal. MRI confirms a joint effusion with a torn medial retinaculum, marrow oedema affecting the anterior aspect of the lateral femoral condyle, and a chondral defect of the medial facet of the patella. What is the most likely injury?

a. lateral collateral ligament tear
b. medial meniscal tear
c. pivot shift injury
d. transient patellar dislocation
e. posterolateral corner syndrome

76) A 50-year-old mechanic with a long history of back pain presents to the spinal clinic complaining of sudden onset of numbness and pain over the right lateral calf and dorsum and sole of the right foot following heavy lifting. Which of the following spinal pathologies is most likely to explain the patient's symptoms?

a. lumbar spinal stenosis
b. paracentral L4−5 disc protrusion
c. paracentral L5−S1 disc protrusion
d. far lateral L4−5 disc protrusion
e. central L5−S1 disc protrusion

77) A patient undergoes skull radiographs for a suspected occipital depressed skull fracture after falling backwards onto the pavement. You receive non-angulated AP frontal and lateral views. Which additional view would you request from the radiographer in order to detect an occipital bone skull fracture?

a. orthopantomogram
b. submentovertical
c. Towne's
d. Caldwell's
e. Water's

78) A 30-year-old man undergoes MRI of the whole of the left lower limb and pelvis for a mid-femoral destructive lytic lesion identified on radiography that is thought to represent a primary bone tumour. MRI shows that the disease is confined to the femur with a 5 cm diaphyseal lesion and a 1 cm proximal metaphyseal skip lesion. No enlarged lymph nodes are identified. CT scans of the chest, abdomen and pelvis show two metastatic nodules in the lower lobe of the left lung. Subsequent biopsy confirms the diagnosis of osteosarcoma. The cancer is correctly staged as which of the following?

a. TI N0 M0
b. TI N0 MIa
c. T2 N0 MIb
d. T3 N0 MIa
e. T3 N0 MIb

79) A young women attempts to commit suicide by jumping from a third-storey window, sustaining a fall of 15 metres. In addition to bilateral lower limb and spinal fractures, she suffers a blunt deceleration injury to the mediastinum. CT findings are of a large mediastinal haematoma and a focal area of irregularity in the contour of the wall of the aorta, which appears otherwise normal. Which segment of the thoracic aorta is most commonly affected by tear or transection?

a. root
b. ascending
c. isthmus
d. arch
e. descending

80) A 72-year-old women presents to the rheumatologist with a long history of shoulder pain affecting her dominant arm that began at night with associated stiffness, but has suddenly worsened over the past few weeks. Radiographs show a superiorly subluxed humeral head forming a pseudarthrosis with the acromion, glenohumeral joint space loss, humeral head collapse with cysts and sclerosis, and periarticular soft-tissue calcification. Ultrasound scan demonstrates an effusion with widespread degeneration of the rotator cuff and a complete tear of the supraspinatus tendon. Examination of aspirated joint fluid shows calcium hydroxyapatite crystals. What is the most likely diagnosis?

a. Milwaukee shoulder
b. pseudogout
c. myositis ossificans progressiva
d. erosive osteoarthritis
e. scleroderma

81) Which of the following is not an appropriate indication for percutaneous polymethylmethacrylate cement vertebroplasty?

a. progressive osteoporotic deformity
b. painful osteoporotic collapse
c. painful haemangioma
d. painful osteoid osteoma
e. painful metastases

82) On MRI of the spine demonstrating vertebral body collapse, which additional feature favours an underlying diagnosis of malignancy rather than osteoporosis?

a. bone fragment retropulsion
b. focal low signal in the vertebral body on T1W images
c. diffuse intermediate signal in the vertebral body on T2W images
d. no enhancement with gadolinium
e. convex posterior border to the vertebral body

83) By the middle of the third decade, the adult pattern of haemato-poietic and fatty marrow distribution is established. Red marrow remains in all but which of the following locations?

a. sternum
b. clavicles
c. ribs
d. proximal humeri
e. distal femora

84) A 35-year-old woman of African origin is admitted to accident and emergency with acute abdominal and back pain with pyrexia. Radiographs of the chest, abdomen and lumbar spine show rib thinning with notching, sclerosis of the right humeral head and biconcave, 'fish-shaped', lumbar vertebral bodies. A subsequent radiograph of the skull reveals widening of the diploë with hair-on-end striations. What is the most likely underlying condition?

a. neurofibromatosis
b. thalassaemia major
c. sickle cell disease
d. syphilis
e. Scheuermann's disease

85) Radiographic arthrography of the shoulder with injection of contrast into the glenohumeral joint is performed for a painful joint with a globally reduced range of movement. Which single finding is most likely to indicate a diagnosis of adhesive capsulitis?

a. pain on injection of contrast
b. small axillary recess
c. contrast tracking along the subscapularis muscle
d. contrast in the subacromial space
e. obliteration of the subcoracoid fat

86) A 45-year-old, right-handed, male mechanic presents to orthopaedic clinic with intermittent ulnar-sided wrist pain that is at its worst while he uses a screwdriver. Radiographs show positive ulnar variance with a normal ulnar styloid. Subsequent MRI reveals a central perforation of the triangular fibrocartilage complex with chondromalacic changes in the lunate. What is the most likely condition?

a. ulnar impingement syndrome
b. ulnar impaction syndrome
c. ulnar styloid impaction syndrome
d. hamatolunate impaction syndrome
e. triangular fibrocartilage tear

87) On plain radiographs of the long bones or the spine, which of the following is not a recognized cause of a 'bone within a bone' appearance?

a. infant physiology
b. sickle cell anaemia
c. nutritional disturbance
d. renal osteodystrophy
e. metastatic disease

88) On radiographs and MRI of the spine performed for lower back pain with clinical signs of radiculopathy, which of the following features favours a diagnosis of discitis rather than degenerative disc disease?

a. vacuum phenomenon in the discs
b. reduced disc space
c. intermediate signal posterior to the vertebral body on T1W images
d. vertebral endplate low signal on T1W images
e. Schmorl's nodes

89) A young man is admitted to accident and emergency following an assault, during which he was struck in the face with a heavy blunt object. Radiographs show multiple midface fractures. Which supporting buttress of the face is disrupted in a Le Fort II fracture, but spared in a Le Fort I fracture?

a. inferior lateral maxillary
b. inferior medial maxillary
c. superior medial maxillary
d. transverse maxillary
e. pterygomaxillary

90) A 30-year-old man visits his general practitioner complaining of recent onset of acne and discharging pustules on his palms. He has a history of several years of pain and swelling at the medial end of his right clavicle. Radiographs of the shoulder demonstrate hyperostosis and early ankylosis of the sternoclavicular joint. What is the most likely diagnosis?

a. SAPHO syndrome
b. suppurative osteomyelitis
c. psoriatic arthritis
d. Reiter's disease
e. recurrent multifocal osteomyelitis

91) A 70-year-old man undergoes CT of the skull for investigation of clinically apparent macrocephaly confirmed on skull radiography. You are asked by the referring clinician to review the images. Which finding is most likely to support a diagnosis of fibrous dysplasia over Paget's disease?

a. widened diploë
b. asymmetrical involvement of the skull
c. sparing of the paranasal sinuses
d. osteoporosis
e. ground-glass medulla

92) Vertebral bone marrow oedema, seen as low signal on T1W and high signal on T2W MR images, occurs typically in all but which of the following conditions?

a. degenerative disc disease
b. multiple myeloma
c. osteoporotic collapse
d. spondylolysis
e. ankylosing spondylitis

93) An elderly man undergoes ^{99m}Tc-labelled diphosphonate bone scintigraphy. There is no uptake of tracer in the soft tissues, urinary tract or appendicular skeleton, but the axial skeleton shows diffuse homogeneous tracer uptake. No focal lesions are seen. What is the most likely cause of these appearances?

a. prostatic metastases
b. renal osteodystrophy
c. Paget's disease
d. mastocytosis
e. myelofibrosis

94) A 65-year-old man undergoes radiographs of the lumbar spine and pelvis for lower back pain. A destructive lytic lesion is identified in the midline of the inferior sacrum with internal areas of calcification. Subsequent MRI reveals a heterogeneous lesion replacing much of the sacrum, which returns moderate low signal on T1W and high signal on T2W images, with a soft-tissue component extending into the presacral soft tissues. The lesion shows patchy moderate enhancement with intravenous gadolinium. What is the most likely diagnosis?

a. metastasis
b. giant cell tumour
c. aneurysmal bone cyst
d. chordoma
e. plasmacytoma

95) A 70-year-old man attends a 6-week follow-up appointment after cemented total hip arthroplasty, complaining of a poor range of motion. Radiographs taken during the appointment show small areas of pericapsular bone, and formation of small bony spurs at the acetabular margin. CT demonstrates these areas to have well-defined mineralization peripherally and indistinct centres. Which of the following processes are responsible?

a. femoral component loosening
b. heterotopic ossification
c. periprosthetic fracture
d. postoperative infection
e. stress shielding

96) A 30-year-old woman in the third trimester of pregnancy complains of a 4-week history of gradual onset of pain in the left hip following minor trauma. Radiographs show a normal-appearing joint space, mild osteopenia of the femoral head and neck, and an indistinct subchondral femoral head. On subsequent MRI, the bone marrow in the affected regions returns patchy but diffuse low signal on T1W and high signal on T2W images. There is a similar small area of marrow abnormality in the acetabulum, and a small hip effusion is seen. What is the most likely diagnosis?

a. septic arthritis
b. infarction
c. reflex sympathetic dystrophy
d. rheumatoid arthritis
e. transient osteoporosis

97) Which of the following can cause a false-negative result in performing an ultrasound scan of the shoulder for suspected rotator cuff tear?

a. rotator interval
b. musculotendinous junction
c. limited joint mobility
d. anisotropy
e. acoustic shadowing

98) Following wrist arthrography by a single-compartment radiocarpal injection technique, contrast seen on MR arthrographic images in the midcarpal compartment can be explained by disruption of which of the following structures?

a. triangular fibrocartilage
b. lunotriquetral ligament
c. dorsal distal radioulnar ligament
d. flexor retinaculum
e. radioscapholunate ligament

99) A young footballer sustains a twisting injury to the right knee in training. He is able to continue practising but complains of moderate medial knee pain. The following morning he wakes with a swollen stiff joint. Radiographs show an effusion only. Subsequent MRI confirms an effusion and reveals a truncated medial meniscus with a 'bow-tie' configuration seen on only a single sagittal image. Sagittal sequences reveal a 'double' appearance of the posterior cruciate ligament. He has not had any previous surgery. What is the most likely injury or combination of injuries?

a. torn medial meniscus
b. torn medial meniscus and anterior cruciate ligament
c. torn medial meniscus and posterior cruciate ligament
d. torn anterior cruciate ligament
e. torn posterior cruciate ligament

100) Plain radiographs of the femur performed for pain reveal a centrally located lucent lesion in the medulla with a partially calcified matrix. Which of the following features favours a diagnosis of chondrosarcoma over enchondroma?

a. arc-and-ring matrix calcification
b. ground-glass matrix
c. multiple lesions
d. deep endosteal scalloping
e. lesion size over 5 cm

Module 2: Musculoskeletal and Trauma: Answers

1) a. **

The vast majority of giant cell tumours occur in patients with closed epiphyses, and although they may originate in the metaphysis, lesions typically involve the epiphysis and abut the subarticular surface. They are classically eccentrically located lesions with a narrow zone of transition, no sclerosis, and no internal matrix mineralization. Giant cell tumours tend to be locally aggressive, with a high recurrence rate after initial treatment. Enchondromas are the commonest benign cystic lesion of the phalanges, though they are also seen in the long bones. However, those in the long bones almost always contain calcified chondroid matrix. Aneurysmal bone cysts are often seen as an eccentric lytic expansile lesion, but patients are nearly all under the age of 30. Monostotic fibrous dysplasia is more commonly seen in the proximal femur than distally, and lesions tend to have a sclerotic margin. Fibrous cortical defects are asymptomatic lesions seen in children, which usually regress spontaneously, so they are only rarely seen after the age of 30. They typically appear as lytic lesions with a thin sclerotic border in the metaphysis of a long bone.

Helms (2005), 13–15.

2) c. ***

Gaucher's disease is the most common lysosomal storage disorder with an incidence of 1:50 000 (100 times more common in Ashkenazi Jews). It is caused by a defect of hydrolase acid β-glycosidase, which results in accumulation of the fatty substance glucosylceremide within macrophages in the reticuloendothelial system. It characteristically causes an Erlenmeyer flask deformity of the distal femur or proximal tibia due to marrow infiltration. Patients may be asymptomatic or present with anaemia, large joint stiffness or bone pain. Diagnosis is by bone marrow aspirate. The mucopolysaccharidoses are a spectrum of lysosomal storage diseases that typically present in infancy with a variety of overt symptoms and signs. Rheumatoid arthritis can present with anaemia and joint stiffness, but marrow infiltration is not a feature on plain film. Musculoskeletal manifestations of Langerhans' cell histiocytosis most commonly affect the skull (50%). Although Erlenmeyer flask deformity is seen in thalassaemia major, presentation is within the first 2 years of life.

Dähnert (2007), 93–4.

3) b. **

The avulsion fracture described is a Segond fracture, which is classically associated with anterior cruciate ligament (ACL) rupture, and represents avulsion of the meniscotibial portion of the middle third of the lateral capsular ligament. Anterior translocation of the tibia occurs in complete ACL rupture, and manifests clinically as the anterior draw sign. Also associated with ACL rupture is an impaction injury of the lateral femoral condyle, which can be seen on radiographs as a deepened lateral femoral condylar sulcus, although sometimes this cannot be identified on acute films.

Remer et al (1992).

4) d. ***

The fracture described is a hangman fracture. This involves either the pedicles or pars interarticularis of C2 bilaterally. The mechanism is usually extension and traction (as caused during hanging). Hyperflexion injuries produce anterior tear-drop or of a vertebral body wedge fractures. Axial loading can produce a burst fracture of C1 (Jefferson's fracture) or a vertebral body elsewhere in the spine. Hyperflexion and extension are associated with longitudinal ligament injury. Hyper-rotation is associated with soft-tissue injury or facet joint dislocation.

Mackintosh & Tucker (2002).

5) c. **

Pulmonary embolism is a common complication following immobility and major surgery, particularly orthopaedic surgery of the pelvis. It typically occurs 7–10 days post-surgery. Chest radiograph findings can be normal but include small effusion, collapse or consolidation, elevation of the hemidiaphragm, a prominent pulmonary artery and hypertransradiance of the affected side (Westermark sign). Fat embolism is preceded by long bone injury in 90% of cases but usually occurs within 36 hours of the injury, and is much less common than pulmonary embolus from deep vein thrombosis even in the context of major trauma. Pneumonia and pneumothorax do of course occur in postoperative patients, but it would be reasonable to expect associated findings on the chest film. Hyperventilation should be a diagnosis of exclusion once other potentially serious causes have been excluded.

Fabian (1993); De Lacey et al (2007), 293.

6) d. ****

The structures of the posterolateral corner of the knee have a very important role in maintaining the rotational stability of the knee joint. The lateral collateral ligament forms the superficial layer, with the remainder of the structures comprising the deep layer. Injury is relatively common and results most frequently from a varus force on an extended joint. The lateral collateral ligament and popliteus tendon are present in all joints, with the popliteofibular ligament being present in approximately 98%. Both the arcuate ligament and fabellofibular ligaments are variable, with the former absent more frequently. Absence of one of these structures is often compensated for by hypertrophy of the other.

Davies et al (2004).

7) a. ***

The spinal injury described is a Chance fracture, a fracture through the vertebral body and pedicles caused by hyperflexion, therefore causing compression of the spine anteriorly and distraction posteriorly. This injury typically occurs in back-seat passengers wearing a lap seat belt during a road traffic collision. In children, there is a 50% incidence of associated intra-abdominal organ injury. Retroperitoneal organs are most vulnerable, being closest to the spine. Duodenal injuries are most common, and have a significant associated mortality. The pancreas is also commonly injured due to its retroperitoneal location.

Vandersluis & O'Connor (1987).

8) e. ***

Osteopoikilosis is a rare condition causing multiple enostoses (bone islands), which are asymptomatic and usually of no clinical significance. They represent deposits of normal cortical bone within the cancellous bone. Osteopathia striata (Voorhoeve's disease) is similar to osteopoikilosis in appearance and is usually asymptomatic, but it consists of linear longitudinal or sunburst striations rather than rounded densities. Osteopetrosis causes generalized increase in bone density, whereas melorrheostosis is a cortical process giving a 'flowing wax' appearance, usually affecting only one side of the affected bone. While metastases are plausible, the patient would probably be symptomatic and have evidence or a history of a primary tumour.

Dähnert (2007), 140–1.

9) e. ***

The findings describe the Buford complex, a normal variant present in 1.5% of the population. It consists of an absent anterior labrum with a thickened cord-like middle glenohumoral ligament. It can be misdiagnosed as a torn or avulsed anterior labrum, resulting in unnecessary shoulder arthroscopy.

Tirman et al (1996).

10) b. ****

Cam is the most common form of femoroacetabular impingement in men, typically presenting in the third or fourth decade. It is often related to a previous slipped upper femoral epiphysis in the teenage years. A change in the rotational axis (increase in the alpha angle) causes the proximal superior femoral neck to impinge upon the superior acetabular margin and labrum, in turn causing intermittent pain, particularly in physically active individuals. Even without a history of slipped femoral epiphysis, an osseous bump on the superior femoral neck obliterating the femoroacetabular sulcus can cause symptoms. Labral or articular cartilaginous tears can follow repetitive microtrauma, leading to persistent pain and locking. The pincer type is more common in women and is caused by an abnormally deep acetabulum.

Pfirrmann et al (2006).

11) e. **

Bilateral lower limb involvement suggests a myelopathy rather than a radiculopathy. The presence of urinary and bowel symptoms and saddle anaesthesia suggests compression of lumbosacral nerve roots. This complex of symptoms is cauda equina syndrome and is considered an orthopaedic emergency because of the likelihood of permanent neurological impairment, particularly affecting the autonomic supply to the bladder or bowel, which can result in permanent incontinence if surgery is delayed. The Royal College of Radiologists recommends proceeding straight to MRI in patients who have 'red flag' signs.

Royal College of Radiologists (2007), 110–11.

12) a. **

The common cancers that typically metastasize to bone are breast, lung, thyroid, renal and prostate. Due to the high prevalence of colon cancer, even though only a relatively small proportion metastasizes to bone, it forms a significant proportion of bone metastases. Prostatic metastases are typically sclerotic, whereas breast deposits are mixed. Colonic bone metastases are usually lytic, with renal metastases typically lytic and expansile due to their highly vascular nature. Other less frequent sources of lytic expansile metastases include thyroid, melanoma and phaeochromocytoma.

Chapman & Nakielny (2003), 18.

13) b. **

The fallen fragment is virtually pathognomonic for a simple bone cyst. It represents a fragment from a pathological fracture through the lesion, which has fallen to lie in a dependent location in the cyst matrix.

Killeen (1998).

14) c. ***

The lesser arc refers to the arc of ligamentous attachments around the lunate. These ligaments become disrupted in a stepwise four-stage fashion. Stage I injury is to the scapholunate ligament, leading to dissociation with rotary subluxation of the scaphoid. Stage II is radiographically characterized by perilunate dislocation, caused by additional injury to the capitolunate joint. The carpus migrates dorsally and the lunate maintains a normal relationship with the radius. Stage III involves the triquetrolunate ligaments, and stage IV is complete disruption of the perilunate ligaments, allowing dislocation and rotation of the lunate. It is this rotation that creates the triangular outline on AP radiographs. Segmental instabilities relate to the spectrum of dynamic scaphoid instability.

Resnick & Kransdorf (2005), 851–3.

15) a. **

New bone formation is the hallmark finding of psoriatic arthritis and is not seen in rheumatoid arthritis. Conversely, periarticular osteoporosis is seen in rheumatoid but is not a feature of psoriatic arthritis. Both conditions may cause soft-tissue swelling (typically a sausage digit in psoriatic arthritis), joint space loss and erosions, which are marginal in psoriatic and marginal and/or central in rheumatoid arthritis. Another distinguishing factor is the distribution of involved joints in the hands, which is typically, but not always, interphalangeal in psoriatic and metacarpophalangeal in rheumatoid arthritis.

Dähnert (2007), 149, 153–6.

16) b. ****

Abnormal disc position and morphology are the earliest and most sensitive signs of derangement, occurring three to five times more commonly in women and usually manifesting by the fourth decade. The cause is often not found but includes trauma, malocclusion, bruxism (teeth grinding) and primary osseous abnormalities. Disc deformity, if unchecked, leads to secondary osseous abnormality. Degenerative arthritis is typically erosive with flattening of the condylar head and anterior osteophytosis. The disc may become biconcave, thickened, folded or torn. On MRI of the joint, the position of the disc should be assessed first on closed-mouth sagittal T1W images. It may become displaced in any direction, with anterior being the most common. In the initial stages the disc may reduce on mouth closing, but with progression it becomes fixed in an anteriorly subluxed position. The temporomandibular joint can also be an involved site in rheumatoid arthritis.

Harms & Wilk (1987); Tomas et al (2006).

17) e. **

The zone of transition relates to the interface between the tumour margin and the host bone. It is an extremely important discriminator, particularly for lytic lesions. Lesions with a well-defined margin (and therefore narrow zone of transition) are described as geographic and are usually non-aggressive, whereas those with a wide zone of transition are termed 'permeative' and are often malignant or aggressive (such as in osteomyelitis). Cortical expansion without destruction is seen in many benign or slow-growing conditions such as fibrous cortical defect and aneurysmal bone cyst. Many bone lesions, both benign and aggressive, are lytic. Periosteal reaction does not indicate an aggressive lesion as such, but the pattern of reaction can do so. Multiplicity is not an indicator of malignancy, as it can be seen in benign and self-limiting processes (such as multiple enchondromatosis and neurofibromatosis). Equally, a solitary lesion may be malignant.

Manaster et al (2006), 407–10.

18) e. ****
The far lateral disc protrusion is the least common type of symptomatic disc herniation. It distinguishes itself from the posterolateral herniation in that the disc ruptures outside the spinal canal, lateral to the root foramen. The disc, instead of tethering the traversing nerve root, compresses the more rostral nerve root that has already exited the root foramen. The neurological symptoms therefore correspond to a lesion at the upper disc level, often leading to confusion in the diagnosis. It is also difficult to diagnose radiologically, as the far lateral location is usually not detected on the sagittal images but only on axial images. STIR is an inversion recovery sequence that suppresses fat and so highlights areas of increased fluid. However, it is not sensitive when the herniation is outside the fluid-filled spinal canal; therefore, the T2W gradient echo sequence is better at detecting far lateral disc herniation.

Maravilla & Cohen (1991), 202.

19) c. **
Chondroid tumour matrix may or may not calcify, but, if it does, the pattern is characteristically in arcs or circles and is sometimes described as 'popcorn'. Osteoid matrix when calcified is usually dense and homogeneous like a cloud. Calcified fibrous matrix has a characteristic ground-glass appearance, whereas a cellular tumour usually does not show matrix calcification. A mixed matrix will show mixed characteristics.

Weissleder et al (2007), 430.

20) d. *
Rickets (vitamin D deficiency) results in failure of normal bone mineralization (osteomalacia) during bone growth and may have a dietary, cultural or metabolic cause. A widened growth plate in a child is due to rickets until proven otherwise. Other features include bowing deformity, metaphyseal cupping and/or fraying, poor epiphyseal mineralization, delayed closure of the fontanelles, enlargement of the costochondral junction (rachitic rosary) and craniotabes. Scurvy is a deficiency of vitamin C and is a primarily a disorder of collagen

production, resulting in osteopenia with dense metaphyseal lines and a sclerotic rim around the epiphysis.

Dähnert (2007), 156–7.

21) e. **

Achondroplasia is the most commonly seen autosomal dominant rhizomelic dwarfism. Rhizomelia refers to relative shortening of the proximal compared with the distal portion of the limbs. Achondroplasia has widespread skeletal manifestations affecting the skull, chest, spine, pelvis and extremities. Intelligence and motor function are normal. The most significant complication is brain-stem or spinal cord compression due to spinal stenosis, which is caused by alignment abnormalities and decreased spinal canal size due to short pedicles with a reduced interpedicular distance. Atlantoaxial instability is defined as a predental space of 3 mm or more in adults and 5 mm or more in children, or where there is considerable change between flexion and extension. It is seen in inflammatory arthritides, in Down's and Morquio's syndromes, and with retropharyngeal abscess in a child.

Resnick & Kransdorf (2005), 1298–1300.

22) b. ***

Pigmented villonodular synovitis is a benign proliferative disorder of the synovium that has a propensity for young to middle-aged adults and typically has a long history. On plain radiographs, joint space and bone mineralization are typically preserved until late in the disease, but soft-tissue swelling or effusion may be apparent early on. Haemorrhage is relatively common and can result in haemarthrosis and blooming artefact seen on gradient echo MRI sequences. Malignant fibrous histiocytoma is the most common soft-tissue sarcoma after age 50. Synovial osteochondromatosis is more common in men and is characterized by proliferation of the synovium with formation of cartilaginous nodules (that often calcify), but does not show haemorrhage. Baker's cyst has synovial fluid characteristics on MRI and is located posterior to the joint.

Sheldon et al (2005).

23) b. ***

Ollier's disease or multiple enchondromatosis is characterized by the presence of benign intraosseous cartilaginous tumours. The estimated prevalence of the disease is 1 in 100 000. The distribution and number of lesions are variable, but are often unilateral and monomelic. Complications include pain, skeletal deformities, limb length discrepancy (including Madelung's deformity) and the potential risk of malignant change to chondrosarcoma in 20–50% of cases. The condition in which enchondromas are associated with haemangiomas is known as Maffucci's syndrome. Neither is usually inherited. Trevor's disease is an epiphyseal dysplasia, whereas Lichtenstein–Jaffé disease is another name for fibrous dysplasia. Morquio's syndrome is one of the lysosomal storage disorders known as the mucopolysaccharidoses.

Pannier & Legeai-Mallet (2008).

24) a. **

Periosteal reactions are usually a radiographic manifestation of underlying bone disease. The term 'soap bubble' refers to expansion of the cortex without destruction by a lytic bone lesion. The intact cortex usually indicates a benign process, whereas cortical destruction is associated with malignant or aggressive lesions. Sunray and hair-on-end reactions are spiculated forms of periosteal reaction that occur following periosteal elevation by tumour, with tumour preventing the subperiosteal space from filling with new bone. Laminated or 'onion-skin' reaction occurs with both malignant and benign processes and indicates an intermittent or cyclical process. Codman's triangles are formed by elevation and then destruction of the periosteum. They are usually related to malignant tumours but can also be formed by aggressive benign processes.

Greenfield et al (1991).

25) e. **

Looser's zones or Milkman's pseudofractures are seen as linear lucencies in the bone due to incomplete fractures that have non-mineralized osteoid deposited within them. The underlying failure of bone to mineralize is termed 'osteomalacia' (which means bone softening), and is most often due to vitamin D deficiency. Rickets is osteomalacia in an immature skeleton. The most common conditions resulting in an osteomalacic process and inadequate bone mineralization include renal osteodystrophy and vitamin D deficiency due to malnutrition/malabsorption of vitamin D or phosphate.

Resnick & Kransdorf (2005), 565–6.

26) d. ***

Diffuse idiopathic skeletal hyperostosis (DISH) is an ankylosing disorder of the spine. It is most commonly seen in the thoracic region but may involve cervical and lumbar regions. Diagnostic criteria are of flowing calcification along the anterolateral border of at least four vertebral bodies, relative preservation of intervertebral disc height, and absence of sacroiliac joint or apophyseal involvement. These three criteria aid differentiation of spondylosis deformans, intervertebral osteochondromatosis and ankylosing spondylitis respectively. Extra-spinal manifestations of DISH include Achilles tendinosis, tennis elbow, calcaneal and olecranon enthesopathy and dysphagia. Whiskering is seen radiographically at tendinous insertions, particularly of the pelvis.

Ramos-Remus et al (1993); Resnick & Kransdorf (2005), 425–33.

27) a. **

The musculoskeletal system is affected in only 1–3% of tuberculous infections, but the spine is the most common skeletal location affected, accounting for 50% of musculoskeletal tuberculosis. Tuberculous spondylitis (or Pott's disease) can result in significant neurological sequelae. A history of pulmonary infection may or may not be present. The infection usually begins in the anterior vertebral body via haematogenous spread. The intervertebral discs are frequently involved, and the loose internal structure of the disc allows the infection to disseminate more widely, often resulting in paraspinal or psoas abscess. Calcification within the abscess is very specific for tuberculosis. The disease process often leads to vertebral collapse with gibbous deformity and obliteration of the disc space. However, elevation of the anterior ligaments by subligamentous abscess allows tracking superiorly and inferiorly, and classically spares the disc. Tuberculosis characteristically results in little reactive sclerosis or periosteal reaction, which helps to distinguish it from pyogenic infections.

Burrill et al (2007).

28) a. **

Paget's disease is a common progressive disorder of osteoclasts and osteoblasts resulting in bone remodelling. It is usually polyostotic and asymmetrical, and affects 10% of those aged over 80. Osteoporosis circumscripta is seen in the initial phase of Paget's disease, which is characterized by an aggressive, predominantly lytic process with intense osteoclastic activity causing bone resorption. Bone marrow is replaced by fibrous tissue with large vascular channels. Geographic osteoporosis is seen in the skull and long bones, where the characteristic feature is a flame-shaped radiolucency beginning in a subarticular location and progressing into the diaphysis. The disease then progresses through a mixed phase to a quiescent inactive late stage where bone turnover is decreased. The skull is involved in 29–65% of cases, most commonly the anterior calvarium.

Dähnert (2007), 144–6.

29) b. ***

Morquio's syndrome is type IV and the most common of the mucopolysaccharidoses, a family of inherited disorders of metabolism. A central vertebral beak is relatively specific for the condition. Other spinal manifestations include odontoid hypoplasia with atlantoaxial subluxation (which can be life threatening), platyspondyly, ovoid vertebral bodies, widened intervertebral disc space and exaggeration of the normal lumbar lordosis. Other skeletal findings include dwarfism, as well as skull, face and appendicular abnormalities. Hurler's syndrome belongs to the same family of disorders but has an inferior vertebral beak, which is also seen in achondroplasia and Down's syndrome. Scheuermann's disease does not show vertebral beaking.

Boström et al (2006).

30) d. ***
High T2 signal in the bone underlying an osteochondral lesion has been described as the most common of four MRI findings indicating instability of an osteochondral fragment, which is the most important factor when considering treatment options. The reported accuracy of this sign for predicting instability varies from 45% to 85%, with one study reporting an increased accuracy when this sign is combined with the second sign of a cartilaginous defect on T1W images. However, another study states that often only a single indicator is present. The other indicators of instability are high signal in the articular cartilage and a cystic lesion in the bed (but this needs to be 5 mm or larger).

De Smet et al (1996).

31) c. *
Metastatic disease, myeloma and lymphoma are the most common malignant spinal tumours, and haemangioma is the most common benign tumour of the spine. The appearances described are characteristic of a vertebral haemangioma. On MRI, these lesions typically appear of mottled low-to-high signal on T1W images depending on the degree of fat present, and of very high signal on T2W images. Other primary osseous lesions of the spine are more unusual but may exhibit characteristic imaging features that can help develop a differential diagnosis. Radiological evaluation of a patient who presents with osseous vertebral lesions often includes radiography, CT and MRI. The complex anatomy of the vertebrae means that CT is more useful than conventional radiography for evaluating lesion location and assessing bone destruction. The diagnosis of spinal tumours is based on patient age, topographic features of the tumour and lesion pattern as seen on imaging.

Rodallec et al (2008).

32) b. ***
Seronegative spondyloarthritis is an umbrella term for inflammatory joint or spinal conditions that are not associated with rheumatoid factor or rheumatoid nodules. There are five described subgroups: ankylosing spondylitis, psoriatic arthritis, arthritis associated with inflammatory bowel disease, reactive arthritis (e.g. Reiter's syndrome) and an undifferentiated subgroup. The subgroups may overlap both clinically and radiologically, and the diagnosis is more easily made on the basis of clinical history and examination. Imaging plays a limited role in differentiation, particularly early in the disease when there can be considerable overlap of appearances. The main exception is the identification of parasyndesmophytes, which are seen almost exclusively

in psoriatic arthropathy. In addition, bone marrow oedema can involve the entire vertebral body in psoriatic arthritis, which may be a further useful distinguishing feature. Undifferentiated spondyloarthritis is diagnosed when there is no clinical or radiological evidence of sacroiliitis. All types may eventually progress to ankylosis.

Hermann et al (2005).

33) e. **

A Galeazzi fracture–dislocation is a pattern of injury sustained by falling on an outstretched hand with a flexed elbow. It most commonly consists of a fracture of the radial diaphysis with dislocation or subluxation of the distal radioulnar joint. It is associated with a high rate of non-union, and one or both components are usually treated with surgical fixation. It is important therefore that the radiologist can recognize potential patterns of injury and radiographically demonstrate their full extent. As a general rule, fractures should be viewed in two orthogonal planes, as should the joint above and below any fracture. The opposite pattern, of an ulnar shaft fracture with dislocation of the proximal radial head, is termed a Monteggia fracture–dislocation. A mnemonic for remembering the two is Glasgow Rangers (Galeazzi, radius) and Manchester United (Monteggia, ulna), which indicates for each injury which of the forearm bones is fractured.

Dähnert (2007), 87.

34) b. *

The Salter–Harris classification originally described five types of growth plate injury. Type I (6–8%) is slip of the epiphysis due to shearing forces, and the fracture line is a cleavage through the growth plate only. Type II is by far the most common (75% of injuries) and is also a shearing injury. The fracture line involves the physis and extends proximally into the metaphysis separating a triangular fragment. Type III (6–8%) occurs in partially closed growth plates, involves the physis and extends distally into the epiphysis, involving the articular surface. Type IV (10–12%) is a fracture that begins in the metaphysis, crosses the physis and also involves the epiphysis. Type V (1%) is a crush injury. The classification indicates progressively poorer prognosis with regard to future growth disturbance. There have been subsequent additions to the classification.

Salter & Harris (1963).

35) c. **

Osteoid osteoma accounts for 12% of benign neoplasms of bone. It is most commonly located in the cortex of long bones (50% in the femur and tibia) with 15% in the spine, typically the pedicle. It rarely exceeds 15 mm in size. Young men are most commonly affected, with pain as the predominant presenting feature due to the extensive inflammatory reaction and vascularity of the lesion. With spinal lesions this results in a painful positional scoliosis, though the majority of patients experience improvement of the pain with salicylates. The lucent central area or nidus represents the underlying pathological process, with the surrounding sclerosis representing reactive inflammatory change in normal bone. Treatment traditionally was surgical curettage, but radiologically guided percutaneous radiofrequency ablation is now used.

Kransdorf et al (1991).

36) a. ****
In trauma, an incomplete spinal cord injury is one in which there is any degree of sparing of motor or sensory function distal to the site of injury, whereas complete cord injury results in complete lack of neurological function distal to the injury. The diagnosis can be made only in the absence of spinal shock, a transient spinal cord concussion. Central cord syndrome is the most common incomplete injury, and is associated with hyperextension injury in middle-aged patients; injury to centrally located grey matter in the cord causes a greater motor neurological deficit in the upper than in the lower extremities. Sensory involvement can be variable, and bowel and bladder function may be affected. Anterior cord syndrome, caused by anterior spinal vascular insufficiency, causes complete motor paralysis with sparing of the posterior columns. SCIWORA is seen in children, when the elastic cervical spine deforms sufficiently to cause cord injury but without any radiological findings. Brown-Séquard syndrome results from hemitransection and causes ipsilateral muscle paralysis and contralateral hyperaesthesia to pain and temperature.

Wheeless (1996).

37) e. ***
The 'rugger jersey spine' appearance refers to sclerotic bands along the superior and inferior endplates of the thoracic and lumbar vertebral bodies. These bands represent accumulation of excess osteoid and result in a striped appearance of the vertebral bodies. Despite being poorly mineralized, the accumulated osteoid appears opaque on plain radiographs because of its increased volume compared with that of normal bone. The 'rugger jersey spine' is said to be almost pathognomonic for the osteosclerosis seen with the secondary hyperparathyroidism of chronic renal failure. Renal osteodystrophy is a term for the constellation of musculoskeletal abnormalities occurring with chronic renal failure. Osteoporosis and Paget's disease are more likely to affect the whole of the vertebrae diffusely. Discitis usually causes a reduction in the intervertebral disc space on radiographs, with indistinct endplates. The mucopolysaccharidoses result in anterior vertebral body beaking rather than sclerosis.

Wittenberg (2004).

38) d. **

Morton's or interdigital neuroma is a benign lesion consisting of perineural fibrosis that entraps a plantar digital nerve. It is frequently asymptomatic and women represent 80% of cases. Clinical presentation is with foot pain exacerbated by walking, and symptomatic lesions are surgically excised. They are not usually demonstrated on plain radiography and are poorly seen on MRI, returning intermediate T1 and low T2 signal (similar to surrounding tissues). Typical ultrasound appearances are of a hypoechoic rounded lesion, larger in the axial than the sagittal plane. Ganglia and cysts would return high signal on T2W images, and pathology arising from the tendon sheath itself can also show high signal. Giant cell tumours are usually painless.

Llauger et al (1998).

39) e. ***

The mandible is best considered as a closed ring, and as such approximately half of all mandibular fractures are bilateral and multiple. The majority occur at the angle, and a significant portion occur at the condylar neck, a common pattern of injury being an ipsilateral body fracture from a direct blow, with a contralateral angle or condylar neck fracture due to transmitted rotation force compressing that side. Fractures of the condylar neck have a limiting effect on the opening and closing of the jaw and can be missed radiographically. Fractures in the midline are also subtle and account for a significant minority. A flail mandible occurs when the anterior support for the tongue is lost due to a bilateral fracture. This injury carries the risk of the tongue prolapsing posteriorly and occluding the airway.

Weissleder et al (2007), 390–1.

40) b. *

The artefact created by metallic prostheses on CT and MRI means that plain radiography has an important role in the evaluation of post-operative arthroplasty joints. Cemented prostheses may normally show a 1–2 mm lucent line at cement interfaces, but definite loosening is diagnosed with progressive widening of this zone. Other specific indicators of loosening in both cemented and uncemented prostheses include migration of components or a new abnormality of alignment. Periosteal reaction and sclerosis can be normal findings, particularly in uncemented prostheses. Serial imaging is often required to confirm the diagnosis of loosening.

Manaster (1996).

41) c. ***

Ewing's sarcoma is a relatively common malignant bone marrow tumour related to, and sharing a common chromosomal translocation with, peripheral neuroectodermal tumours. It is a very aggressive tumour that is expressed in the radiological findings of permeative osteolysis, cortical erosion, periostitis and a soft-tissue mass. It principally affects the lower half of the skeleton, with the most frequent location being metadiaphyseal in the femur, ilium, tibia, humerus, fibula and ribs. Both radio- and chemotherapy are used in treatment. Sclerosis within several months of treatment usually indicates bone healing or disease recurrence/persistence. Radiation-induced osteonecrosis is mainly an effect on the osteoblasts and is dose dependent (deterministic). It may be seen within the mandible within 1 year, but in other sites the latent period is longer and can be a number of years.

Resnick & Kransdorf (2005), 1192–5.

42) a. **

Osteochondromas are the commonest bone tumours and are considered developmental exostoses rather than true neoplasms. They represent 20–50% of benign and 10–15% of all bone tumours. They are made up of cortical and medullary bone and an overlying cartilage cap. The cortex and medulla of the osteochondroma are continuous with the underlying host bone. They are typically orientated away from an adjacent distal joint. Lesions are frequently solitary, but multiple lesions are seen in hereditary multiple exostoses, an autosomal dominant syndrome. Malignant transformation occurs in 1% of solitary lesions and in 3–5% of patients with hereditary multiple exostoses. After skeletal maturity, continued lesion growth, particularly of the cartilage cap, is suggestive of malignant transformation. Although benign lesions may reach 10 cm in size, the cartilage cap should not exceed 1.5 cm after skeletal maturation. Any bone that develops by enchondral ossification may develop an osteochondroma, the long bones of the lower extremity being most frequently affected.

Murphey et al (2000).

43) b. **

In MRI of the spine in postoperative discectomy patients with recurrent or persistent radiculopathy, a T1W sequence with intravenous gadolinium enhancement is added to distinguish between postoperative epidural fibrosis (or scarring) and recurrent disc herniation. Both can have similar, low-signal appearances on unenhanced T1W and T2W images, but fibrosis will show enhancement with gadolinium whereas recurrent disc prolapse will not. Difficulties arise where both conditions exist concurrently, and fibrosis that is not causing nerve root irritation may also enhance. The importance of distinguishing between the two is that surgical treatment is indicated for recurrent disc herniation but is of no value in treating postoperative fibrosis, also known as failed back syndrome.

Hueftle et al (1988).

44) d. **

First rib fracture is considered a harbinger of major trauma, with approximately two-thirds of fractures being associated with major chest injury and carrying a significant mortality. The anatomy of the first rib is such that it is protected from the minor insults that often break other ribs, and fracture of the first rib usually indicates violent blunt trauma to the thorax. Associated local injuries include damage to the brachial plexus, major vascular structures and the underlying lung and heart. There is also an association with significant abdominal injury, but the major cause of death in patients with a first rib fracture is an associated head injury. It is rare for a first rib fracture to be an isolated finding.

Richardson et al (1975).

45) e. **

Extradural (or epidural) haematoma is the accumulation of blood in the potential space between the inner table of the skull and the dura. Ninety per cent of cases are associated with a fracture of the temporal bone which traverses and ruptures the middle meningeal artery (in 60–90%) or vein. In children, vascular injury may occur here without a fracture. In half of cases, there is a lucent interval between injury and the onset of deteriorating consciousness level, as opposed to diffuse axonal injury where coma is immediate. CT appearances are of an extra-axial, biconvex, high-attenuation collection. A subdural haematoma is caused by shearing forces on small bridging veins and is not necessarily associated with a fracture of the calvarium, although this may coexist. It differs from an extradural haematoma not in radiographic location but in that it has a crescentic rather than a biconvex shape.

Grossman & Yousem (2003), 247–8.

46) b. **

The Boutonnière deformity is commonly caused by injury or inflammatory conditions such as rheumatoid arthritis, and more commonly affects the index than middle fingers. It consists of four stages. Stages 1 and 2 are mild and moderate, passively correctable extension lag, whereas stages 3 and 4 are mild and advanced flexion contractures. The proximal flexion deformity is due to disruption of the central slip of the extensor tendon, with the proximal phalanx herniating through the defect and the lateral slips lying on either side. The position of the proximal phalanx stretches the lateral slips and pulls the distal phalanx into extension. Swan-neck deformity has similar causes but the opposite configuration, with extension at the proximal interphalangeal joint and flexion distally. Mallet (or baseball) fingers have a passively correctable flexion deformity of the distal interphalangeal joint caused by avulsion of the extensor digitorum tendon by a hyperflexion injury. Z-deformity is the name given to a Boutonnière-type deformity seen in the thumb.

Apfelberg et al (1978).

47) d. *****
Catterall described four radiographic signs that indicate a femoral 'head at risk' of avascular necrosis (Perthes' disease), in an attempt to predict those cases in which considerable collapse of the femoral head may occur. Gage's sign is a radiolucent V-shape seen in the lateral side of the epiphysis on frontal pelvis radiographs. Calcification lateral to the epiphysis indicates a small area of lateral head collapse. The third sign is lateral subluxation, best seen as an increased inferomedial joint space, which when seen in conjunction with the first two worsens the prognosis. Finally, in some individuals the normal growth plate is more horizontally orientated, which results in normal weight-bearing forces exerting a shearing force on the growth plate, rather than a compressive force as seen in the more common transversely orientated growth plate. A horizontal growth plate is therefore considered a further poor prognostic sign in Perthes' disease.

Catterall (1971).

48) d. ***
The Maisonneuve fracture is a spiral fracture of the upper third of the fibula associated with a tear of the distal tibiofibular syndesmosis and the interosseous membrane. The medial component of the injury may be an associated fracture of the medial malleolus or rupture of the deep deltoid ligament. The ankle joint is effectively a bony ring that extends up to the knee. Interruption of the ring in this way allows lateral displacement of the fibula and so disruption of the congruence of the ankle mortise, resulting in an unstable ankle injury that requires surgical fixation.

Raby et al (2005), 222–4.

49) d. ***
MRI is valuable in the diagnosis of a number of musculoskeletal conditions of the ankle, including osteochondral lesions of the talus, bone infarcts and bruising, stress fractures, osteoid osteoma and tarsal coalition. Forty-five per cent of tarsal coalition occurs at the calcaneonavicular joint, with a further 45% at the subtalar joint, most commonly involving the middle facet. Radiographic findings include joint space narrowing, indistinct articular margins, elongation of the anterior calcaneus, a hypoplastic talus and reactive sclerosis of the involved bones. It is commonly associated with pes planus. Treatment options include physical supports, anti-inflammatory medication, local steroid injection, and surgical resection or arthrodesis.

Kier et al (1991).

50) c. **
O'Donoghue's unhappy triad consists of injuries to the anterior cruciate and medial collateral ligaments and the medial meniscus, and is an injury associated with contact sports. The mechanism is indirect trauma

causing deceleration, hyperextension and twisting forces. The combination of external rotation of the tibia on the femur, knee flexion and valgus stress can produce an anterior cruciate ligament injury combined with additional medial collateral ligament injury. The meniscus and collateral ligament medially are attached to one another, unlike their lateral counterparts, resulting in a higher frequency of concordant injury to the other medial structure when one is injured.

O'Donoghue (1964).

51) e. *
Osteonecrosis may be caused by two mechanisms: interruption of arterial supply, and intra- or extra-osseous venous insufficiency. Interruption of vascular supply is usually associated with a fracture, as seen in the proximal scaphoid following waist fractures. Femoral head osteonecrosis can occur with subcapital fractures, or without fracture as in Legg–Calvé–Perthes disease. Other common locations that may develop osteonecrosis without overt fracture include the medial tibial condyle (Blount's disease), metatarsal head (Freiberg's infraction) and the lunate (Kienbock's disease). Radiographic findings often lag several months behind the injury or onset of symptoms, and MR is the most sensitive imaging modality. Radiographic signs include focal radiolucencies, sclerosis, bone collapse and loss of joint space.

Weissleder et al (2007), 474–6.

52) a. **
Acetabular fractures are common in multiple or major trauma patients, particularly those involved in road traffic collisions, and are classified according to the Letournel classification. Fractures are often complex and require accurate delineation with CT, often following limited or suboptimal initial radiographic investigation with or without oblique pelvic (Judet) views. Isolated posterior rim or wall fractures are the most common type (27%) and are associated with a high frequency of posterior dislocation of the femoral head causing sciatic nerve injury. If the entire posterior column is involved in the fracture, there is a lower incidence of sciatic nerve injury, as the femoral head may not be dislocated. Anterior injuries are uncommon (5%) and may be associated with anterior femoral head dislocation and iliac wing fracture. Transverse fractures account for 9%.

Martinez et al (1992).

53) c. **
Osteosarcoma is the second most common primary malignancy of bone after multiple myeloma, accounting for 15% of all primary bone tumours. It usually affects those aged 10–30. Ninety-five per cent are of the primary osseous type and, of these, paraosteal osteosarcoma has the most favourable 5-year survival rate of 80%. Other osteosarcomas of the primary osseous type include periosteal (5-year survival rate 50%)

and telangiectatic (less than 20%). Multicentric refers to synchronous osteoblastic osteosarcomas at multiple sites. It occurs exclusively in children aged 5–10, and carries an extremely poor prognosis. The soft-tissue type is rare, representing only 1.2% of all soft-tissue tumours. These lesions are primary soft-tissue tumours with no attachment to bone. Death occurs within 3 years in the majority of cases, tumour size being the major predictor of outcome.

Dähnert (2007), 141–4; Weissleder et al (2007), 433–5.

54) c. *****
Bizarre paraosteal osteochondromatous proliferation (also known as Nora's lesion) is a rare condition usually seen in adults in the third and fourth decades of life. Osteochondroma-like lesions are seen most commonly at the proximal and middle phalanges, followed by the metacarpals and metatarsals. A relationship to trauma has been suggested but not proven. Other locations that may be affected include the long bones (especially those of the upper extremity), skull and jaw. It is thought to be a similar process to that which gives rise to lesions in myositis ossificans, reactive periostitis and subungual exostosis. On plain radiographs, a well-defined bony mass is seen attached to the surface of the parent bone. Features differentiating this from osteochondroma are the absence of angulation away from the nearby physis and a wide base.

Murphey et al (2000); DeGroot (2001).

55) b. ***
The axillary nerve is a large terminal branch of the posterior cord of the brachial plexus that passes into the posterior aspect of the upper arm via the quadrilateral space, where it winds around the surgical neck of the humerus to supply the deltoid and teres minor muscles. It has a cutaneous distribution called the 'regimental badge area' over the lateral aspect of the deltoid (where a soldier may wear his regimental badge). Due to its intimate relationship with the humerus and its passage through the relatively small quadrilateral space, the axillary nerve is by far the most commonly injured nerve with shoulder dislocation or fractures. As loss of abduction may be caused by pain rather than deltoid paralysis, it is good practice to assess the sensation in the cutaneous distribution of the axillary nerve before and after any attempted shoulder reduction.

Visser et al (1999).

56) d. ***
Hypertrophic pulmonary osteoarthropathy (HPOA) is a clinical syndrome of osteitis of the long bones, arthritis and digital clubbing of the fingers and toes. It is most commonly associated with lung cancer (affecting 3–10% of patients) or other chronic pulmonary or pleural disease. The underlying mechanism has not been established with certainty, but autonomic nervous or endocrine stimulation by tumours

is postulated, with hormones such as oestrogen, adrenocorticotrophic hormone and growth hormone implicated. In patients presenting with HPOA, approximately 80% have an underlying lung cancer, 10% a pleural tumour and 5% another intrathoracic malignancy. Other causes include chronic, suppurative, pulmonary inflammatory disease and congenital cyanotic heart disease. Typical radiographic appearances are of a lamellar periosteal reaction affecting the diametaphyseal regions of the long bones, particularly the dorsal and medial aspects. Bone symptoms and radiographic signs frequently regress following treatment of the underlying cause.

Mito et al (2001).

57) d. **
The use of eponymous names for fractures allows quick and accurate identification and communication of bone injuries while simultaneously alerting clinicians to the potential complications associated with a given fracture pattern. This is also particularly useful when describing complex radiographic appearances to someone remote from the images. The full value of such eponyms depends on accurate use and understanding of their meaning: Barton's fracture–dislocation is an intra-articular fracture of the dorsal margin of the distal radius with dorsal dislocation of the radiocarpal joint; Segond's fracture is an avulsion fracture of the proximal lateral tibia; Jones' fracture is a transverse fracture of the base of the fifth metatarsal, at the junction of the diaphysis and metaphysis; Smith's fracture is a distal radial fracture with ventral displacement; and Hutchinson's fracture is a triangular fracture of the radial styloid.

Hunter et al (2000).

58) e. ***
Even or eccentric joint space reduction representing cartilage loss is seen in both types of arthritis and not a distinguishing diagnostic feature. Although osteoarthritis is said to be classically eccentric, this is difficult to assess accurately on many hip radiographs, as they are not routinely taken in the upright, weight-bearing position. Subchondral sclerosis and cysts are typically associated with degenerative osteoarthritis. Although soft-tissue swelling is a feature of rheumatoid arthritis, the depth of the hip joint and the copious surrounding soft tissues mean that any synovial swelling is unlikely to be appreciated clinically or radiologically. Subtle osteophytes (in osteoarthritis) or erosive change/osteoporosis (in rheumatoid arthritis) can distinguish between the two entities. An inflammatory cause should be considered in young adults with hip pain and, if protrusio or other abnormalities are found, the sacroiliac joints should be examined.

Manaster (2000).

59) a. ****

The association of fibrous dysplasia and soft-tissue myxoma is well established and is commonly termed Mazabraud's syndrome. The key is identifying the relationship between the bone and soft-tissue pathology, with the osseous features of fibrous dysplasia usually preceding the formation of a soft-tissue mass. The condition is non-familial and more commonly affects women, the thigh being the most common location. Typical MRI appearances are of a well-defined lesion with signal intensity similar to water, and often a fat rind or adjacent muscle high signal on T2W images is seen. Although uncommon, there have been reported cases of malignant change into osteosarcoma.

Kransdorf & Murphey (1999).

60) c. **

The lateral third of the clavicle is the most common location for post-traumatic osteolysis. It is usually preceded by a fairly severe injury to the shoulder, typically dislocation or subluxation of the acromioclavicular joint. Changes may be evident radiographically after as little as 1 month. If no bone loss was apparent on radiographs at the time of injury, the diagnosis is unequivocal. However, if no such comparison can be made, then other causes of lateral clavicular osteolysis include rheumatoid arthritis, scleroderma and hyperparathyroidism. Other sites affected are the pubic and ischial rami, distal portions of the radius or ulna, the carpus and femoral neck. Widespread idiopathic osteolysis is termed Gorham's or vanishing bone disease.

Jacobs (1964).

61) b. ***

Posterior shoulder dislocation is much rarer than anterior dislocation, accounting for only 5% of dislocations. It can be caused by direct or indirect force and is most commonly seen following seizure or electrocution. The internal rotators of the shoulder are stronger than the external rotators, resulting in internal rotation of the arm if all the shoulder muscles contract simultaneously. This internal rotation predisposes to posterior dislocation in the same way that external rotation does for anterior dislocation. Radiographic findings may be subtle on the AP projection, and include superior position of the humeral head relative to the glenoid, external rotation (the humeral head appears symmetrical like a light bulb), a sharp angle to the scapulohumeral arc and a compression fracture of the anterior humeral head (a reverse Hill–Sachs lesion).

Weissleder et al (2007), 393–4.

62) c. **

Carpal fractures in general are much less common than fractures to the distal radius. The two bones most commonly injured are the scaphoid (75%) followed by the triquetrum (14%), and these provide a greater diagnostic challenge radiographically than distal radial fractures. Triquetrum fractures generally occur on the dorsal surface due to avulsion of the dorsal radiocarpal ligament, or shearing forces from impaction with the ulnar styloid or hamate in hyperextension. Less commonly, the body of the bone can fracture in a transverse pattern. A posterior chip fragment can often be seen with dorsal surface fractures, but is only visualized on the lateral view. Such an injury may be a primary triquetrum injury (such as avulsion) or related to a perilunate fracture–dislocation.

Goldfarb et al (2001).

63) e. **

A Malgaigne fracture of the pelvis is a fracture of the ischiopubic rami and an ipsilateral sacroiliac joint (or para-articular) fracture, and occurs due to high-energy blunt trauma. It represents complete disruption of the pelvic ring and therefore an unstable fracture. In such fractures, distortion and disruption of the pelvic soft tissues and vascular injury involving the rich blood supply in the pelvis will not be tamponaded by the bony ring, as the pelvis will expand to accommodate ever-increasing haematoma. Mortality rate from major pelvic trauma is 10%; other common causes of death include multiorgan failure and sepsis, the latter expected to take several days to evolve.

Failinger & McGanity (1992).

64) a. **

Contusions are traumatic injuries to the cortical grey matter of the brain and make up approximately half of primary intra-axial traumatic lesions. They are often multiple and bilateral, with the most common locations being the inferior frontal lobes and temporal poles. Diffuse axonal injury results from rotational shearing forces on cerebral white matter and common locations are white matter-rich areas, such as the corticomedullary junction, centrum semiovale, corpus callosum and cerebellum. In comparison to diffuse axonal injury, contusions tend to be larger and more superficial, with a higher proportion being haemorrhagic due to the increased vascularity of grey compared with white matter. Local or widespread oedema can be seen in both conditions.

Gentry (1994).

65) b. **

Post-arthrography pain due to sterile chemical synovitis is the most common complication of the procedure, typically beginning after 4 hours and peaking at 12 hours. Other, less common, immediate and short-term complications include allergic contrast reaction (rare in intra-articular injections), introduction of infection and vasovagal reaction.

Weissleder et al (2007), 423.

66) d. ***
CREST syndrome represents the limited form of the autoimmune connective tissue disorder scleroderma. Five-year survival rate is 50–67%. The two other types of scleroderma are generalized (also called systemic sclerosis) and localized (morphoea). Common findings are digital soft-tissue oedema with sclerodactyly (tapered soft tissues), acro-osteolysis (autoamputation) and calcinosis. There may be associated arthritis that shows erosions (also seen in the ribs) or terminal phalanx resorption, with joint space narrowing a late sign. Osteoporosis is not usually a feature except in the context of disuse.

Dähnert (2007), 863–5.

67) b. **
The spine can be divided anatomically into three columns: the anterior column contains the anterior longitudinal ligament, anterior half of the vertebral body and anterior annulus fibrosus; the middle column contains the posterior half of the vertebral body, posterior longitudinal ligament and the posterior annulus fibrosus; and the posterior column contains the posterior elements of the spine, facet joint capsule and interspinous ligaments. Two intact columns are required for intrinsic spinal stability. Disruption of two columns can therefore be used to infer instability. Usual traumatic patterns are anterior and middle, or posterior and middle, disruption. Isolated middle column interruption can occur after trauma or surgery, or as a congenital abnormality, and is also considered potentially unstable.

Denis (1983); Slone et al (1993).

68) e. ***
Marrow reconversion is the repopulation of yellow (fatty) marrow with haematopoietic cells, reconverting the fatty marrow to red marrow. This occurs when the haematopoietic capacity of the existing red marrow in an adult is insufficient. This can result from increased physiological requirement (long distance running), chronic anaemia (sickle cell disease) and chemotherapeutic treatment with granulocyte–macrophage colony-stimulating factor. The pattern of reconversion is predictable and it is the reverse of the age-related physiological conversion of red to yellow marrow. Reconversion begins in the axial skeleton and progresses distally through the appendicular skeleton, to end in the hands and feet. Knowledge and recognition of this pattern are important because neoplastic infiltration of adult yellow marrow in malignant disease may have similar MR appearances. However, malignant marrow replacement tends to have a more random

distribution than reconversion; it may enhance with intravenous gadolinium, can cause cortical destruction and may extend into the soft tissues.

Siegel (2008), 169–79.

69) e. **

Rickets is a deficiency of vitamin D in a child that results in osteomalacia of the immature skeleton. Scurvy is a deficiency of vitamin C and is a disorder of collagen synthesis that can occur in children or adults. Pathological fractures may be seen in both conditions. Ground-glass osteoporosis is characteristic of scurvy, with other features including a sclerotic line in the metaphyseal zone of preparatory calcification (white line of Fränkel), a radiolucent zone immediately to the diaphyseal side of the white line (Trümmerfeld's zone), corner fractures (Parke's corner sign) and a sclerotic ring around the epiphysis (Wimberger's sign). In addition, bleeding diathesis is seen in scurvy; therefore, subperiosteal haematoma and haemarthrosis are also features.

Dähnert (2007), 160–1.

70) d. **

Fracture sites that have a poor blood supply, either as a result of the original injury or due to subsequent surgical treatment, may go on to develop atrophic non-union where the bone ends become osteoporotic, thin and pointed (osteolysis) with no evidence of fracture healing. A fracture site that is very mobile may develop hypertrophic non-union where there is attempted healing denoted by excessive callus formation, but the fracture cleft persists. Open fractures are often high energy, with soft-tissue damage and comminution of fracture fragments, and are prone to infection, all of which predispose to non-union. Osteomyelitis in any fracture can result in delayed, non- or malunion. Non-union in most skeletal locations should not be diagnosed radiographically until 6 months have passed, particularly in the presence of complicating factors.

Russell et al (2004), 356.

71) c. ****

Sinus tarsi syndrome is a common complication of ankle sprains, but may also result from an inflammatory arthropathy. It is associated with abnormalities of one or more structures in the tarsal sinus and tarsal canal that lead to pain and a feeling of instability of the hindfoot. Most patients with this syndrome present in the third or fourth decade of life with persistent lateral foot pain, though the pathogenesis of the condition is poorly understood. Conventional radiography generally is not valuable, but on MRI there is alteration of the fat signal, the most common changes being diffuse low-signal-intensity infiltration on both T1W and T2W images. Other common MR findings include synovial thickening and diffuse enhancement of the tarsal sinus following intravenous gadolinium.

Lektrakul et al (2001).

72) c. ****
The hypoperfusion complex is a marker of severe injury and is an important prognostic indicator related to radiological signs on CT following blunt abdominal trauma. The features are of hypovolaemia, with small arterial and collapsed venous vessels indicating reduced circulating volume. Hyperenhancement of the kidneys, adrenal glands, pancreas and bowel wall is seen, but the spleen may be small and hypodense. If injury to the vascular pedicle is not present, non-enhancement of the spleen could be secondary to severe vasoconstriction and poor perfusion.

Dähnert (2007), 807.

73) b. ***
Haemochromatosis is excess iron deposition in the tissues and can be either primary (autosomal recessive genetic disorder) or secondary to ineffective erythropoiesis or iron overload. Skeletal manifestations include osteoporosis (which is proportional to the extent of iron deposition), small subchondral cysts, arthropathy (50%), concentric joint space narrowing, chondrocalcinosis, and characteristic hooked osteophytes on the radial aspect of the metacarpal heads. Other organs can be affected by iron deposition, most commonly the brain, liver, pancreas and spleen.

Dähnert (2007), 100–1.

74) a. *****
Fractures of the hook of the hamate are the most frequent type of hamate fracture, and most often occur from the repetitive stress of swinging a bat, club or racket, or from the direct blow of a club on the ground. This may result in ulnar nerve compression at the wrist in Guyon's canal, which is particularly exacerbated in the context of non-union due to secondary osteoarthritis or loose bodies in the pisotriquetral joint. Other causes of ulnar nerve compression at the wrist include adjacent masses, anomalous muscles and tendons, fibrous palmar arch, ulnar artery aneurysm, primary osteoarthritis of the pisotriquetral joint, os hamuli proprium and dislocation of the pisiform bone.

Blum et al (2006).

75) d. **
Transient patellar dislocation always occurs laterally and was originally thought to be an injury confined to teenage girls with abnormal

patellofemoral anatomy, but is now considered a potential injury in anyone who partakes in athletic activity. The most common finding is effusion and lateralization of the patella with or without an abnormally shallow femoral sulcus. Other findings seen on MRI are contusions of the lateral femoral condyle and medial patella with potential osteochondral defects, and disruption or sprain of the medial retinaculum. Less specific findings include loose bodies and associated ligamentous or meniscal injury.

Kirsch et al (1993).

76) b. ****
Degenerative disc disease of the spine is one of the leading causes of functional incapacity and chronic disability in the working population, affecting both men and women. Although there is no universally established nomenclature for describing disc herniation, 'protrusion' is commonly used if the herniation is broader than it is deep and 'extrusion' if it is deeper than it is broad. A disc 'bulge' is used to describe a herniation that is very broad based and may even be circumferential, with a generalised disc bulge being one that affects at least half of the periphery. As a result of the strong posterior longitudinal ligament, posterior disc herniation is often paracentral, i.e. to the side of the midline. This can result in compression of the transiting nerve root in the lateral recess, which is the one that will exit at the level below. A lateral disc herniation narrowing the neural foramen compresses the exiting nerve root. Therefore, for a given intervertebral disc, a paracentral herniation will affect the nerve that exits one level below, whereas a lateral protrusion affects the nerve root at that level.

Modic & Ross (2007).

77) c. ***
In modern radiology departments with the widespread availability of CT, the indications for skull radiograph are few, and it has little place in the evaluation of brain injury. Standard practice will usually comprise a lateral and a PA frontal view. The frontal view may be angled to show different areas of anatomy. Towne's view is an AP projection through the frontal and occipital bones (30° caudal tube tilt) and is mainly used to show the occipital bone. The Caldwell view is a similar AP projection but with only 15° of caudal tube tilt to allow evaluation of the orbits. An occipitomental (and therefore PA, unlike Towne's or the Caldwell) projection is called Water's view. It is used to demonstrate the facial bones and sinuses and may be angulated to highlight the zygomatic arches. Further angulation results in a submentovertical view, which is also used to evaluate the zygomatic arches. This requires extension of the neck and is therefore contraindicated in patients with suspected cervical spinal injuries. The orthopantomogram is a panoramic view of

the mandible used primarily in dental radiography and to evaluate the whole of the mandible in a single exposure.

Hemker (1999).

78) d. ****
Complete staging of primary bone sarcomas is unusual in that it also incorporates the histological staging once tissue diagnosis via biopsy or surgical resection is available. The local TNM classification is T1 (single lesion less than 8 cm), T2 (single lesion over 8 cm) or T3 (skip lesions of any size). Nodal staging is N0 (no nodes) or N1 (any number of metastatic nodes). Metastatic spread is staged, accordingly, as M0 (no metastases), M1a (metastases to lung) or M1b (any other distant site). Once histology is available, tumours can be staged I–IV.

Hricak et al (2007), 276–82.

79) c. ***
Ninety per cent of traumatic thoracic aortic injuries occur at the aortic isthmus, just distal to the origin of the left subclavian artery. The isthmus is the section between the origin of the left subclavian and the attachment of the ligamentum arteriosum, and is about 1.5 cm in length in a normal adult. The mechanism is usually rapid deceleration (but it can be due to direct trauma) as in a fall from a height or a road traffic collision. The isthmus is thought to be particularly vulnerable to the shearing forces that occur with deceleration compared with the descending aorta, as it is relatively mobile and can be bent over the left bronchus main stem and left pulmonary artery. A more recent theory is that this part of the aorta is particularly vulnerable to being crushed by the surrounding bony thorax (manubrium, clavicle and first rib) at the point of maximum deformation during high-energy injury. The ascending aorta is the site for injury in only 5% of those who survive to reach hospital, but is more prevalent in cadaveric studies due to the high association of fatal cardiac injuries. The mechanism here is thought to be torsional forces or a water-hammer effect (a sudden increase in intrathoracic pressure).

Creasy et al (1997).

80) a. ****
Milwaukee shoulder is a crystal deposition disease of basic calcium phosphate, predominantly affecting elderly women and resulting in a dysfunctional shoulder from destruction of the rotator cuff. It is often bilateral but always involves the dominant side. Radiographic findings include superior subluxation of the humerus due to loss of the superior rotator cuff, often forming a pseudarthrosis with the clavicle or acromion. Glenohumeral degeneration manifests as sclerosis and collapse of the humeral head, joint space narrowing and osteophyte formation. Erosion at the site of rotator cuff insertion and periarticular soft-tissue calcification is also a feature. Examination of effusion fluid is stereotypical, revealing spheroid-shaped aggregates of hydroxyapatite

crystals. The condition is also seen in the knee, where, unlike osteoarthritis, it predominates in the lateral compartment.

McCarty (1991).

81) d. ****
Percutaneous cement vertebroplasty is a treatment for vertebral compression fractures that involves the injection of acrylic bone cement into the vertebral body in order to relieve pain, stabilize fractured vertebrae or, in some cases, restore vertebral height. Current guidelines from the National Institute for Health and Clinical Excellence (NICE), regarding the use of vertebroplasty in the UK, state that it may be used for pain relief in patients with severe painful osteoporosis with loss of height, compression fractures of the vertebral body, symptomatic vertebral haemangioma and painful vertebral body tumours (metastases or myeloma). Review of current evidence indicates some level of pain relief in 58–97% of patients.

NICE (2003).

82) e. ***
A convex bulge involving the whole posterior border of the vertebral body strongly suggests vertebral body expansion by tumour invasion, and is only very rarely a feature of osteoporosis. Other findings on MRI suggestive of malignancy include a soft-tissue mass, involvement of the pedicles, and heterogeneous high signal on T1W post-contrast or T2W images. Retropulsion of bone fragments, focal T1 low signal or an isointense appearance on T1W or T2W images suggests osteoporotic collapse.

Cuénod et al (1996).

83) e. ***
MRI is superior to other imaging modalities in evaluating red (haematopoietic) and yellow (fatty) bone marrow, as a result of its very high sensitivity for lipid, which is present in significantly higher concentrations in yellow marrow than in red. At birth, haematopoietic marrow is present throughout the entire skeleton. A predictable sequence of conversion of red to yellow marrow begins distally in the hands and feet, and migrates proximally (over a period of 20 years) until red marrow remains only in the axial skeleton and the proximal humeral and femoral metaphyses. Reversal of this process is called reconversion. Appreciation of the areas of remaining red marrow in an adult is important, because malignant marrow infiltration can have a similar appearance to haematopoietic marrow, with location being a major discriminator.

Hwang & Panicek (2007).

84) c. **

Sickle cell disease is a haemoglobinopathy that results from the presence of abnormal β-globin chains within haemoglobin, which may manifest as anaemia, infarction and superimposed infection. It is much more prevalent in those of African–Caribbean origin. Over time, the disease produces musculoskeletal abnormalities as a result of chronic anaemia, such as marrow proliferation (which produces the characteristic changes in the skull), marrow reconversion and extramedullary haematopoiesis. Other common skeletal complications include bone softening, infection or infarction.

Ejindu et al (2007).

85) b. ***

Adhesive capsulitis or frozen shoulder is clinically characterized by restriction of both active and passive elevation and external rotation. Patients are commonly 40–70 years old and predominantly female. It may be idiopathic, preceded by trauma, or associated with diabetes mellitus or other conditions. Patients have been shown to have a significantly thickened coracohumeral ligament and joint capsule, and an axillary recess significantly reduced in volume. Obliteration of the fat triangle between the coracohumeral ligament and the coracoid process is specific when seen on MR arthrography. Treatment options include physiotherapy, intra-articular corticosteroid injection, manipulation under anaesthetic and surgical capsulotomy.

Mengiardi et al (2004).

86) b. ***

Ulnar-sided wrist pain is often caused by one of the spectrum of conditions known as impaction syndromes. These include ulnar impaction syndrome (most common), ulnar impingement syndrome, ulnocarpal impaction syndrome secondary to non-union of the ulnar styloid process, ulnar styloid impaction syndrome and hamatolunate impingement syndrome. Ulnar impaction syndrome is a degenerative condition secondary to excessive loading across the wrist and characteristically shows a positive ulnar variance that is accentuated in pronation and during a firm grip. MRI is used to identify complications such as triangular fibrocartilage complex tear or bone marrow oedema.

Cerezal et al (2002).

87) d. ***

'Bone within a bone' is a term used to describe a radiographic appearance in which one bone appears to arise within another. It can be a physiological finding in a neonate or infant due to new bone formation. Pathological conditions that can cause the appearance include periosteal new bone formation, cortical splitting, subcortical osteopenia, altered bone growth, impairment of osteoclastic activity, altered bone metabolism, crystal deposition, and iatrogenic and technical radiological factors. It is not a feature of renal osteodystrophy but is seen in hypervitaminosis D and in healing rickets.

Williams et al (2004).

88) c. **

Intermediate signal in the extradural space on T1W images is the most common appearance of extradural abscess formation. The most common primary focus of infection is discitis, but abscess formation may also be spontaneous. Patients particularly at risk are those with a history of diabetes mellitus, intravenous drug use, trauma, haemodialysis or recent surgery (particularly dental). MRI features of extradural abscess include iso- or slight hyperintensity on T1W images when compared with the spinal cord. High signal on T2W and proton density sequences makes it difficult to differentiate abscess from CSF, but these sequences are useful, as osteomyelitis and paravertebral abscess are well visualized as high-signal lesions. Administration of intravenous gadolinium contrast characteristically demonstrates diffuse enhancement of the solid component of the abscess.

Numaguchi et al (1993).

89) c. *****

Le Fort fractures involve separation of all or part of the maxilla from the skull base. For this to occur, the posterior vertical maxillary (pterygomaxillary) buttress at the junction of the posterior maxillary sinus with the pterygoid plates of the sphenoid must be disrupted. The remaining facial buttresses are inspected to determine the class of Le Fort fracture. A Le Fort I fracture involves the inferior portions of both the lateral and medial maxillary buttresses, resulting in the maxillary arch floating free from the face. In a Le Fort II fracture, the inferior lateral maxillary buttress is similarly injured, but, unlike type I, it is associated with fracture of the superior portion of the medial maxillary buttresses, resulting in dissociation of the entire maxilla from the skull base. A Le Fort III fracture results in the whole face floating free from the skull with disruption of the superior portions of both the lateral and medial maxillary buttresses and upper transverse maxillary buttress.

Hopper et al (2006).

90) a. ***

Synovitis, acne, pustulosis, hyperostosis and osteitis (SAPHO) syndrome is a term encompassing several disease entities that demonstrate an association between rheumatological and cutaneous lesions. There may be a delay of several years between the onset of osseous symptoms and cutaneous manifestations. It is thought to be similar to chronic recurrent multifocal osteomyelitis in children.

The dominant radiographic abnormality is new and bizarre bone proliferation, with the sternoclavicular joint affected in 70–90% of cases.

Suei et al (2003).

91) e. **

A ground-glass appearance is characteristic of fibrous dysplasia and is the most useful discriminating factor. Other features of fibrous dysplasia of the skull that can help distinguish it from Paget's disease are symmetry of distribution, presence of a soft-tissue mass, cyst-like changes, thickness of the cranial cortices, and involvement of the paranasal sinuses, maxilla, sphenoid, orbits and nasal cavity.

Tehranzadeh et al (1998).

92) b. **

Multiple myeloma is a malignant condition of plasma cells that commonly shows infiltration of the bone marrow, best seen on MRI. Patterns of infiltration can be classified as focal, diffuse or variegated. Although marrow infiltration returns similar signal to marrow oedema on T1W and T2W images, infiltration will show diffuse enhancement following administration of intravenous gadolinium. The pattern of infiltration also differs. Infiltration will be patchy and randomly distributed throughout the vertebral bone. In contrast, bone oedema occurs adjacent to its cause, being linear at the endplates in the case of degenerative disc disease, and linear with a fracture line in osteoporotic collapse, in the pedicles adjacent to spondylolysis or at the entheses in ankylosing spondylitis.

Moulopoulos et al (1994).

93) a. **

The resulting pattern following diffuse uptake of ^{99m}Tc-labelled diphosphonates in the axial skeleton, with little or no uptake of tracer in the soft tissues or urinary tract, is frequently referred to as a superscan. When there is little uptake in the limbs, the cause is most likely to be diffuse metastases in the axial skeleton, most commonly prostatic or breast. Uptake in metabolic bone disease is more uniform in appearance, and extends into the distal appendicular skeleton. Intense calvarial uptake disproportionate to that in the remainder of the skeleton may also be seen. The most important factor is to recognize the scan as abnormal in the absence of focal lesions. The lack of renal uptake (absent kidney sign) is a useful discriminator.

Love et al (2003).

94) d. **

Chordomas arise from notochordal rests and therefore almost always occur in the midline. They are the most common primary malignant sacral tumour and account for 2–4% of all malignant tumours of bone. They are found at all ages but most commonly occur in the fourth to seventh decades of life. Approximately half develop in the sacrococcygeal region. There is usually a large soft-tissue component and the tumour may extend across the intervertebral disc space or sacroiliac joint. Overall, the most common sacral lesion is metastasis due to the high red marrow content, but other primary malignant lesions include myeloma, Ewing's sarcoma and lymphoma. The most commonly found benign tumours are giant cell tumours and aneurysmal bone cysts. Despite being relatively common in the rest of the spine, haemangiomas and osteoid osteomas are rare.

Diel et al (2001).

95) b. ***
Heterotopic ossification, also known as myositis ossificans, is a benign, self-limiting process of ossification occurring within skeletal muscle. Seventy-five per cent of cases are due to trauma (including iatrogenic trauma), with other causes including paralysis, burns, tetanus and intramuscular haematoma. The areas of new bone are surrounded by fibrotic connective tissue, which can be seen as a soft-tissue mass on MRI. Some heterotopic ossification is seen in half of all total hip replacements, with one-third considered clinically significant. It is classified radiographically according to the Brooker classification.

Dähnert (2007), 126–7.

96) e. ****
Transient osteoporosis of the hip is part of the bone marrow oedema syndromes that also encompass migratory regional osteoporosis and transient bone marrow oedema. The condition is spontaneous and self-limiting, clinical recovery occurring in several weeks to months with no specific treatment, although radiographic changes lag behind. It is seen in pregnant women in the third trimester and middle-aged men. The radiographic hallmark is the loss of subchondral cortex in the femoral head, and marrow oedema is seen on MRI with intense uptake of ^{99m}Tc-labelled diphosphonates on bone scintigraphy. The aetiology is uncertain, but speculation has been made that the bone marrow oedema syndromes are related to reflex sympathetic dystrophy. The appearance of transient osteoporosis of the hip may be mimicked by osteonecrosis.

Hayes et al (1993).

97) c. **
A false-negative result in this context is failure to identify pathology and to report incorrectly the ultrasound examination as normal. Limited shoulder mobility will not permit correct positioning of the shoulder for best interrogation of the whole of each tendon and may lead to non-visualization of a tear. Other causes of false negatives include technical

factors such as using an incorrect transducer (should be at least 7.5 MHz), poor focusing and poor transducer handling. There are also anatomical causes, including non-diastasis of the tendon fibres, scar tissue, bursitis, tendinosis and massive tear, with complete retraction of the tendon ends preventing their visualization. Anisotropy, poor transducer positioning or misinterpretation of the rotator interval, musculotendinous junction, supraspinatus–infraspinatus interface, acoustic shadowing and fibrocartilaginous insertion can all give rise to false-positive findings.

Rutten et al (2006).

98) b. **

The two most important intercarpal ligaments are the scapholunate and lunotriquetral ligaments. These are crescent shaped with strong anterior and posterior zones and a relatively thin middle membrane. Disruption of either of these will result in communication of the radiocarpal compartment proximally with the midcarpal compartment distally. Contrast material seen in the distal radioulnar joint indicates disruption to the triangular fibrocartilage complex or distal radioulnar ligaments. Some authors advocate selective midcarpal injection as superior in delineating injury to the scapholunate and lunotriquetral ligaments, and a sequential technique of three injections has also been described.

Steinbach et al (2002).

99) a. *

Truncation of a meniscus may be due to previous injury or surgical resection, but in the absence of a relevant history it suggests meniscal tear with displacement of the body of the meniscus. On sagittal sequences, one would normally expect to see a full 'bow-tie'-shaped meniscus on three or more contiguous images, as the meniscal body is approximately 11 mm in thickness (this of course will depend on slice thickness). Any fewer suggests a meniscal body tear with displacement of the fragment. The fragment often flips into the intercondylar groove of the femur to lie anterior and parallel to the posterior cruciate ligament, giving the impression of two similar structures. This injury is known as a bucket-handle tear.

Mesgarzadeh et al (1993).

100) d. ***

Distinction of enchondroma and intramedullary chondrosarcoma in the appendicular skeleton proximal to the metacarpals/-tarsals is difficult radiologically. A series of 187 patients showed that chondrosarcoma was associated with endosteal scalloping, with scalloping involving more than two-thirds of the extent of the lesion being strongly suggestive of malignancy. Other powerful discriminating factors identified as favouring chondrosarcoma were cortical destruction, soft-tissue mass, periosteal reaction, radionuclide uptake at scintigraphy and pain associated with the lesion. Chondrosarcoma also tended to be larger with a mean size of 10 cm compared with 6.7 cm for enchondroma. A ground-glass matrix with arcuate calcification is characteristic of both types of cartilaginous lesion. Multiple lesions may be seen in both malignancy and enchondromatosis (Ollier's disease).

Murphey et al (1998).

MODULE 3
GASTROINTESTINAL

1) A 46-year-old woman with a multisystem disorder presents with dysphagia and heartburn. Barium swallow reveals a dilated oesophagus with aperistalsis of the lower two-thirds of the oesophagus, a patulous lower oesophageal sphincter and gastro-oesophageal reflux. Which other organ system is most likely to be affected?

   a. respiratory
   b. cardiovascular
   c. skin
   d. central nervous
   e. renal

2) A 70-year-old hospitalized male patient presents with watery diarrhoea and abdominal pain. CT of the abdomen demonstrates marked circumferential bowel wall thickening involving the entire colon, with minimal pericolonic stranding and a small amount of ascites. The small bowel appears normal. What is the most likely diagnosis?

   a. Crohn's disease
   b. ischaemic colitis
   c. diverticulitis
   d. pseudomembranous colitis
   e. ulcerative colitis

3) A 65-year-old man undergoes endoscopy for dysphagia, during which an ulcerated mass is seen in the distal oesophagus. Biopsy confirms oesophageal adenocarcinoma. What is the most accurate imaging modality for local staging of oesophageal cancer?

   a. endoscopic ultrasound
   b. CT
   c. ^{18}FDG PET/CT
   d. MRI
   e. barium swallow

4) A 64-year-old man undergoes a barium meal examination for upper abdominal pain. A 10 mm ulcer is demonstrated at the gastric antrum. Which radiological feature would favour a diagnosis of malignant rather than benign gastric ulcer?

   a. round ulcer shape
   b. ulcer crater confined within the gastric contour
   c. gastric folds identified up to the edge of the ulcer crater
   d. associated duodenal ulcer disease
   e. uniform mucosal collar around a centrally located ulcer

5) A 34-year-old woman with a history of steatorrhoea and weight loss undergoes a small bowel follow-through examination that demonstrates dilatation of the proximal small bowel with flocculation and segmentation of the barium column. Fold thickness is normal. What is the most likely diagnosis?

a. Crohn's disease
b. Zollinger–Ellison syndrome
c. coeliac disease
d. small bowel lymphoma
e. Whipple's disease

6) A 44-year-old man undergoes ultrasound of the abdomen during which the liver is incidentally noted to be of diffusely increased echogenicity, with attenuation of the ultrasound beam and poor visualization of the intrahepatic architecture. Which of the following imaging features is most likely in this condition?

a. liver echogenicity less than that of renal cortex on ultrasound scan
b. relatively hypoattenuated intrahepatic vessels on unenhanced CT
c. liver attenuation 10 HU greater than that of the spleen on unenhanced CT
d. absolute liver attenuation of >40 HU on contrast-enhanced CT
e. loss of liver signal intensity on out-of-phase gradient echo MR images

7) A 54-year-old woman with a sensation of incomplete evacuation on defecation undergoes conventional defecography. Following introduction of barium paste into the rectum, in which position should the patient be placed for imaging?

a. supine
b. prone
c. left lateral
d. right lateral
e. sitting

8) A 68-year-old woman presents with small bowel obstruction, and undergoes contrast-enhanced CT of the abdomen. This demonstrates dilated small bowel to the level of the mid-ileum, where a herniated loop of small bowel is seen emerging inferolateral to the left pubic tubercle. What is the most likely cause of small bowel obstruction in this patient?

a. femoral hernia
b. indirect inguinal hernia
c. direct inguinal hernia
d. spigelian hernia
e. obturator hernia

9) A 34-year-old man presents with acute left lower quadrant pain following unaccustomed exercise. CT of the abdomen demonstrates a 2.5 cm oval lesion with attenuation value of -60 HU abutting the sigmoid colon, with surrounding inflammatory changes. The sigmoid colon itself appears normal. What is the most likely diagnosis?

a. omental infarction
b. diverticulitis
c. epiploic appendagitis
d. liposarcoma
e. appendicitis

10) A 65-year-old woman undergoes CT of the abdomen. An incidental finding of a well-defined 5 cm mass in the head of the pancreas is noted. It has a mean attenuation value of 5 HU, and contains multiple tiny cysts with a central nidus of calcification. There is no pancreatic duct dilatation. What is the most likely diagnosis?

a. mucinous cystadenoma
b. main duct intraductal papillary mucinous tumour
c. serous cystadenoma
d. pancreatic pseudocyst
e. pancreatic insulinoma

11) Which venous structure divides the liver into the right and left lobes?

a. right hepatic vein
b. middle hepatic vein
c. left hepatic vein
d. left portal vein
e. right portal vein

12) What is the primary imaging investigation for staging of colon cancer diagnosed at colonoscopy?

a. CT of the abdomen and pelvis
b. CT of the thorax, abdomen and pelvis
c. abdominal ultrasound scan
d. double-contrast barium enema
e. ^{18}FDG PET/CT

13) A 65-year-old man presents with a several-week history of lower abdominal pain and diarrhoea. On examination he has tenderness and guarding in the left lower quadrant. On contrast-enhanced CT, the inferior mesenteric vein is dilated, with a thin rim of enhancement around a central area of low density. What is the most likely additional pathology demonstrated on the CT?

a. sigmoid diverticulitis
b. appendicitis
c. Crohn's disease
d. pancreatitis
e. caecal malignancy

14) A 47-year-old woman presents with progressive abdominal distension. CT of the abdomen demonstrates loculated collections of very low-attenuation fluid in the peritoneal cavity containing scattered curvilinear calcifications, and a scalloped contour to the liver. What is the most likely diagnosis?

a. pancreatic pseudocysts
b. ascites due to liver cirrhosis with portal hypertension
c. peritoneal metastases
d. pseudomyxoma peritonei
e. peritoneal mesothelioma

15) A 50-year-old woman presents with recurrent episodes of hypoglycaemia. Biochemistry confirms endogenous insulin hypersecretion, and she undergoes multiphasic CT of the abdomen. Which of the following is the most likely finding in the pancreas?

a. 1.5 cm arterially enhancing, solid mass in the head
b. 5 cm arterially enhancing, cystic mass in the tail
c. 1.5 cm arterially enhancing, cystic mass in the body
d. 1.5 cm non-enhancing, solid mass in the tail
e. 5 cm non-enhancing, cystic mass in the body

16) A previously well, 28-year-old man recently returned from the Far East becomes acutely unwell with fever and right upper quadrant pain. Ultrasound scan demonstrates a well-defined, rounded, 7 cm hypoechoic lesion in the right lobe of the liver contiguous with the liver capsule, with fine homogeneous, low-level internal echoes and acoustic enhancement. What is the most likely diagnosis?

a. pyogenic abscess
b. amoebic abscess
c. fungal abscess
d. hydatid disease
e. incidental simple hepatic cyst

17) A 64-year-old woman presents to the dermatologist with erythematous maculopapular lesions on her legs, buttocks and face, and is diagnosed with necrolytic migratory erythema. Which initial imaging investigation is most appropriate?

a. no imaging
b. mammography
c. CT of the brain
d. chest radiograph
e. CT of the abdomen

18) A 70-year-old man presents with fresh bleeding per rectum. He undergoes resuscitation, receiving 5 units of blood over the following 24 hours. Colonoscopy is unsuccessful in detecting the source of the bleeding, and he continues to pass fresh blood, although he remains haemodynamically stable. What is the most appropriate next investigation?

a. ^{99m}Tc-labelled red blood cell radionuclide imaging
b. CT angiography
c. repeat colonoscopy
d. digital subtraction mesenteric angiography
e. abdominal ultrasound scan

19) A 70-year-old man with a history of several months of dysphagia undergoes double-contrast barium swallow. This demonstrates a moderately dilated oesophagus with reduced peristalsis and smooth tapering of the distal oesophagus. What is the most likely diagnosis?

a. primary achalasia
b. gastric carcinoma
c. scleroderma
d. oesophageal carcinoma
e. presbyoesophagus

20) A 25-year-old woman presents with cramping abdominal pain and bleeding per rectum. On examination she has mucocutaneous pigmentation of her mucous membranes and face. A small-bowel follow-through examination demonstrates small-bowel intussusception. Which other finding is most likely to be demonstrated?

a. separation and displacement of small bowel loops
b. localized outpouching of the antimesenteric border of the distal ileum
c. generalized irregular fold thickening
d. multiple filling defects in the small bowel
e. generalized dilatation of the small bowel

21) A 65-year-old woman, with a history of previous partial gastrectomy 10 years earlier, presents with upper abdominal pain and early satiety. She undergoes a double-contrast barium meal, which demonstrates a 4 cm intraluminal, mottled filling defect in the gastric remnant with no fixed attachment to the gastric wall. What is the most likely diagnosis?

a. suture granuloma
b. trichobezoar
c. phytobezoar
d. gastric carcinoma
e. villous adenoma

22) A 23-year-old man with dysphagia undergoes a double-contrast barium swallow, which demonstrates a smooth, well-defined, 12 cm submucosal lesion in the distal oesophagus causing deformity of the lumen. CT demonstrates coarse calcification within the mass. What is the most likely diagnosis?

a. oesophageal lipoma
b. oesophageal duplication cyst
c. oesophageal carcinoma
d. oesophageal varices
e. oesophageal leiomyoma

23) A 54-year-old man with known metastatic malignant melanoma presents with epigastric pain and haematemesis. What is the most likely finding in the stomach on double-contrast barium meal?

a. multiple submucosal nodules with central ulceration
b. solitary ulcerated mass in the gastric antrum
c. linitis plastica
d. solitary, well-defined, pedunculated filling defect
e. thickened tortuous gastric folds

24) A 56-year-old man presents acutely with chest pain after a night out. On examination he is febrile, tachycardic and hypotensive. Chest radiograph demonstrates extensive pneumomediastinum, with left pleural effusion and left lower lobe atelectasis. What is the most likely diagnosis?

a. acute pulmonary embolism
b. spontaneous oesophageal rupture
c. aortic dissection
d. lobar pneumonia
e. acute pancreatitis

25) A 43-year-old woman is incidentally found to have a well-defined, rounded, low-density, 2 cm lesion in the liver on unenhanced CT. Contrast-enhanced CT demonstrates peripheral nodular arterial enhancement with complete fill-in on delayed images. What is the most likely diagnosis?

a. hepatic haemangioma
b. hepatocellular carcinoma
c. simple hepatic cyst
d. focal fatty infiltration
e. focal nodular hyperplasia

26) A 78-year-old man presents with abdominal pain. A plain abdominal radiograph demonstrates a distended, inverted U-shaped loop of bowel devoid of haustra, extending from the left iliac fossa inferiorly to just beneath the left hemidiaphragm superiorly. What is the most likely diagnosis?

a. caecal volvulus
b. sigmoid volvulus
c. paralytic ileus
d. large bowel obstruction due to distal malignancy
e. small bowel malrotation and volvulus

27) A 46-year-old man presents with severe abdominal pain. An erect chest radiograph shows free intraperitoneal air below the diaphragm. What is the most likely cause?

a. perforated anterior wall duodenal ulcer
b. perforated posterior wall duodenal ulcer
c. perforated gastric ulcer
d. perforated appendix
e. diverticulitis with perforation

28) A 20-year-old woman with anorexia nervosa presents with intermittent abdominal pain and vomiting relieved by lying prone. Barium meal examination reveals a vertical band-like narrowing of the third part of the duodenum, with proximal duodenal dilatation and vigorous to-and-fro peristalsis. What is the most likely diagnosis?

a. duodenal duplication cyst
b. annular pancreas
c. Ladd's bands
d. superior mesenteric artery syndrome
e. duodenal atresia

29) A 34-year-old woman presents with bloody diarrhoea and abdominal pain. Which feature on barium enema favours a diagnosis of ulcerative colitis rather than Crohn's disease?

   a. thickened ileocaecal valve
   b. circumferential wall involvement
   c. fistula formation
   d. skip lesions
   e. normal rectum

30) A 68-year-old man presents with acute abdominal pain. As well as other pathology, CT of the abdomen reveals multiple linear branching structures with an attenuation value of −1000 HU in the liver extending to the periphery. What are these appearances most likely to represent?

   a. gas in the portal venous system
   b. gas in the biliary tree
   c. portal venous thrombosis
   d. intrahepatic biliary dilatation
   e. fatty infiltration of the liver

31) A 23-year-old man presents with acute lower abdominal pain. An abdominal radiograph demonstrates a rounded, laminated calcific density projected over the right lower quadrant. What is the approximate likelihood of a diagnosis of acute appendicitis?

   a. 10%
   b. 30%
   c. 50%
   d. 70%
   e. 90%

32) A 64-year-old man with known sigmoid adenocarcinoma diagnosed at endoscopy undergoes staging CT. A solitary, well-defined, rounded, homogeneous, 1 cm mass of mean attenuation value identical to the spleen is seen near the splenic hilum. What is the most likely diagnosis?

   a. metastatic lymph node
   b. wandering spleen
   c. splenic artery aneurysm
   d. polysplenia
   e. accessory spleen

33) A 45-year-old woman with pleuritic chest pain and breathlessness undergoes CT pulmonary angiogram for suspected acute pulmonary embolism, which demonstrates multiple irregular areas of relatively poor enhancement in the visualized portion of the spleen. What is the most likely cause?

a. normal arterial-phase enhancement
b. splenic infarction
c. splenic clefts
d. splenosis
e. spontaneous splenic rupture

34) A 26-year-old man known to have AIDS presents with a 2-week history of difficult and painful swallowing. He undergoes double-contrast barium examination of the oesophagus, which demonstrates multiple, small, superficial, round ulcers in the mid-oesophagus. The intervening mucosa is normal and no plaques are seen. What is the most likely diagnosis?

a. HIV oesophagitis
b. cytomegalovirus oesophagitis
c. reflux oesophagitis
d. candida oesophagitis
e. herpes simplex oesophagitis

35) A 72-year-old man attends for a barium enema examination. He has no known allergies. In considering administration of intra-venous hyoscine-N-butylbromide (Buscopan), which factor in his medical history is it most important to be aware of?

a. prostatism
b. type I diabetes
c. glaucoma
d. migraine
e. unstable cardiac disease

36) A 67-year-old man presents with abdominal pain, distension and vomiting. Multiple dilated loops of small bowel are seen on plain abdominal radiograph. A contrast-enhanced CT of the abdomen and pelvis is performed, which shows small bowel dilatation to the terminal ileum, where there is a nodular calcified mass with surrounding desmoplastic reaction. What is the most likely cause of small bowel obstruction?

a. adhesions
b. carcinoid tumour
c. Crohn's disease
d. previous irradiation
e. small bowel lymphoma

37) A 45-year-old man presents with dysphagia and undergoes a double-contrast barium swallow. This demonstrates a smooth oblique indentation on the posterior wall of the oesophagus. What is the most likely cause of these appearances?

a. enlarged left atrium
b. aberrant right subclavian artery
c. aberrant left pulmonary artery
d. right-sided aortic arch
e. coarctation of the aorta

38) A 30-year-old woman on the oral contraceptive pill undergoes unenhanced CT of the abdomen, which demonstrates a well-circumscribed, slightly hypoattenuating mass in the liver. Which additional radiological finding would favour a diagnosis of hepatic adenoma rather than focal nodular hyperplasia?

a. measured lesion size of 3 cm
b. accompanying acute subcapsular haematoma
c. transient arterial-phase enhancement
d. normal uptake on ^{99m}Tc-labelled sulphur colloid scan
e. hypodense central stellate scar

39) A 25-year-old man presents with jaundice and malaise. Ultrasound scan demonstrates a general decrease in liver echogenicity and a well-distended gallbladder with a wall thickness of 4 mm. No gall-stones are seen and the intra- and extrahepatic bile ducts appear normal. What is the most likely diagnosis?

a. acute cholecystitis
b. cirrhosis
c. fatty liver
d. acute viral hepatitis
e. primary sclerosing cholangitis

40) Which anatomical structure separates the right and left subphrenic spaces?

a. gastrohepatic ligament
b. foramen of Winslow
c. falciform ligament
d. Morison's pouch
e. lesser omentum

41) A 74-year-old man presents with severe abdominal pain and is admitted under the surgical team with suspected perforation. He is too unwell to undergo an erect chest radiograph. What is the most appropriate alternative plain film to detect the presence of free intraperitoneal gas?

a. supine chest
b. erect abdomen
c. supine abdomen
d. left lateral decubitus abdomen
e. right lateral decubitus abdomen

42) A 64-year-old woman presents with jaundice. An abdominal ultrasound scan demonstrates the intrahepatic biliary ducts to be of similar calibre to the adjacent portal veins. The extrahepatic common bile duct measures 5 mm in diameter. No gallstones are seen. What is the most appropriate further imaging investigation?

a. CT of the abdomen
b. endoscopic ultrasound scan
c. MRCP
d. ERCP
e. no imaging indicated as normal findings

43) The gastroduodenal artery normally has its origin from which vessel?

a. superior mesenteric artery
b. common hepatic artery
c. left gastric artery
d. coeliac axis
e. aorta

44) A 45-year-old patient with cirrhosis is found to have a focal liver lesion on ultrasound scan, clinically suspected to be hepatocellular carcinoma. What would be the expected appearances of the lesion on T2W MR images following infusion of superparamagnetic iron oxide particles?

a. increased signal intensity compared with rest of liver
b. decreased signal intensity compared with rest of liver
c. lesion signal intensity unchanged; rest of liver increased signal intensity
d. lesion signal intensity unchanged; rest of liver decreased signal intensity
e. no effect on appearances on T2W images

45) A 35-year-old woman on the oral contraceptive pill presents with right upper quadrant pain, shortness of breath and leg oedema. Ultrasound scan of the abdomen demonstrates hepatosplenomegaly and ascites. The hepatic veins are not visualized on Doppler ultrasound scan. What is the most likely diagnosis?

a. acute Budd–Chiari syndrome
b. primary biliary cirrhosis
c. passive hepatic congestion
d. hepatic veno-occlusive disease
e. viral hepatitis

46) An 86-year-old, otherwise well woman is admitted with abdominal pain and undergoes plain abdominal radiography. This demonstrates a normal bowel gas pattern, but the liver and spleen are noted to be of increased density with a stippled appearance. What is the most likely cause?

a. haemochromatosis
b. thorotrastosis
c. amiodarone therapy
d. sickle cell anaemia
e. glycogen storage disease

47) A 40-year-old woman undergoes abdominal ultrasound scan, which demonstrates three small, rounded, echogenic structures in relation to the anterior wall of the gallbladder. There is no posterior acoustic shadowing, and appearances remain constant with variation in patient position. The remainder of the gallbladder and biliary tree appear unremarkable. What is the most likely diagnosis?

a. gallstones
b. cholesterol polyps
c. adenomyomatosis
d. gallbladder carcinoma
e. strawberry gallbladder

48) A 51-year-old man with alcoholic cirrhosis presents with jaundice. CT of the abdomen reveals an encapsulated, 20 mm focal area of low density in the liver, which demonstrates arterial-phase enhancement and rapid washout on delayed imaging. What is the most likely diagnosis?

a. regenerative nodule
b. dysplastic nodule
c. hepatocellular carcinoma
d. hepatic haemangioma
e. focal fatty sparing

49) A 36-year-old man with ulcerative colitis develops progressive jaundice and pruritis. CT of the abdomen demonstrates multiple areas of dilatation and stenosis of tortuous intrahepatic bile ducts, with wall thickening and contrast enhancement of the extrahepatic bile ducts. What is the most likely diagnosis?

a. primary sclerosing cholangitis
b. choledocholithiasis
c. primary biliary cirrhosis
d. ascending cholangitis
e. chronic pancreatitis

50) A 73-year-old man presents with lower abdominal pain and a change in bowel habit. A contrast enema demonstrates a stricture in the sigmoid colon. Which feature would favour a diagnosis of colorectal carcinoma rather than diverticulitis?

a. long (>10 cm) segment of involvement
b. mucosal ulceration
c. presence of a colovesical fistula
d. multiple diverticula in the sigmoid colon
e. smoothly tapered stricture margins

51) A 45-year-old man undergoes barium swallow for dysphagia, which demonstrates multiple flask-shaped outpouchings of barium arranged in longitudinal rows paralleling the long axis of the oesophagus. Which of the following is a commonly associated condition?

a. scleroderma
b. rheumatoid arthritis
c. chronic obstructive airway disease
d. AIDS
e. diabetes

52) What is the most common cause of varices affecting the upper third of the oesophagus?

a. portal hypertension due to cirrhosis
b. splenic vein thrombosis
c. inferior vena caval obstruction
d. superior vena caval obstruction
e. hepatic vein obstruction

53) A 66-year-old woman with a known large para-oesophageal hiatus hernia presents with sudden onset of severe epigastric pain and vigorous retching without production of vomitus. Passage of a nasogastric tube is unsuccessful. Plain abdominal radiograph demonstrates a markedly distended stomach in the left upper quadrant extending into the chest. What is the most likely diagnosis?

a. pyloric stenosis
b. 'cup-and-spill' stomach
c. acute gastric volvulus
d. acute gastric dilatation
e. paraduodenal hernia

54) Which of the following may improve the detection of Meckel's diverticulum on a [^{99m}Tc] pertechnetate study?

a. prior administration of cimetidine
b. prior administration of laxatives
c. prior administration of potassium perchlorate
d. maintenance of a full bladder
e. barium follow-through prior to study

55) A 60-year-old woman presents with weight loss and diarrhoea. CT of the abdomen demonstrates multiple, enlarged, low-attenuation mesenteric lymph nodes containing fat–fluid levels and splenic atrophy. What is the most likely diagnosis?

a. tuberculosis
b. coeliac disease
c. Whipple's disease
d. lymphoma
e. metastatic squamous cell carcinoma

56) A 27-year-old woman presents with upper abdominal pain and is found to have a palpable right upper quadrant mass on examination. CT demonstrates a low attenuation lesion in the right lobe of the liver. Which imaging feature would favour a diagnosis of fibrolamellar carcinoma of the liver rather than focal nodular hyperplasia?

a. calcifications within a central scar
b. lesion size of 3 cm
c. multiple lesions
d. increased uptake on sulphur colloid scan
e. central scar hyperintense on T2W images

57) In patients with cystic fibrosis, which gastrointestinal pathology may occur as a result of high-dose lipase supplementation?

a. rectal prolapse
b. fibrosing colonopathy
c. pneumatosis intestinalis
d. gastro-oesophageal reflux
e. meconium ileus equivalent syndrome

58) A 45-year-old man undergoes ultrasound scan of the abdomen 2 days following orthotopic liver transplantation, which demonstrates periportal oedema and a small fluid collection at the hilum of the liver. What is the most likely diagnosis?

a. graft rejection
b. hepatic arterial thrombosis
c. portal vein stenosis
d. bile leak
e. normal post-transplantation findings

59) A transjugular intrahepatic portosystemic shunt lies between the portal vein and which vessel?

a. hepatic vein
b. inferior vena cava
c. aorta
d. common hepatic artery
e. left gastric vein

60) In a 67-year-old female patient with jaundice and gallbladder wall thickening on ultrasound scan, which feature on CT favours a diagnosis of xanthogranulomatous cholecystitis rather than gallbladder carcinoma?

a. pericholecystic fat infiltration
b. intramural hypoattenuating nodules throughout the gallbladder
c. biliary obstruction
d. hepatic extension
e. regional lymphadenopathy

61) A 76-year-old woman presents with dysphagia and regurgitation of undigested food. She undergoes barium swallow, which demonstrates a barium-filled pouch extending from the posterior oesophageal wall at the level of C5–6 that is causing oesophageal compression. What is the most likely diagnosis?

a. intramural pseudodiverticulum
b. epiphrenic diverticulum
c. lateral pharyngeal diverticulum
d. interbronchial diverticulum
e. Zenker's diverticulum

62) A 68-year-old man undergoes barium swallow for dysphagia. During the examination the patient has an episode of coughing, and barium is noted to enter the larynx and proximal trachea. What is the appropriate management?

a. no action needed
b. physiotherapy
c. prophylactic antibiotics
d. chest radiograph in 48 hours
e. admission to hospital for observation

63) During MRCP, which substance may be administered to improve visualization of the pancreatic ducts?

a. glucagon
b. secretin
c. cholecystokinin
d. gastrin
e. Buscopan

64) A 64-year-old man undergoes renal ultrasound scan and is incidentally noted to have a well-defined, rounded, 3 cm lesion in the spleen. It has a thin wall with curvilinear rim calcification and contains low-level internal echoes. What is the most likely diagnosis?

a. post-traumatic (false) cyst
b. epidermoid cyst
c. echinococcal cyst
d. pyogenic abscess
e. pancreatic pseudocyst

65) Which is the most appropriate contrast medium for a barium follow-through examination of the small bowel?

a. 100 ml of 250% w/v barium sulphate
b. 135 ml of 250% w/v barium sulphate
c. 300 ml of 100% w/v barium sulphate
d. 1500 ml of 20% w/v barium sulphate
e. 500 ml of 115% w/v barium sulphate

66) A 40-year-old man with hyperpigmentation, arthalgia and diabetes mellitus is clinically suspected to have primary haemochromatosis. What are the most likely findings on liver MRI in this condition?

a. normal appearances of the liver
b. decreased signal intensity on T1W and T2W images
c. decreased signal intensity on T1W and increased signal intensity on T2W images
d. increased signal intensity on T1W and decreased signal intensity on T2W images
e. increased signal intensity on T1W and T2W images

67) A 58-year-old man with recurrent episodes of upper abdominal pain undergoes MRCP, which demonstrates pancreatic atrophy and marked dilatation of the main pancreatic duct, which contains high T2-signal material. A low T2-signal nodular filling defect is also identified within the dilated duct. ERCP demonstrates thick mucus protruding from a bulging papilla. What is the most likely diagnosis?

a. intraductal papillary mucinous tumour
b. chronic pancreatitis
c. mucinous cystadenoma
d. pancreatic pseudocyst
e. acute pancreatitis

68) On contrast-enhanced CT of the abdomen, what is the most common abnormality of the spleen seen in sarcoidosis?

a. capsular calcification
b. multiple low-attenuation nodules
c. splenomegaly
d. splenic rupture
e. multiple cystic lesions

69) A 54-year-old woman undergoes CT of the abdomen and pelvis for weight loss and is found to have multiple, irregular, calcified, low-attenuation lesions in the liver, suggestive of metastases. What is the most likely primary lesion?

a. invasive ductal carcinoma of the breast
b. mucinous adenocarcinoma of the gastrointestinal tract
c. osteosarcoma
d. non-small-cell lung carcinoma
e. carcinoid

70) A 68-year-old woman presents with abdominal pain, distension and vomiting. Plain abdominal radiograph demonstrates bowel obstruction, gas within the biliary tree, and an ectopic, calcified, 3 cm gallstone. What is the most likely site of bowel obstruction?

a. pylorus
b. duodenum
c. proximal ileum
d. terminal ileum
e. sigmoid

71) Which structure marks the transition from squamous oesophageal to columnar gastric epithelium?

a. A-ring
b. B-ring
c. Z-line
d. oesophageal vestibule
e. gastro-oesophageal junction

72) A 45-year-old woman undergoes abdominal ultrasound scan. The portal vein measures 16 mm in diameter and demonstrates continuous monophasic flow without respiratory variation. Portal vein flow velocity is hepatopetal and is measured to be 7 cm/s. What is the most likely diagnosis?

a. normal findings
b. Budd–Chiari syndrome
c. portal hypertension
d. cavernous transformation of the portal vein
e. portal vein thrombosis

73) A 73-year-old woman presents with intermittent lower gastrointestinal bleeding and iron deficiency anaemia. She is clinically suspected to have angiodysplasia. What are the most likely findings on barium enema?

a. normal appearances
b. multiple small polyps in the colon
c. multiple shallow ulcers in the colon
d. multiple, serpiginous, filling defects in the colon
e. a focal, irregular, circumferential narrowing in the colon

74) A 50-year-old woman undergoes CT colonography for a change in bowel habit, which demonstrates a well-defined, broad-based, 3 cm submucosal mass of density −40 HU in the ascending colon. It is noted to change shape between prone and supine images. What is the most likely diagnosis?

a. adenomatous polyp
b. endometriosis
c. primary pneumatosis coli
d. lipoma
e. enteric duplication cyst

75) A 48-year-old man presents with epigastric pain, weight loss and peripheral oedema. Blood tests demonstrate hypoalbuminaemia. At barium meal the stomach is well distended, but there is poor mucosal coating. Markedly enlarged and tortuous gastric rugae are seen in the fundus and body of the stomach, with sparing of the antrum. What is the most likely diagnosis?

a. lymphoma
b. Ménétrièr's disease
c. gastric carcinoma
d. Zollinger−Ellison syndrome
e. eosinophilic gastroenteritis

76) On a barium meal examination, the incisura angularis marks the border between which structures?

a. lesser and greater curvatures of the stomach
b. antrum and pylorus of the stomach
c. fundus and body of the stomach
d. body and antrum of the stomach
e. oesophagus and the stomach

77) At abdominal ultrasound scan, when scanning the abdomen in a transverse plane at the level of the pancreas, which of the following structures may normally be seen lying between the superior mesenteric artery and the aorta?

a. splenic vein
b. left renal vein
c. neck of the pancreas
d. inferior vena cava
e. common bile duct

78) A 67-year-old man undergoes Whipple's procedure for adeno-carcinoma of the head of the pancreas. Which finding is of most concern on CT of the abdomen performed 4 days postoperatively for persistent pyrexia?

a. free intraperitoneal gas
b. aerobilia in the left intrahepatic ducts
c. oral contrast within the afferent jejunal loop
d. small thin-walled fluid collection in Morison's pouch
e. gas-containing fluid collection in the pancreatic bed

79) A 45-year-old man is admitted after a road traffic accident in which he sustained abdominal injuries. After fluid resuscitation he under-goes CT of the abdomen and pelvis with intravenous contrast. This demonstrates a serpiginous area of attenuation value 130 HU at the splenic hilum with surrounding lower-attenuation material. What is this most likely to represent?

a. active arterial extravasation
b. acute clotted blood
c. acute unclotted blood
d. splenic arterial calcification
e. ascites

80) In the staging of rectal cancer by MRI, which sequence provides optimum visualization of the tumour?

a. T1W
b. contrast-enhanced T1W
c. T2W
d. FLAIR
e. proton density

81) A 41-year-old woman with morbid obesity presents with a plateau in weight loss 12 weeks after laparoscopic gastric banding. She undergoes a contrast swallow, which demonstrates concentric dilatation of the neostomach with a widely patent stoma. What is the most appropriate management?

a. no action necessary
b. nutritional advice
c. prompt decompression of the stoma by the radiologist
d. fluoroscopically guided band inflation
e. surgical replacement of the gastric band

82) A 67-year-old man presents with a sensation of incomplete evacuation and passage of thick mucus per rectum. Serum electrolytes demonstrate hypokalaemia and hyponatraemia. He undergoes barium enema, which demonstrates a broad-based, papillary, 2 cm lesion in the rectum with poor mucosal coating of barium. What is the most likely diagnosis?

a. lipoma
b. tubular adenoma
c. villous adenoma
d. colorectal carcinoma
e. solitary rectal ulcer syndrome

83) What is the most common site of involvement in tuberculosis of the gastrointestinal tract?

a. stomach
b. duodenum
c. ileocaecal region
d. splenic flexure
e. rectum

84) A 45-year-old woman with a previous history of treatment for advanced carcinoma of the cervix 8 years earlier presents with constipation and rectal bleeding. She undergoes CT of the abdomen and pelvis, which demonstrates a narrowed rectum with symmetrical wall thickening, perirectal inflammatory changes, thickening of the perirectal fascia and an increase in the AP diameter of the presacral space. What is the most likely diagnosis?

a. colorectal carcinoma
b. ulcerative colitis
c. radiation injury of the rectum
d. Hirschsprung's disease
e. lymphoma

85) Which of the following best describes the intravenous iodinated contrast agent iodixanol (Visipaque)?

a. ionic, high-osmolar, monomeric
b. non-ionic, iso-osmolar, dimeric
c. ionic, low-osmolar, dimeric
d. non-ionic, low-osmolar, monomeric
e. ionic, high-osmolar, dimeric

86) A 26-year-old man with AIDS presents with weight loss. He is noted to have multiple raised purple skin lesions on examination. Contrast-enhanced CT of the abdomen and pelvis demonstrates multiple, subcentimetre, low-attenuation nodules within the liver, as well as high-attenuation lymphadenopathy at the porta hepatis, retrocaval and aortocaval regions. What is the most likely diagnosis?

a. fungal infection
b. multiple haemangiomas
c. lymphoma
d. Kaposi's sarcoma
e. mycobacterial disease

87) A patient undergoes ^{111}In-labelled white blood cell scintigraphy for investigation of suspected occult sepsis. Which of these would be regarded as abnormal on imaging at 4 hours?

a. uptake in the large bowel
b. splenic uptake greater than that of the liver
c. uptake in the bone marrow
d. diffuse uptake in the lungs
e. uptake in the thymus in children

88) In the assessment of tumour response to treatment, what method of tumour measurement is used in the RECIST (Response Criteria in Solid Tumours) criteria?

a. unidimensional (long axis dimension)
b. unidimensional (short axis dimension)
c. bidimensional (product of longest diameter and greatest perpendicular diameter)
d. bidimensional (product of longest diameter and shortest diameter)
e. volumetric

89) A 69-year-old man undergoes staging of gastric carcinoma diagnosed at upper gastrointestinal endoscopy. CT of the abdomen demonstrates focal gastric wall thickening with extension into the perigastric fat, but no invasion of adjacent structures. Five local lymph nodes measuring 10–12 mm in short axis diameter are identified. There is no distant metastatic disease. What is the TNM staging of the tumour?

a. T2 N0 M0
b. T2 N1 M0
c. T2 N2 M0
d. T3 N1 M0
e. T3 N2 M0

90) In normal anatomy, the portal vein is usually formed by the confluence of which vessels?

a. left and right portal veins
b. inferior and superior mesenteric veins
c. superior mesenteric and splenic veins
d. inferior mesenteric and splenic veins
e. left, middle and right hepatic veins

91) A 45-year-old woman undergoes a follow-up staging CT of the chest, abdomen and pelvis after treatment for metastatic breast cancer. Compared with her initial staging scan, there is a generalized decrease in the attenuation value of the liver. No focal liver lesion or other new feature is seen. What is the most likely cause?

a. diffuse metastatic disease
b. fatty liver related to chemotherapy
c. hepatic venous congestion
d. amyloidosis
e. Budd–Chiari syndrome

92) During double-contrast barium enema, a prone overcouch film with the tube angled 45° caudally, centred 5 cm above the posterior superior iliac spines, is performed to optimally visualize which segment of the large bowel?

a. caecum
b. hepatic flexure
c. transverse colon
d. splenic flexure
e. sigmoid colon

93) For relief of malignant biliary obstruction by percutaneous stenting, which factor is an advantage of using a metallic rather than a plastic stent?

a. higher long-term patency rates
b. lower cost
c. easily removed if infection develops
d. does not shorten following deployment
e. higher surface area

94) At endoscopic ultrasound scan for staging of an oesophageal carcinoma, the tumour is seen extending into the hypoechoic fourth layer of the oesophagus but not beyond this. What is the T staging of the tumour?

a. Tis
b. T1
c. T2
d. T3
e. T4

95) For a standard portal-phase spiral CT of the abdomen and pelvis, after what period of time following commencement of the intravenous contrast injection should image acquisition begin?

a. 0 seconds
b. 10–15 seconds
c. 25–30 seconds
d. 65–70 seconds
e. 120–180 seconds

96) What is the most common side effect associated with administration of superparamagnetic iron oxide particles as a contrast agent during MRI?

a. urticarial skin rash
b. back pain
c. nephrotoxicity
d. nausea
e. headache

97) A 47-year-old woman with dysphagia undergoes barium swallow, which demonstrates a persistent smooth posterior bulge at the pharyngo-oesophageal junction at the level of C5–6 with mild proximal pharyngeal dilatation. What is the most likely diagnosis?

a. normal findings
b. impaired cricopharyngeus relaxation
c. pharyngeal web
d. anterior cervical osteophytes
e. thyroid enlargement

98) A 22-year-old woman with known medullary sponge kidney presents with recurrent upper abdominal pain and jaundice. Cholangiography demonstrates segmental saccular dilatation of the intrahepatic bile ducts and ectasia of the extrahepatic ducts. What is the most likely diagnosis?

a. choledochocele
b. choledochal cyst
c. primary sclerosing cholangitis
d. Caroli's disease
e. polycystic liver disease

99) A 65-year-old man presents with early satiety and bloating, and undergoes barium meal. This demonstrates a smoothly marginated, 15 cm mass in the body of the stomach, making an obtuse angle with the gastric wall. CT demonstrates peripheral enhancement of the mass with central areas of low attenuation and extragastric extension into the lesser sac. There is no associated lymphadenopathy. What is the most likely diagnosis?

a. gastrointestinal stromal tumour
b. gastric carcinoma
c. gastric lymphoma
d. adenomatous polyp
e. gastric carcinoid

100) From which vessel does the majority of the arterial supply to the pancreas derive?

a. splenic artery
b. left gastric artery
c. superior pancreaticoduodenal artery
d. right hepatic artery
e. superior mesenteric artery

Module 3: Gastrointestinal: Answers

1) c. ***
The patient is suffering from systemic sclerosis, a multisystem connective tissue disorder of unknown aetiology, classified by extent of skin involvement and overlap with other autoimmune disorders. The skin is the most commonly involved organ, demonstrating thickening, atrophic changes and fibrosis. The gastrointestinal system is the next most commonly affected, with around 50% of patients having symptomatic disease. The oesophagus is most frequently involved, with fibrosis of the circular layer of smooth muscle resulting in a dilated oesophagus with absent or reduced peristalsis in the lower two-thirds. The lower oesophageal sphincter is wide, in contrast to the tapered narrowing seen in achalasia. Patients suffer from reflux that predisposes to Barrett's oesophagus and distal strictures. The cardiovascular, respiratory, central nervous and renal systems may all be affected in systemic sclerosis, though less commonly than the skin and gastrointestinal systems.

Madani et al (2008).

2) d. ***
Pseudomembranous colitis is an acute infectious colitis caused by *Clostridium difficile* and its toxins A and B; this pathogen has become increasingly common largely due to widespread use of broad-spectrum antibiotics. The commonest CT finding is of colonic wall thickening (due to mural oedema and the presence of pseudomembranes), which is typically greater than in other causes of colitis apart from Crohn's disease. Pericolonic inflammatory changes are disproportionately mild relative to the marked wall thickening. Ascites is common, and this, together with the lack of small bowel involvement, can help to distinguish pseudomembranous colitis from Crohn's colitis. Ischaemic colitis demonstrates a lesser degree of wall thickening, and is usually segmental, tending to affect the watershed areas of the colon.

Ramachandran et al (2006).

3) a. ***
CT is the most commonly used imaging investigation for staging of oesophageal cancer. However, the overall accuracy of T staging is poor, particularly with T1 and T2 tumours, and CT also tends to overestimate tumour length. Endoscopic ultrasound scan is the most accurate imaging method for local staging, but is limited in its assessment of nodal and metastatic disease. [18]FDG PET/CT is useful in evaluation of nodal and metastatic disease, particularly in patients being considered for surgical resection, but has limited resolution for T staging and often fails to demonstrate T1 lesions. MR is useful in characterization of

indeterminate liver lesions seen on CT. Barium swallow is not used in the staging of oesophageal cancer.

Hricak et al (2007), 16–18.

4) b. ****
Many distinguishing features of gastric ulceration have been proposed in an attempt to classify gastric ulcers as benign or malignant, but there is significant overlap between the two categories. One reliable sign of a benign ulcer is the projection of the ulcer outside the gastric contour in profile, due to excavation into the mucosal wall. In contrast, a malignant ulcer occurring within a tumour mass does not usually extend beyond the confines of the gastric wall. Other features indicative of benignity include a round, centrally located ulcer with a uniform collar of oedematous mucosa, gastric folds extending to the edge of the ulcer crater and associated duodenal ulcer disease.

Halpert (2006), 82–5.

5) c. ***
Coeliac disease is characterized by malabsorption due to intolerance to the alpha-gliadin component of gluten, which causes small intestinal villous atrophy. Typical findings are of dilatation of the proximal small bowel, together with dilution of the barium column due to hypersecretion of fluid. Artefacts such as segmentation (breaking up of the barium column) or flocculation (clumping of disintegrated barium) were traditionally classic features of coeliac disease, but are less often seen nowadays with improved barium suspensions. In Whipple's disease the small bowel is typically non-dilated, and shows moderate fold thickening. Crohn's disease usually causes nodular fold thickening, and predominantly involves the distal small bowel. Zollinger–Ellison syndrome results in dilatation of proximal small bowel due to hypersecretion, but typically causes thickened folds. Small bowel lymphoma is usually associated with fold thickening.

Halpert (2006), 111–13.

6) e. ***
Fatty liver describes a spectrum of conditions characterized by triglyceride accumulation within hepatocytes. It is common, affecting around 15% of the general population, but is more prevalent among those with obesity, hyperlipidaemia and high alcohol consumption. Fatty liver may be diagnosed on ultrasound scan if liver echogenicity exceeds that of renal cortex, with attenuation of the ultrasound beam, loss of definition of the diaphragm and poor visualization of the intrahepatic architecture. CT features include absolute attenuation of less than 40 HU on contrast-enhanced CT and, on unenhanced CT, liver attenuation at least 10 HU less than that of spleen, and relatively hyperattenuating liver vasculature. Chemical shift gradient echo imaging is the most widely used MR technique for assessment of fatty liver, demonstrating

signal intensity loss on out-of-phase images compared with in-phase images.

Hamer et al (2006).

7) e. **
Conventional defecography is used in the imaging evaluation of obstructed defecation. Barium paste is instilled into the rectum with a Foley catheter, with the patient in the left lateral position. Prior opacification of the small bowel, bladder, vagina or peritoneum may also be performed to aid diagnosis. With the patient sitting on a commode placed on the footrest of a standard fluoroscopic table, static images are first obtained at rest and with contraction of the pelvic floor muscles. A cine-loop of evacuation is then obtained until the rectum is empty or three 30-second attempts at evacuation have been made. A variety of conditions may be demonstrated, including rectocele, enterocele, rectal intussusception and anismus.

Ganeshan et al (2008).

8) a. ****
External hernias are the second most common cause of small bowel obstruction after adhesions. A femoral hernia protrudes through the femoral ring, lying medial to the femoral vein, which may be compressed. On CT the hernia is seen inferolateral to the pubic tubercle, in contrast to inguinal hernias, which usually lie superomedial to the tubercle, though differentiation may be difficult in non-incarcerated cases. Femoral hernias are more prone to incarceration due to the inflexible margins of the femoral ring. Inguinal hernias may be classified as indirect (passing down the inguinal canal, seen lateral to the inferior epigastric vessels) or direct (protruding directly through the lower abdominal wall medial to the inferior epigastric vessels). A spigelian hernia protrudes through a defect in the inferolateral anterior abdominal wall. Obturator hernias protrude through the obturator foramen, between the pectineus and external obturator muscles.

Suzuki et al (2007).

9) c. ****
Acute epiploic appendagitis is thought to result from torsion of one of the fatty epiploic appendages arising from the serosal surface of the colon. It usually occurs in young men, presenting as acute lower quadrant pain, and is associated with obesity and unaccustomed exercise. Typical CT findings are of an oval pericolonic fat density lesion of <5 cm, with surrounding inflammatory changes, most commonly in the sigmoid, descending or right hemicolon. Right-sided epiploic appendagitis may be mistaken clinically for appendicitis. Omental infarction typically appears as a larger, heterogeneous lesion, usually affecting the caecum or ascending colon. Acute diverticulitis usually occurs in older patients, and is associated with colonic diverticula and

wall thickening. Liposarcoma is rare, but is included in the differential of a fat-containing intra-abdominal mass.

Singh et al (2005a).

10) c. ****
Serous cystadenomas are benign neoplasia of the pancreas most commonly seen in older women and are frequently asymptomatic. Typical appearances are of a cystic lesion measuring up to 20 cm in size, containing innumerable small cysts, though these may be difficult to discriminate, giving the appearance of a solid mass. They may occur in any part of the pancreas but are slightly more common in the pancreatic head and neck. Characteristic features include a central stellate scar containing dystrophic calcification. Mucinous cystadenomas usually occur in the pancreatic tail (90%) and, when multilocular, contain larger cysts of >2 cm in diameter. Pancreatic pseudocysts are usually unilocular and occur following a history of pancreatitis. Intraductal papillary mucinous tumours of the main duct are typically associated with dilatation of the main pancreatic duct. Insulinomas are usually small (<2 cm) solid tumours that produce symptoms early due to recurrent hypoglycaemia.

Planner et al (2007).

11) b. ***
The functional segmental anatomy of the liver is based on the distribution of the three major hepatic veins. The middle hepatic vein divides the liver into left and right lobes. The left hepatic vein divides the left lobe into medial and lateral segments. The right hepatic vein divides the right lobe into anterior and posterior segments. In addition, the four sections are further subdivided in a transverse plane by an imaginary line drawn between the right and left portal veins. Segments run in a clockwise fashion, with segments III, IV(b), V and VI lying below the portal veins and segments VII, VIII, IV(a) and II lying above. The caudate lobe (segment I) lies posterior and to the right of the inferior vena cava.

Dähnert (2007), 684–5.

12) b. **
Patients with colon cancer diagnosed endoscopically or suspected following barium enema should be imaged for staging purposes. Objectives of staging include determination of size and local extent of tumour, assessment of the extension of tumour into adjacent structures, and detection of local and distant nodal involvement and presence of metastatic disease. Abdominal ultrasound scan alone is not considered sufficient, and CT of the chest, abdomen and pelvis with oral and intravenous iodinated contrast medium is the primary imaging investigation. The liver is the commonest site of distant metastases, but pulmonary metastases occur in 5–50% of patients. [18]FDG PET/CT is

not used in initial staging but is particularly useful for detecting recurrent disease.

Royal College of Radiologists (2006), 70–1.

13) a. ***

The inferior mesenteric vein provides venous drainage for the rectum, sigmoid and descending colon, and is a potential route of spread of neoplastic and inflammatory conditions. Inferior mesenteric vein thrombosis may occur secondary to an inflammatory process, most commonly diverticulitis, or malignancy. Other potential causes include hypercoagulable states, surgery, trauma and bowel obstruction. Appearances are of an enlarged vein with rim enhancement surrounding central low-density thrombus. Superior mesenteric vein thrombosis is much more common (95% of mesenteric venous thrombosis) and may follow an inflammatory or neoplastic process affecting the small intestine, caecum, and ascending and transverse colon.

Akpinar et al (2008).

14) d. ****

Pseudomyxoma peritonei results from rupture of a benign or malignant mucin-producing tumour, most commonly of the appendix or ovary, but also of the pancreas, stomach and colon. Typical findings are of large-volume mucinous ascites, which appears on CT as very low-attenuation (mucinous) fluid collections in the omentum, mesentery and peritoneal cavity, often loculated and containing curvilinear or punctuate calcifications. A characteristic feature is scalloping of the contour of the liver and splenic margins, which distinguishes mucinous from serous ascites. Peritoneal metastases may also demonstrate loculated peritoneal fluid collections, but there are typically nodular peritoneal densities and thickening of the greater omentum (omental cake). Peritoneal mesothelioma usually presents with thickened mesentery, omentum, peritoneum and bowel wall, with a disproportionately small amount of ascites.

Dähnert (2007), 866.

15) a. ****

Insulinomas are rare tumours of the islet cells of the pancreas, which present at an early stage with hypoglycaemic episodes. Diagnosis is made biochemically, by demonstrating fasting hyperinsulinaemia, and the main purpose of imaging is to detect and localize accurately the tumours, which tend to be small (<2 cm) at presentation. Tumours may occur anywhere in the pancreas, with 2–5% in an ectopic location. CT is considered the first-line investigation, but newer techniques such as MR and functional imaging are being increasingly used. On CT, insulinomas are typically solid and highly vascular, and are best visualized on arterial-phase imaging, when they demonstrate marked enhancement.

McAuley et al (2005).

16) b. ***
Pyogenic abscesses are the commonest type of liver abscess in developed countries, and are most frequently due to ascending cholangitis from benign or malignant obstructive biliary disease. They are often poorly defined with irregular walls on ultrasound scan, and may contain debris or demonstrate intense hyperechogenicity when containing gas. Amoebic abscesses tend to occur in younger, more acutely unwell patients from high prevalence areas or with a history of recent travel. They are treated medically whereas pyogenic abscesses usually require percutaneous or surgical drainage. Fungal abscesses are usually multiple and occur in immunosuppressed individuals. Hydatid disease tends to be asymptomatic or present with biliary colic. Characteristic ultrasound scan features include daughter cysts and detachment of the endocyst, giving rise to 'floating membranes' within the cyst cavity.

Doyle et al (2006).

17) e. ***
Necrolytic migratory erythema is a rare dermatological condition with a strong association with glucagonoma, an islet-cell tumour of the pancreas derived from alpha cells. Over 70% of patients with glucagonoma demonstrate the condition, and they may also complain of weight loss, diarrhoea and diabetes. The association is considered strong enough to warrant thorough investigation for pancreatic malignancy. Glucagonomas typically occur in the pancreatic body or tail, and are large (2.5–25 cm) hypervascular tumours with solid and necrotic components. They have a high rate of malignant transformation, and around 50% of patients have liver metastases at the time of diagnosis.

Rutherford et al (2007).

18) b. ****
Several imaging methods are available for use in those patients in whom endoscopy fails to detect the source of bleeding in gastrointestinal haemorrhage. Radionuclide imaging is non-invasive and very sensitive, detecting bleeding rates as low as 0.1–0.5 ml/min. Images are acquired over several hours, enabling detection of intermittent and venous bleeding, but anatomical localization can be insensitive and variable. Conventional angiography is invasive and requires active bleeding at the time of both imaging and contrast injection. Higher bleeding rates of 0.5–1 ml/min are required, and motion artefact from bowel peristalsis may be problematic, but it provides superior localization of the bleeding site and options for therapeutic intervention. However, CT angiography

is advocated as the most appropriate investigation, due to its wide availability, minimal invasiveness and high sensitivity, detecting bleeding rates as low as 0.3 ml/min in animal models. In addition, it enables assessment of a pathological lesion causing bleeding, which may be helpful in planning further management.

Anthony et al (2007).

19) b. ****
Primary achalasia is an abnormality of the myenteric plexus resulting in reduced or absent peristalsis and failure of relaxation of the lower oesophageal sphincter. The oesophagus is typically markedly dilated with absent primary peristalsis and a smooth tapered narrowing at the contracted lower oesophageal sphincter. It usually presents in young adults with long-standing dysphagia. In contrast, secondary achalasia due to malignancy usually presents in older patients with a short duration of dysphagia. Decreased peristalsis and distal oesophageal tapering in these patients result from tumour infiltration of the myenteric plexus of the distal oesophagus by gastric carcinoma, lymphoma or metastatic disease. Distal oesophageal carcinoma tends to give rise to irregular, asymmetrical narrowing. Scleroderma typically appears as a dilated oesophagus with a patulous lower oesophageal sphincter. Presbyoesophagus is a disorder of oesophageal motility, characterized by oesophageal dilatation and repetitive, non-peristaltic, tertiary contractions in the distal oesophagus.

Halpert (2006), 20–6.

20) d. ***
Peutz–Jegher syndrome is characterized by multiple benign hamartomatous intestinal polyps and mucocutaneous pigmentation. It is familial in 50% of cases, with an autosomal dominant inheritance, and sporadic in 50%. It is the most common polyposis syndrome to involve the small intestine, and frequently presents with intussusception. Typical findings are of multiple hamartomatous polyps in the small bowel, and less commonly the colon and stomach. Patients are at increased risk of gastrointestinal malignancy, but also of tumours of the pancreas, breast, ovary, endometrium and testis.

Dähnert (2007), 862–3.

21) c. ****
Bezoars are masses of accumulated ingested material forming in the stomach or intestines. Phytobezoars are the commonest type, composed of poorly digested fibre and vegetable matter. They are seen particularly in patients with previous gastric surgery, probably due to diminished gastric emptying. Patients may be asymptomatic or present with early satiety or symptoms of gastritis, as phytobezoars are irritant. Occasionally, they may obstruct the stomach with a ball–valve mechanism. They are seen as relatively mobile filling defects, the

interstices of which are filled with barium. Trichobezoars are composed of hair, and are usually larger, and found in younger patients, particularly those with a psychiatric history. Gastric carcinoma, villous adenoma and suture granuloma are all causes of gastric filling defects but have a constant relationship to the gastric wall.

Halpert (2006), 52–3.

22) e. ***

Leiomyomas are benign tumours of smooth muscle, and represent the most common benign neoplasm of the oesophagus. They are often asymptomatic but may present with dysphagia and rarely haematemesis. They appear on barium swallow as large, well-defined, intramural masses causing luminal deformity. A characteristic finding is of coarse calcifications – leiomyoma is the only calcifying oesophageal tumour. Oesophageal lipomas and duplication cysts also appear as well-defined submucosal lesions (of fat and of water density respectively on CT), but are less common, and internal calcification is not a feature. Oesophageal carcinoma usually appears as an irregular ulcerated stricture. Oesophageal varices are seen as serpiginous filling defects.

Dähnert (2007), 849.

23) a. ***

GI tract metastases are seen in 4–8% of patients with malignant melanoma. The small intestine is most commonly affected, followed by the colon and stomach. Typical features are of multiple submucosal nodules, with a target appearance due to central ulceration. This appearance is particularly seen with malignant melanoma metastases but may also be seen with gastric metastases from breast, lung and renal cell carcinoma. Other common appearances of gastric metastases include linitis plastica in 20%, most typically from breast cancer, and a solitary mass in 50%.

Dähnert (2007), 852–3.

24) b. **

Iatrogenic injury is the most common cause of oesophageal rupture, but, in 15% of cases, rupture is spontaneous and occurs during vomiting (Boerhaave's syndrome). Patients present with pain and dysphagia, and rapidly develop sepsis. Characteristic chest radiograph findings are of extensive pneumomediastinum and subcutaneous emphysema, pleural effusion or hydropneumothorax, and left lower lobe atelectasis. Widening of the mediastinum may accompany the development of mediastinitis. Pleural effusion and atelectasis may be seen in acute pulmonary embolism, acute pancreatitis and aortic dissection, but pneumomediastinum is not a recognized feature of these conditions. Other common causes of pneumomediastinum include asthma, chest trauma and perforation of a hollow viscus with extension of gas via the retroperitoneum.

Dähnert (2006), 828–9.

25) a. ***
Haemangiomas are the most common benign liver tumour. They are often asymptomatic but may present with hepatomegaly or rarely spontaneous haemorrhage. Typical CT features of a hepatic haemangioma are of a well-defined hypodense mass on unenhanced CT, with early peripheral enhancement after intravenous contrast followed by complete fill-in on delayed images. Hepatocellular carcinoma is seen as a hypodense mass and usually demonstrates contrast enhancement during the arterial phase, but enhancement decreases on delayed images. Focal fatty infiltration usually has a geographic distribution, and, like simple hepatic cysts, does not demonstrate contrast enhancement. Focal nodular hyperplasia is usually isodense on unenhanced CT and, although it tends to show intense transient arterial phase enhancement, is often isodense during the portal phase. A central scar, if present, may demonstrate enhancement on delayed images.

Brant & Helms (2007), 765.

26) b. **
Sigmoid volvulus usually occurs when the sigmoid loop twists around its mesenteric axis, creating a closed loop obstruction. Typical features are of an inverted U-shaped loop converging on the left side of the pelvis. The bowel loop is usually markedly distended, appears ahaustral, and may overlap the lower border of the liver (liver overlap sign) or the haustrated dilated descending colon (left flank overlap sign). The apex of the volvulus usually lies under the left hemidiaphram with its apex above the level of T10. Caecal volvulus occurs when the caecum is on a mesentery, and involves the caecum either twisting and inverting so the caecal pole lies in the left upper quadrant, or twisting in an axial plane so that the caecum remains right sided or central. Appearances are of a large, gas-distended viscus, usually with haustral markings, and occasionally the gas-filled appendix may be identified.

Sutton (2002), 676–8.

27) a. ***
The commonest cause of a free intraperitoneal perforation is an anterior wall duodenal ulcer. However, free peritoneal air is only apparent on an erect chest radiograph in 60% of perforated duodenal ulcers. Possible causes include sealing of the perforation, adhesions preventing the gas reaching the subphrenic space or insufficient time being allowed for gas to collect under the diaphragm. Anterior wall gastric ulcers also perforate into the peritoneal cavity but are a less common cause of pneumoperitoneum. Posterior wall duodenal and gastric ulcers perforate into the lesser sac or retroperitoneal region

rather than the peritoneal cavity. Perforated appendix and diverticulitis may produce localized collections of extraluminal gas, but pneumoperitoneum is rare.

Sutton (2002), 585.

28) d. ****
The third part of the duodenum is bounded posteriorly by the aorta, and anteriorly by the root of the mesentery carrying the superior mesenteric artery. In superior mesenteric artery syndrome, the third part of the duodenum is compressed by the superior mesenteric artery, and the angle between it and the aorta narrows to $10-22°$ (normal $45-65°$). The condition is associated with severe weight loss, prolonged bedrest (particularly in a body cast), lumbar lordosis and pregnancy. Patients report intermittent abdominal pain and vomiting, relieved by lying prone or in the knee–elbow position. Duodenal atresia causes complete obstruction usually distal to the ampulla of Vater, and presents in neonates with a 'double-bubble' sign on plain abdominal radiograph. Annular pancreas is usually asymptomatic but may present with abdominal pain and vomiting, and barium meal demonstrates narrowing of the second part of the duodenum. Duodenal duplication cysts cause extrinsic compression of the first and second portions of the duodenum. Ladd's bands are congenital peritoneal bands occurring in association with malrotation that may cause obstruction of the second part of the duodenum, but presentation is usually in infants and children.

Dähnert (2007), 871.

29) b. ***
Ulcerative colitis and Crohn's disease are idiopathic inflammatory diseases of the bowel. Ulcerative colitis predominantly involves the mucosa and submucosa, and characteristically produces continuous, circumferential involvement of the colon. Crohn's disease produces transmural inflammation, may affect the entire gastrointestinal tract, and is characterized by eccentric and discontinuous involvement. Typical features of ulcerative colitis include predominantly left-sided colonic involvement with rectosigmoid involvement in 95% of cases, a patulous ileocaecal valve and shallow ulceration. Typical features of Crohn's disease include skip lesions (discontinuous disease), terminal ileal involvement with a thickened ileocaecal valve and fistula formation.

Dähnert (2007), 873–4.

30) a. ***
Portal venous gas is identified on CT as linear branching structures of air density extending to the periphery of the liver, presumably due to the direction of portal venous flow. The commonest cause in adults is mesenteric infarction, when it is a poor prognostic sign. In infants the commonest cause is necrotizing enterocolitis, when it does not necessarily imply a poor outcome. In contrast, gas within the biliary tree

is central and does not extend into the peripheral 2 cm of the liver. In portal venous thrombosis, a focal hypodensity is seen within the portal vein on contrast-enhanced CT. Intrahepatic biliary dilatation appears as dilated branching ductal structures of fluid density. In fatty infiltration of the liver, vessels may appear hyperattenuating on unenhanced CT in contrast to the hypodense liver.

Brant & Helms (2007), 763–4.

31) e. ***
A laminated calcified appendicolith is seen in only 7–15% of patients with acute appendicitis. However, the presence of acute abdominal pain with an appendicolith on abdominal plain film indicates a 90% probability of acute appendicitis, and also indicates a high probability of gangrene/perforation. Other plain film signs of acute appendicitis include caecal wall thickening, small bowel obstruction and focal extraluminal gas collections.

Dähnert (2007), 803–5.

32) e. ***
Accessory spleen (splenunculus) is seen in 10–30% of the population and results from developmental failure of fusion of the mesodermal buds that form the spleen. They appear as small (usually < 10 mm), well-defined masses with identical attenuation and enhancement characteristics as the spleen, and are most commonly located near the splenic hilum. Following splenectomy for haematological disorders, an accessory spleen may undergo hypertrophy and result in recurrence of the original disorder. Regional lymph nodes from colorectal cancer extend along the course of the main vessels supplying the segment of bowel. Wandering spleen refers to a normal spleen positioned in an abnormal location within the abdomen due to laxity of the splenic ligaments. Splenic artery aneurysms are focal dilatations of the splenic artery, which may be intra- or extrasplenic and are frequently calcified. Polysplenia is a rare congenital disorder associated with situs ambiguous, and characterized by multiple small spleens usually in the right abdomen.

Dähnert (2007), 692.

33) a. ***
A CT pulmonary angiogram is performed during pulmonary arterial phase enhancement. During arterial phase enhancement, variable rates of flow through the splenic parenchyma result in heterogeneous enhancement, which may appear as alternating bands of high and low attenuation, or give the impression of irregular, low-density mass lesions. Enhancement becomes homogeneous in the portal venous phase. Splenic infarction is the most common cause of (true) focal splenic defects, and typically appears as single or multiple, wedge-shaped, peripheral, low-attenuation defects. Clefts in the splenic

contour are common normal variants, appearing as smoothly contoured, medially located defects, and should not be mistaken for lacerations. Splenosis is the implantation of splenic tissue in ectopic sites following traumatic rupture or splenectomy, and appears as multiple, small, homogeneous, enhancing masses that may mimic peritoneal deposits. Spontaneous splenic rupture is rare, though it may be delayed following trauma or be associated with splenomegaly. Appearances may include low-density, linear, parenchymal lacerations and areas of mottled parenchymal enhancement representing contusions.

Dähnert (2007), 691.

34) e. *****

Candida oesophagitis is the commonest cause of infectious oesophagitis and is particularly seen in immunosuppressed individuals. It is frequently associated with oral thrush. It tends to affect the upper half of the oesophagus, and typical appearances are of linear, longitudinally oriented filling defects representing heaped-up areas of mucosal plaques consisting of necrotic debris and fungal colonies. In contrast, a normal intervening mucosa in oesophagitis is suggestive of a viral aetiology. Findings in cytomegalovirus and HIV oesophagitis are similar, with typical appearances of one or more large flat ulcers seen in the distal oesophagus. Distinction between the two is made by brushings or biopsy at endoscopy. In herpes simplex infection, the typical features of multiple, small, superficial ulcers are similar at all sites of potential involvement, including the oesophagus, oral cavity, rectum and anus.

Pantongrag-Brown et al (1995).

35) e. ****

Buscopan is commonly used in radiological practice as a smooth muscle relaxant. As a non-selective muscarinic antagonist, it produces other autonomic responses including pupillary dilatation and tachycardia, and may potentially precipitate an attack of acute angle-closure glaucoma that requires prompt treatment to prevent permanent visual loss. However, most glaucoma is of the open-angle form, which is unaffected by Buscopan, and it is therefore advised that routine enquiry about a history of glaucoma is unnecessary. Instead patient information leaflets should advise all patients to attend hospital immediately should they develop painful, blurred vision. Routine enquiry about prostatism, porphyria and myasthenia gravis is also not recommended. However, in patients with unstable cardiac disease, the tachycardia and slight increase in diastolic blood pressure caused by Buscopan carry the potential risk of arrhythmia. The presence of unstable cardiac disease is therefore deemed to be the only potential reason to withhold Buscopan.

Dyde et al (2008).

36) b. ***
The commonest cause of small bowel obstruction in adults is adhesions, which are diagnosed on CT when there is an abrupt calibre transition without an associated mass, surrounding inflammatory changes or bowel wall thickening. Carcinoid tumours comprise 25% of all tumours of the small bowel. They are commonly asymptomatic but may present with pain or obstruction, or with carcinoid syndrome in 7% of patients. Most occur in the ileum, and typical appearances are of a calcified mass with surrounding desmoplastic reaction, retraction of the mesentery and thickening of surrounding loops of bowel. Small bowel obstruction complicates Crohn's disease in approximately 15% of patients, due to thickening and submucosal oedema of the bowel wall. Previous irradiation may result in adhesions and fibrotic changes in the mesentery that can cause bowel obstruction. Lymphomatous involvement of the small bowel causes circumferential bowel wall thickening, but this rarely results in obstruction.

Sinha & Verma (2005).

37) b. ***
A number of anomalies of the major vessels can cause extrinsic impressions upon the oesophagus. The commonest aortic anomaly is a right-sided aortic arch, which produces an indentation on the right lateral oesophageal wall in the absence of the normal left aortic arch impression. An aberrant right subclavian artery originates from the aortic arch just distal to the left subclavian artery, and passes upwards and to the right, behind the oesophagus, giving rise to an oblique posterior oesophageal indentation. In aortic coarctation, the pre- and post-stenotic dilatations of the aorta produce a characteristic reversed-3 impression upon the left wall of the oesophagus. An enlarged left atrium and an aberrant left pulmonary artery both cause anterior indentations upon the oesophagus.

Sutton (2002), 573.

38) b. *****
Focal nodular hyperplasia (FNH) is a benign hamartomatous malformation commonest in young women. Lesions are usually smaller than 5 cm, and contain a central stellate scar in up to one-third of cases. Hepatic adenomas are benign tumours averaging 8–10 cm in size, seen predominantly in young women and related to oral contraceptive use. Lesions have a propensity for spontaneous haemorrhage, presenting as subcapsular haematoma or haemoperitoneum. FNH, though highly vascular, rarely undergoes spontaneous haemorrhage. FNH usually contains sufficient functioning Kupffer cells to demonstrate normal or increased uptake on ^{99m}Tc-labelled sulphur colloid scan, whereas hepatic adenoma, composed of hepatocytes and non-functioning Kupffer cells, appears as a focal photopenic lesion. Both lesions

demonstrate transient arterial enhancement following intravenous contrast.

Dähnert (2007), 713–15, 719–20.

39) d. ***
Acute hepatitis results in a diffuse decrease in liver echogenicity on ultrasound scan, with increased brightness of the portal triads resulting in a 'starry sky' appearance. Other imaging features include oedema of the gallbladder fossa and gallbladder wall thickening. Gallbladder wall thickening (anterior wall thickness >3 mm in a non-contracted gallbladder) may be seen in a wide range of intrinsic and extrinsic conditions. The commonest intrinsic cause is cholecystitis (acute and chronic), whereas common extrinsic causes include hepatitis, hypoalbuminaemia, heart failure and renal failure.

Chapman & Nakielny (2003), 291.

40) c. ****
The right subphrenic space is in communication around the liver with the anterior subhepatic and posterior subhepatic (Morison's pouch) spaces. The right subphrenic and subhepatic spaces communicate freely with the right paracolic gutter and via this with the pelvic peritoneal cavity. The left subphrenic space communicates with the left subhepatic space but is separated from the right subphrenic space by the falciform ligament and from the left paracolic gutter by the phrenicocolic ligament. The falciform ligament is a sickle-shaped fold of peritoneum that attaches the ventral surface of the liver to the anterior abdominal wall. It extends in a parasagittal plane from the umbilicus to the diaphragm and carries the ligamentum teres in its free inferoposterior margin. The lesser sac is an isolated peritoneal compartment between the stomach and pancreas, which communicates with the rest of the peritoneal cavity (greater sac) only through the foramen of Winslow (epiploic foramen). The lesser omentum is composed of the gastrohepatic and hepaticoduodenal ligaments and suspends the stomach and duodenal bulb from the inferior liver surface.

Brant & Helms (2007), 733–6.

41) d. ***
An erect chest radiograph is best for demonstrating a small pneumoperitoneum, enabling the identification of as little as 1 ml of free intraperitoneal gas. It is superior to an erect abdomen, as the X-ray beam penetrates the diaphragmatic region almost tangentially, whereas, in an erect abdomen, the divergent beam penetrates this area obliquely. However, if the patient is too unwell to sit erect, the most appropriate projection is a left lateral decubitus abdominal radiograph, performed with the patient lying on the left side, using a horizontal X-ray beam. In this position, air will preferentially leave a perforated duodenal or antral ulcer, and any free gas in the lesser sac will enter the main abdominal

cavity. The supine abdominal radiograph may demonstrate free gas in about 56% of patients with pneumoperitoneum. Characteristic features include gas outlining both inner and outer walls of a bowel loop (Rigler's sign), triangular collections of gas between bowel loops, and outlining of the falciform ligament and other peritoneal reflections by free gas. The supine chest radiograph is not useful in the detection of free intraperitoneal gas.

Sutton, 663–7.

42) c. ****
Intrahepatic bile ducts are considered dilated when they exceed 40% of the diameter of the adjacent portal veins. The upper limit of normal for the extrahepatic common bile duct is 5 mm in adults (increasing after age 60 by approximately 1 mm/decade). Appearances here are indicative of biliary obstruction at the level of the hilum, and MRCP is the investigation of choice after ultrasound scan in these circumstances. MRCP reliably demonstrates the extent of ductal involvement, allowing planning of surgery or treatment; with malignant causes, it may provide further staging information. CT is the investigation of choice when ultrasound scan indicates obstruction below the hilum. If ultrasound scan demonstrates ductal stones, ERCP is the investigation of choice for confirmation and therapeutic intervention. Endoscopic ultrasound scan is particularly useful for detecting small ductal stones and periampullary tumours. Percutaneous transhepatic cholangiography is reserved for cases when ERCP is not possible.

Royal College of Radiologists (2007), 98–9.

43) b. ***
In 75% of cases, the gastroduodenal artery arises from the common hepatic artery before its division into right and left branches. Less common origins include the left hepatic artery (4–11%), the right hepatic artery (7%) and the superior mesenteric artery via a replaced hepatic trunk (4–11%). The artery descends behind the first part of the duodenum, lying anterior to the pancreas and to the left of the common bile duct. At this site, erosion of the posterior duodenal wall by an ulcer may produce life-threatening haemorrhage if the gastroduodenal artery is involved. Its main branches are the posterior and anterior superior pancreaticoduodenal arteries, and the right gastroepiploic artery.

Butler et al (1999), 229–30.

44) d. ****
Superparamagnetic iron oxide (SPIO) particles are iron-based particles of 30–150 nm, which, when administered as an infusion 1–4 hours prior to imaging, act as a negative MR contrast agent. They target the reticuloendothelial system, being taken up by macrophages throughout the body, but are preferentially accumulated by the Kupffer cells of the liver. Their superparamagnetic properties result in T2 and T2*

shortening of the tissues that accumulate the particles, which show reduced signal intensity on T2W, T2*W and, to a lesser extent, T1W images. Most liver tumours do not exhibit uptake, as they are deficient in Kupffer cells. However, as the rest of the liver accumulates SPIO and darkens preferentially, the tumour appears of increased conspicuity. SPIO particles are particularly used, in combination with gadolinium, to improve detection of hepatocellular carcinoma in cirrhotic patients, in whom the parenchymal changes of fibrosis and regenerative nodules make detection with gadolinium alone difficult.

Gandhi et al (2006).

45) a. ***

Budd–Chiari syndrome is caused by obstruction of hepatic venous outflow, which may, in turn, be caused by membranous obstruction of the suprahepatic IVC by a congenital web, or hepatic venous thrombosis due to hypercoagulable state, tumour or trauma. Patients develop hepatosplenomegaly and intractable ascites. Doppler ultrasound scan demonstrates non-visualization of, or thrombus within, one or more hepatic veins. CT findings reflect severely impaired blood flow to the liver, with a 'flip-flop' enhancement pattern after contrast administration. Early images show prominent central liver enhancement with poor peripheral enhancement, whereas delayed images show central washout with peripheral enhancement. The caudate lobe is typically spared because of its separate venous drainage directly into the IVC, and enhances normally. Passive hepatic congestion complicates heart failure, and results in distended hepatic veins and IVC. Hepatic veno-occlusive disease refers to occlusion of small centrilobular hepatic veins following radio- and chemotherapy in bone-marrow transplant recipients, or related to alkaloid consumption. The main hepatic veins and IVC are normal. Hepatic venous involvement is not a feature of viral hepatitis or primary biliary cirrhosis.

Brant & Helms (2007), 762–3.

46) b. ***

Thorotrast (thorium dioxide), an alpha-emitting radioactive isotope of atomic number 90 and long half-life, was used as a contrast agent until the mid-1950s, predominantly for cerebral angiography and reticuloendothelial imaging. It is retained indefinitely by the reticuloendothelial system, and results in increased density of the liver, spleen and lymph nodes with a characteristic stippled appearance. It is associated with delayed malignancies, including angiosarcoma, cholangiocarcinoma and hepatocellular carcinoma. Haemochromatosis may result in diffusely increased density of the liver and spleen, but usually presents earlier in life. Amiodarone may result in increased liver attenuation of 95–145 HU (normal 30–70 HU), but splenic involvement is not usually a feature. Sickle cell anaemia can result in a shrunken calcified spleen, but again is unlikely in this age group. Glycogen storage disease can result in a generalized increase or decrease in hepatic density on CT, but increased splenic density is not a feature.

Dähnert (2007), 750.

47) b. ****

Cholesterolosis is a form of hyperplastic cholecystosis in which triglycerides, cholesterol precursors and cholesterol esters accumulate within the lamina propria of the gallbladder wall. Most cases are of the planar type, termed 'strawberry gallbladder' after the resemblance of the gallbladder mucosa to the surface of a strawberry, and produce no detectable ultrasound changes. In a minority of cases, cholesterol polyps are formed, which are the commonest type of gallbladder polyp. They are generally small, multiple echogenic lesions adjacent to the gallbladder wall. Non-mobility and a lack of posterior acoustic shadowing helps to distinguish polyps from gallstones. Small size and multiplicity distinguishes them from gallbladder malignancy, though, rarely, metastatic disease may produce multiple polypoid lesions, particularly malignant melanoma. Adenomyomatosis, the other form of hyperplastic cholecystosis, results in mucosal hyperplasia and thickening of the muscular layer of the gallbladder. It is characterized by bright reflections and comet-tail artefacts from the gallbladder wall on ultrasound scan.

Middleton et al (2004), 41–3.

48) c. ****

Nodules are a common finding in cirrhosis, and differentiation of benign nodules from hepatocellular carcinoma (occurring in 7–12% of patients) is vital. Most nodules are regenerative nodules, representing reparative attempts by hepatocytes in response to liver injury. These are typically under 10mm in size and appear isodense to liver parenchyma on CT, unless they contain iron deposits (siderotic nodules), in which case they may be slightly hyperdense. Dysplastic nodules are proliferative premalignant lesions found in 15–25% of cirrhotic livers. They resemble regenerative nodules on CT but are usually larger than 10mm. Hepatocellular carcinomas usually appear as encapsulated hypodense masses that demonstrate rapid arterial enhancement and early washout of contrast on delayed images. Hepatic haemangioma usually appears as a low-density mass, but has different enhancement characteristics, demonstrating peripheral enhancement with complete fill-in on delayed images. Focal fatty sparing appears as an area of normal density in a generally hypodense liver and does not demonstrate contrast enhancement.

Brant & Helms (2007), 760–2.

49) a. ****

Primary sclerosing cholangitis is an idiopathic, progressive, fibrosing, inflammatory disorder of the biliary tree, causing multifocal strictures, cholestasis and biliary cirrhosis. There is an association with inflammatory bowel disease and autoimmune conditions. In most cases, both intra- and extrahepatic ducts are involved, and classic appearances on cholangiography are of a 'string-of-beads' appearance with alternating segments of dilatation and stenosis. Biliary cirrhosis develops in up to 49% of cases, and there is an increased risk of cholangiocarcinoma. In primary biliary cirrhosis, disease is limited to the intrahepatic bile ducts. In ascending cholangitis, there may be biliary dilatation and pneumobilia, but multifocal strictures are not a feature. CT features of choledocholithiasis include biliary dilatation and visualization of a stone in the bile duct, but again strictures are not a feature. Chronic pancreatitis may result in a smooth inflammatory stricture of the intrapancreatic portion of the common bile duct.

Dähnert (2007), 699–700.

50) b. ****

The differentiation between complicated diverticular disease and a perforating colorectal carcinoma may be difficult. Both may appear as a focal area of eccentric luminal narrowing on contrast enema. A longer segment of involvement favours diverticulitis, as well as other inflammatory causes of colitis. In addition, stricture margins in diverticulitis tend to be smoothly tapered rather than the abrupt narrowing of carcinoma. Mucosal ulceration occurs in most cases of colorectal carcinoma, and is not a particular feature of diverticulitis. Fistula formation may occur in both conditions, most commonly between the colon and the bladder, though this is more commonly seen in diverticulitis. The presence of diverticula does not exclude the possibility of colorectal carcinoma, and the two conditions may coexist, as both are common in elderly people.

Brant & Helms (2007), 850–1, 859–60; Dähnert (2007), 813–15, 822.

51) e. ***

Oesophageal intramural pseudodiverticulosis is a condition causing dilatation of the ducts of the submucosal glands of the oesophagus. These appear on barium meal as multiple, tiny, flask-shaped collections of barium arranged in longitudinal rows. They may appear to 'float' outside the oesophagus, as the connection to the lumen may not be appreciated. Associated strictures in the distal oesophagus are common. The condition is commonly associated with diabetes and chronic alcoholism, but may also occur with severe oesophagitis of any cause. *Candida* may be cultured in around half the cases, but this may be a secondary infection due to stasis of secretions within the glands.

Sutton (2002), 559–60; Dähnert (2007), 828.

52) d. ****

Oesophageal varices are dilated submucosal veins, which may be classified by their direction of flow as uphill or downhill varices. Uphill varices occur in the lower oesophagus and represent collateral blood flow conveying portal venous blood to the azygos vein. They usually result from portal hypertension due to liver cirrhosis, but may also occur with splenic vein thrombosis, and obstruction of the hepatic veins or IVC. Downhill varices result from obstruction of the SVC. If it is obstructed superior to the entry of the azygos vein, varices will be confined to the upper third of the oesophagus. If the SVC is obstructed below the entry of the azygos vein, the varices convey all of the systemic venous blood from the upper half of the body into the portal vein and IVC, and they will run the entire length of the oesophagus. SVC obstruction is most commonly due to lung cancer or lymphoma.

Sutton (2002), 571–3; Dähnert (2007), 829.

53) c. ***

Acute gastric volvulus is abnormal rotation of one part of the stomach around another part, which may be classified as organoaxial, mesenteroaxial or combination type, depending on the axis of rotation. Predisposing factors include ligamentous laxity, hiatus hernia and diaphragmatic eventration. The classic presentation is with the Borchardt triad of sudden severe epigastric pain, intractable retching with no vomitus produced, and inability to pass a nasogastric tube into the stomach. Other plain film findings include unexpected location of the gastric bubble and air–fluid levels in the mediastinum or upper abdomen, but definitive diagnosis is by barium meal. The condition is a surgical emergency, as it may result in gastric ischaemia or perforation. Acute gastric dilatation and pyloric stenosis may result in gastric distension on plain film, but would not present with intractable retching or difficulty with nasogastric tube passage. A 'cup-and-spill' stomach is an anatomical variant on barium meal, which may simulate an organoaxial volvulus. A paraduodenal hernia usually presents acutely as small bowel obstruction.

Sutton (2002), 600; Dähnert (2007), 836.

54) a. ****

Cimetidine, a histamine H_2-receptor antagonist, may be used to increase uptake of $[^{99m}Tc]$ pertechnetate by inhibiting its secretion from gastric mucosa. Pentagastrin and glucagon have also been used to improve visualization, by stimulating uptake and decreasing peristalsis respectively. Procedures such as colonoscopy and use of laxatives should be avoided prior to the scan, as they may cause mucosal irritation. Potassium perchlorate should not be used to block thyroid uptake, as it also blocks uptake of pertechnetate by the gastric mucosa. The patient normally fasts for 3–4 hours and voids prior to the study, as a full stomach or bladder may obscure an adjacent Meckel's diverticulum. Barium studies should be avoided for 3–4 days prior to the study, as attenuation by the barium may hamper interpretation.

Zeissman et al (2006), 375–7.

55) b. ****
Cavitating mesenteric lymph node syndrome is a rare complication of coeliac disease, in which multiple enlarged lymph nodes are seen in the jejunoileal mesentery. The nodes have central low attenuation and may contain fat or fluid, or fat–fluid levels. Splenic atrophy is usually seen, and jejunal or duodenal biopsy confirms villous atrophy of the small bowel mucosa. Low-attenuation lymphadenopathy may also be seen in tuberculosis, Whipple's disease, lymphoma and necrotic metastases, but fat–fluid levels have been reported only in coeliac disease.

Reddy et al (2002).

56) a. ****
Fibrolamellar carcinoma of the liver is an uncommon variant of hepatocellular carcinoma, typically presenting as a large, 5–20 cm liver mass in a young patient with no risk factors. Typical features are of an encapsulated mass with a prominent central fibrous scar. The scar often contains areas of calcification, and appears hypointense on T1- and T2-weighted images. Focal nodular hyperplasia (FNH) is a hamartomatous malformation also most commonly seen in young woman. However, lesion size is usually <5 cm and, although a central fibrous scar is also a common feature, this usually appears hyperintense on T2-weighted images due to vascular channels and oedema, and calcifications within it are extremely rare. Both pathologies may result in multiple lesions, with FNH being multiple in 20% and fibrolamellar carcinoma demonstrating satellite lesions in 10–15%. FNH is the only liver lesion with sufficient Kupffer cells to cause normal or increased uptake on sulphur colloid scan.

Dähnert (2007), 713–15, 726.

57) b. ****
Fibrosing colonopathy is a condition causing progressive submucosal fibrosis predominantly affecting the proximal colon. It was first described in 1994 in children with cystic fibrosis taking high-dose lipase supplementation to relieve the symptoms of exocrine pancreatic insufficiency. It causes stricturing and longitudinal shortening of the right colon, and patients present with obstruction. Overall, the gastrointestinal tract is affected in 85–90% of patients with cystic fibrosis, and all of the above pathologies may occur, though only fibrosing colonopathy is associated with high-dose lipase supplementation.

Dähnert (2007), 489.

58) e. ****

Orthotopic liver transplantation is the treatment of choice for patients with end-stage liver disease for which no other therapy is available. Surgery involves one arterial anastomosis (hepatic artery), at least two venous anastomoses (portal vein and IVC) and a biliary anastomosis, and complications may occur at any of these sites. Vascular complications are the most frequent cause of graft loss, and most commonly involve the hepatic artery, with portal venous and IVC complications being relatively infrequent. Biliary complications occur in up to 34% of cases, and are the second most common cause of liver dysfunction after graft rejection. They include leak, stricture and obstruction. Other complications include fluid collections, infection and malignancy. Normal findings following liver transplantation include a small amount of free intraperitoneal fluid in the perihepatic region, especially at the hilum, or in the fissure for the ligamentum teres, which usually resolves within a few weeks. Other normal findings are a right fluid pleural effusion, and periportal oedema, attributed to lymphatic channel dilatation due to lack of normal lymphatic drainage.

Quiroga et al (2001).

59) a. ****

A transjugular intrahepatic portosystemic shunt (TIPSS) is an endovascular procedure performed to create a portosystemic shunt between the portal venous and hepatic venous systems, for decompression of portal hypertension, particularly in patients with variceal bleeding uncontrollable by endoscopic management. The shunt is normally formed between the right hepatic vein and right portal vein. The right internal jugular vein is accessed, and via this the right hepatic vein. Curved needle passes are made in an anterior direction to access the right portal vein. The portosystemic pressure gradient is measured and portal venography is performed to enable planning of stent placement. A stent is deployed following balloon dilatation of the stent tract. The goal is to decrease the portosystemic gradient to below 12mmHg and to see no significant filling of varices. Portosystemic shunts require close follow-up, as there is a high incidence of shunt stenosis and occlusion.

Brant & Helms (2007), 722–5.

60) b. ****

Xanthogranulomatous cholecystitis (XGC) is an uncommon inflammatory disease of the gallbladder, which is characterized by multiple intramural nodules and proliferative fibrosis. It is thought to result from rupture and extravasation of bile and mucus following the occlusion of Rokitansky–Aschoff sinuses. There is considerable overlap between the clinical and radiological features of XGC and gallbladder carcinoma. Pericholecystic infiltration, biliary obstruction, regional lymphadenopathy and hepatic involvement may be seen in both conditions, and the difference in incidence between the two conditions is not statistically significant. Only the presence of multiple intramural hypoattenuating nodules (representing xanthogranulomas) occupying a large area of the thickened gallbladder wall allows a diagnosis of XGC to be made with any degree of certainty. Similar hypoattenuating intramural nodules (representing haemorrhage and necrosis) may be seen less commonly in gallbladder carcinoma, but these tend to occupy a much smaller proportion of the thickened gallbladder wall.

Chun et al (1997).

61) e. ***
A Zenker diverticulum is a herniation of the mucosa and submucosa through the midline of the posterior oesophageal wall at the cleavage plane between the oblique and transverse fibres of cricopharyngeus (Killian's dehiscence) at the level of C5−6. The diverticulum is narrow necked and extends caudally, resulting in trapping of undigested food and compression of the adjacent oesophagus. Epiphrenic diverticula are rare, usually occurring on the right lateral wall of the distal oesophagus in association with hiatus hernia. Lateral pharyngeal diverticula are herniations of pharyngeal mucosa through the lateral pharyngeal wall, which occur most commonly in wind instrument players, reflecting increased intrapharyngeal pressure. An interbronchial diverticulum is a traction diverticulum that occurs in the interbronchial segment of the oesophagus in response to adjacent fibrous adhesions following lymph-node infection (usually tuberculous). Intramural pseudodiverticula represent dilated excretory ducts of mucosal glands, which appear as multiple flask-shaped outpouchings and are commonly seen in association with candidiasis.

Brant & Helms (2007), 805−6.

62) b. ***
Barium aspiration is a recognized complication of barium swallow, and may occur particularly in patients with swallowing disorders or recent oesophageal surgery. It is usually clinically insignificant, but complications have been reported, especially with aspiration of larger amounts of barium, and include pneumonitis and granuloma formation. Physiotherapy is the only treatment recommended. Of the water-soluble contrast agents, Gastrografin (ionic and hyperosmolar) may cause pulmonary oedema if aspirated. Gastromiro (non-ionic and iso-osmolar) is safe to use if aspiration is a significant possibility.

Chapman & Nakielny (2001), 51.

63) b. ****
Secretin is a hormone normally secreted by the duodenal mucosa in response to acid within the lumen. It has many physiological effects on the gastrointestinal tract, including stimulation of pancreatic secretions and a transient increase in tone of the sphincter of Oddi. When given intravenously immediately prior to imaging, it results in distension of the

pancreatic ductal system and can significantly improve visualization of the pancreatic main and branch ducts on MRCP, as well as provide information about the secretory reserve capacity of the pancreas. Effects on the biliary tree are less pronounced and not usually appreciable on imaging. Side effects include abdominal pain, bloating and diarrhoea. Glucagon increases bile flow and has been suggested to improve visualization of the biliary tree at MRCP. Cholecystokinin stimulates gallbladder contraction, and is sometimes used in hepatobiliary scintigraphy. Buscopan is widely used in imaging for its inhibition of intestinal motility.

Akisik et al (2006).

64) a. ****
Approximately 80% of all splenic cysts are post-traumatic cysts (also known as false cysts or non-pancreatic pseudocysts), which represent the cystic end stage of trauma, infection or infarction. They are not true cysts, as they lack an epithelial wall. They often contain internal echoes from debris and cyst wall calcification. True cysts may be parasitic (echinococcal) or non-parasitic (epithelial). The spleen is involved in 0.9–8% of cases of echinococcal disease. Features include daughter cysts, and multiple internal dependent echogenic foci resulting in a 'snowstorm' sign. Epidermoid cysts are congenital cysts with the same appearance as post-traumatic cysts, but they are rarer, and rim calcification is less commonly seen. Pyogenic abscesses tend to appear as irregular hypoechoic areas on ultrasound scan, and hyperechoic gas bubbles may be visible. Intrasplenic pancreatic pseudocysts are seen in up to 5% of patients with pancreatitis.

Dähnert (2007), 680–1.

65) c. ***
The recommended contrast is 300 ml of 100% w/v barium sulphate. Transit time may be reduced by the addition of 10 ml of Gastrografin to the barium. Non-ionic, water-soluble contrast media may be used as an alternative where barium is contraindicated. The recommended concentrations and volumes for the other gastrointestinal contrast examinations are barium swallow (a), barium meal (b), small bowel enema (d) and double-contrast barium enema (e).

Chapman & Nakielny (2001), 49–51.

66) b. ***
In primary haemochromatosis, there is increased duodenal absorption and parenchymal retention of dietary iron, which is accumulated within the liver, pancreas, heart and pituitary gland. Intracellular iron deposits within hepatocytes result in a paramagnetic susceptibility effect, leading to marked shortening of T1 and T2 relaxation times of adjacent protons.

This manifests as a marked reduction in liver signal intensity on T2W and T2*W images, and a moderate loss of signal intensity on T1W images.

Dähnert (2007), 717.

67) a. ***
Intraductal papillary mucinous tumour (IPMT) of the pancreas is characterized by a mucin-producing tumour with dilatation of the main or branch ducts of the pancreas due to copious secretions. They may arise in the main duct or branch duct. Main duct tumours typically cause dilatation of all or part of the duct, which is filled with mucinous secretions, appearing hyperintense on T2W images. A T2-hypointense intraductal filling defect may be identified, which may represent the tumour or concretions of mucin. Chronic pancreatitis may result in parenchymal atrophy and duct dilatation, with intraductal filling defects due to calculi or debris, but a bulging papilla at ERCP makes IPMT more likely. The branch duct type usually consists of conglomerated communicating cysts or a unilocular cyst in the uncinate process; these appearances may be mimicked by mucinous cystadenoma and pancreatic pseudocyst.

Lim et al (2001).

68) c. ****
Although symptoms directly referable to the spleen are unusual, autopsy studies have demonstrated the spleen to be involved in 38–77% of patients with sarcoidosis. The commonest abnormality demonstrated on imaging is splenomegaly, occurring in up to 60% of patients. Multiple hypoattenuating nodules measuring up to 3 cm may be seen distributed diffusely throughout the spleen in around 15% of cases, and may occur in the absence of splenomegaly. The lesions appear hypointense on all sequences at MRI and are best seen on T1W or early phase, gadolinium-enhanced, T2W fat-suppressed sequences. Abdominal or systemic symptoms are more frequent in patients with nodular hepatosplenic sarcoidosis. Spontaneous splenic rupture in sarcoidosis has been described but is very rare. Capsular calcification and multiple cystic lesions are not features of the disease.

Warshauer & Lee (2004).

69) b. ***
Calcified liver metastases represent up to 3% of liver metastases, and are most commonly seen with mucinous carcinomas of the gastrointestinal tract. They are also seen in osteosarcoma, breast cancer, lung cancer and carcinoid, but these are less common.

Dähnert (2007), 730.

70) d. ***

Gallstone ileus accounts for up to 5% of intestinal obstruction, increasing in prevalence with age. It involves erosion of a large gallstone from the gallbladder or common bile duct into the bowel, which goes on to cause obstruction. The classic appearance on plain film (Rigler's triad) is only seen in 10% of cases, and consists of partial or complete intestinal obstruction (usually small bowel), gas in the biliary tree and an ectopic calcified gallstone. The most common site of fistulous communication is between the gallbladder and the duodenum, seen in 60%, and this may be demonstrated on barium meal as a contrast collection lateral to the first part of the duodenum representing barium within the gallbladder. Fistulas occur less commonly between the common bile duct and duodenum, gallbladder and colon. The ectopic gallstone most often causes obstruction at the terminal ileum (60–70%), followed by the proximal ileum, distal ileum, pylorus, sigmoid and duodenum.

Dähnert (2007), 832.

71) c. ****

The transition from squamous oesophageal epithelium to columnar gastric epithelium is marked by the Z-line, an irregular zigzag line. It is not a reliable indicator of the gastro-oesophageal junction, however, and may lie some distance above it if there is columnar transformation of the distal oesophagus, as seen in Barrett's oesophagus. The gastro-oesophageal junction may be identified by a thin, shelf-like ring known as the B-ring. It is visible on barium swallow only when the gastro-oesophageal junction lies above the diaphragmatic hiatus. Approximately 2–4 cm above this is a thicker ring produced by active muscle contraction known as the A-ring. The oesophageal vestibule is the saccular termination of the lower oesophagus, which lies between the A-ring and the B-ring, and corresponds with the lower oesophageal sphincter.

Sutton (2002), 554–5.

72) c. ****

The normal portal vein measures up to 13 mm in diameter when measured in the AP direction where the portal vein crosses the inferior vena cava during quiet respiration in a supine patient. Portal venous flow is normally 12–30 cm/s and demonstrates respiratory variation but little or no pulsatility, though this may be seen in thin patients. Normal flow is hepatopetal (anterograde flow into the liver). Portal hypertension is defined as an increase in portal venous pressure above 10 mmHg, and is most commonly caused by cirrhosis in the western world. As portal pressure increases, portal vein diameter increases, and portal flow loses its respiratory fluctuation and becomes slow and turbulent. Reversed (hepatofugal) flow may occur in 8% of patients and is generally associated with a reduced portal vein diameter. Other findings include portosystemic collaterals, splenomegaly and ascites. In portal vein thrombosis, portal vein diameter increases, but no flow is seen on

Doppler ultrasound scan. Echogenic thrombus may be seen within the lumen. Cavernous transformation of the portal vein may occur with chronic portal vein thrombosis, representing a conglomerate of collateral veins. Budd–Chiari syndrome affects the hepatic veins.

Middleton et al (2004), 71–8.

73) a. ***

In angiodysplasia, there is degenerative dilatation of the normal vessels in the submucosa of the bowel wall. It is associated with increasing age, and in about 20% of cases with aortic stenosis. It occurs most commonly in the right colon and presents with intermittent, low-grade bleeding. Barium enema shows no abnormality, as the lesion is submucosal, but increased tracer accumulation may be seen at the site of haemorrhage on ^{99m}Tc-labelled red cell scanning. Angiography, if performed, may demonstrate a cluster of vessels along the antimesenteric border during the arterial phase and early opacification of the draining ileocolic vein.

Dähnert (2007), 802.

74) d. **

The colon is the commonest site for gastrointestinal lipomas. They typically appear as a broad-based mass, but may develop a short pedicle as a result of repeated peristaltic activity. They are soft lesions, and a change in shape or size may be noted on compression. At CT colonography, endoluminal features are non-specific, but the demonstration of fat attenuation on 2D images is diagnostic. Primary pneumatosis coli usually appears as a cluster of air-filled cysts in the left colon. These may mimic polyps at endoscopy or on endoluminal CT colonography, but the demonstration of air attenuation on 2D images is again diagnostic. Endometriosis and enteric duplication cyst are causes of submucosal lesions but are of soft-tissue and fluid density respectively. Adenomatous polyps are mucosal lesions of soft-tissue density.

Dähnert (2007), 850.

75) b. *****

Ménétrièr's disease is characterized by mucosal hypertrophy of the fundus and body of the stomach, with excessive mucus secretion and a protein-losing enteropathy. There may be associated gastric ulceration. Barium meal shows impaired mucosal coating due to hypersecretion and marked gastric fold thickening, though the stomach distends normally. The stomach is the commonest site for gastrointestinal lymphoma, which may be polypoid, ulcerating or infiltrative. The infiltrative form may cause pronounced thickening of gastric folds, with preserved stomach distensibility, but hypersecretion is not a feature. Infiltrating gastric carcinoma may also cause thickened gastric folds, but associated desmoplastic reaction results in a rigid, poorly distensible stomach. Zollinger–Ellison syndrome results in hypersecretion of gastric acid, which impairs mucosal coating of barium, and is associated with ulceration and enlargement of rugal folds, but hypoproteinaemia is not a feature. Eosinophilic gastroenteritis may cause enlarged gastric folds and be associated with protein-losing enteropathy if the small bowel is involved. However, the antrum is most commonly involved.

Sutton (2002), 580.

76) d. ***
The stomach is divided into the fundus, body, antrum and pylorus. The fundus is that part of the stomach extending superiorly and to the left of the cardiac orifice. The body extends from the cardiac orifice to the incisura angularis, which is a constant notch at the lower end of the lesser curvature marking the border between the body and the antrum of the stomach. The antrum extends from the incisura angularis to the proximal pylorus.

Butler et al (1999), 211.

77) b. ***
Ultrasound scan of the pancreas may be difficult and vascular landmarks are important in its identification. In the transverse plane, the splenic vein can be seen coursing from the splenic hilum towards the liver, and the body and tail of the pancreas lie immediately anterior to this. The neck of the pancreas lies immediately anterior to the confluence of the splenic and superior mesenteric veins, and the head and uncinate process of the pancreas lie around this confluence, anterior to the inferior vena cava. At this level, the left renal vein can be seen entering the inferior vena cava, passing between the superior mesenteric artery and aorta.

Brant & Helms (2007), 941–2.

78) e. ****
The two main indications for Whipple's procedure (radical pancreaticoduodenectomy) are tumour in the periampullary region, and chronic pancreatitis involving the head and uncinate process of the pancreas. Surgery is complex and involves gastrojejunostomy, pancreaticoenterostomy and choledochojejunostomy. Common post-operative findings include retroperitoneal fat stranding and transient, thin-walled fluid collections, which may be in the pancreatic bed, perianastomotic or in Morison's pouch. Free gas is common and aerobilia is seen in around 70% of cases, more commonly in the left intrahepatic ducts. Filling of the afferent jejunal loop with contrast is normal and occurs in up to 44% of patients. The commonest complications are delayed gastric emptying, pancreaticojejunal leak and sepsis. Anastomotic failure can occur at any of the sites, but the pancreaticoenterostomy is most important because of the risk of leakage of pancreatic secretions. Anastomotic leak is associated with increased free gas, perianastomotic fluid and ascites. Focal septic

collections can occur anywhere, and complex or gas-containing areas are considered suspicious. Other early complications include vascular injury and thrombosis, *Clostridium difficile* colitis and pancreatitis of the pancreatic remnant.

Smith et al (2008).

79) a. ****
In the evaluation of haemoperitoneum by CT, attenuation values can help differentiate ascites, unclotted blood, active bleeding and haematoma. Blood usually has a higher measured attenuation than other body fluids, but its appearance depends on the age, extent and location of haemorrhage. Unclotted blood has an attenuation value of 30–45 HU, but this may be lower in patients with a lower serum haematocrit and if the haemorrhage is more than 48 hours old. Clotted blood has an attenuation value of 45–70 HU, and identification of the area of highest-attenuation haematoma (sentinel clot) on CT indicates the site of bleeding. Active arterial extravasation is seen as an area of higher attenuation resembling that in the aorta, ranging from 85 HU to 370 HU. It may be surrounded by lower-attenuation haematoma. This finding indicates the need for urgent embolization or surgical treatment.

Lubner et al (2007).

80) c. ****
MR is a highly accurate method of local staging of rectal cancer, with better assessment of locoregional nodal involvement than CT and clear depiction of the mesorectal fascia, allowing accurate prediction of whether the circumferential resection margin will be tumour free. T2W images provide optimal visualization of the tumour, which appears as an intermediate signal-intensity mass. Contrast-enhanced T1W images result in enhancement of the normal bowel wall as well as the tumour, which may lead to upstaging. FLAIR sequences are not routinely used for rectal cancer staging.

Hricak et al (2007), 30–1.

81) b. ****
Laparoscopic gastric banding involves laparoscopic placement of an inflatable gastric band across the proximal stomach, forming a small fundal neostomach or pouch. The band is connected to a subcutaneous port that can be accessed percutaneously to allow inflation or deflation of the band and adjustment of stomal width and degree of hold-up. The commonest postoperative complication is dilatation of the pouch. Three main types are described. (1) Acute concentric pouch dilatation is due to band overinflation, and is seen as a prestenotic dilatation proximal to an obstructed stoma. It presents as acute dysphagia and requires prompt decompression of the stoma. (2) Chronic concentric pouch dilatation with a widely patent stoma is seen in patients who continue to overfill their neostomach after surgery. Nutritional advice is

required. (3) Eccentric pouch dilatation occurs due to slippage of the band, and requires complete decompression and surgical replacement of the band. A plateau in weight loss may also be due to loss of effect of band tightening. At fluoroscopy, fluid may be injected to tighten the band to achieve an optimal stomal width of 3–4 mm.

Roy-Choudhury et al (2004).

82) c. ***
Villous adenomas are a histological subtype of adenomatous polyps with predominantly villous elements, representing 10% of adenomatous polyps. Typical appearances are of a broad-based lesion often over 2 cm in diameter, with frond-like surface projections. They have a higher malignant potential than the other subtypes of adenomatous polyp (tubular and tubulovillous adenomas), which increases further with the size of the adenoma. Lesions under 5 cm have a 9% risk of malignant transformation to adenocarcinoma, whereas lesions over 10 cm have a 100% risk. Villous adenomas are associated with excretion of large amounts of thick mucus, which may result in diarrhoea and electrolyte depletion, as well as poor mucosal coating at barium enema. Lipomas are typically seen as smooth, rounded, submucosal masses. Tubular adenomas are usually < 10 mm and, like lipomas, are not associated with electrolyte depletion. Solitary rectal ulcer syndrome may appear as polypoid lesions in the rectum and be associated with mucus secretion; however, it is normally associated with ulceration and is usually seen in young women.

Dähnert (2007), 874.

83) c. **
Tuberculosis of the gastrointestinal tract may occur through ingestion of infected sputum, or by haematogenous spread to submucosal lymph nodes from a pulmonary tuberculous focus. It most commonly affects the ileocaecal region due to its abundance of lymphoid tissue and relative stasis of gut contents. Typical features at this site include circumferential thickening of the terminal ileum and caecum, a thickened ileocaecal valve and ulceration following the orientation of lymphoid follicles (longitudinal in the terminal ileum and transverse in the colon). Marked enlargement of adjacent mesenteric lymph nodes with central areas of low attenuation may be seen.

Dähnert (2007), 871.

84) c. ***
Gastrointestinal complications following external radiotherapy are becoming more frequent as survival rates of patients with abdominal cancer improve, and they may present up to 15 years following irradiation. The colon and rectum are commonly affected following irradiation for pelvic and genitourinary tract malignancies. Chronic radiation colitis usually presents with strictures, whereas rectal injury

manifests as a narrowed, thickened, poorly distensible rectum, with proliferation of the perirectal fat and thickening of the perirectal fascia. There is an increased incidence of colorectal carcinoma following pelvic irradiation, but a short irregular segment of narrowing would be more likely. Inflammatory bowel disease may result in circumferential rectal wall thickening with widening of the presacral space but is less likely given this history. Hirschsprung's disease usually presents in early childhood. The rectum is an uncommon site for gastrointestinal lymphoma.

Boudiaf et al (2000).

85) b. ***

Modern water-soluble, iodinated, intravenous contrast media are based on the six-carbon ring structure tri-iodobenzoic acid. Earlier contrast agents were ionic and high-osmolar, but the toxicity of these agents prompted further development. In order to decrease osmolality while maintaining an acceptable iodine concentration, the ratio between the number of iodine atoms and the number of particles in solution has been decreased either by combining two tri-iodinated benzene rings or by producing compounds that do not ionize in solution, or, more recently, by both methods. The most recent agents such as iodixanol (Visipaque) and iotrolan (Isovist) are non-ionic dimers with six iodine atoms per molecule in solution, enabling satisfactory iodine concentrations to be obtained at iso-osmolality.

Chapman & Nakielny (2001), 27–30.

86) d. **

Kaposi's sarcoma is a low-grade tumour of the blood and lymphatic vessels that primarily affects the skin but may cause disseminated disease in other organs. It is an AIDS-defining illness and is the most common AIDS-related neoplasm. The commonest manifestation is of multiple raised purplish skin lesions, but lymphadenopathy is the second commonest feature in AIDS-related Kaposi's sarcoma. Typical appearances are of abdominopelvic lymph nodes that enhance after intravenous contrast due to high vascularity, appearing to be of higher attenuation than skeletal muscle. Liver involvement occurs in 34% of cases at autopsy, and typically causes multiple 5–12mm nodules that are hyperechoic on ultrasound scan and of low attenuation on CT. Skin lesions are present in most cases, and help to distinguish Kaposi's sarcoma from other conditions such as fungal microabscesses and multiple haemangiomas, which may have similar appearances on CT. Mycobacterial disease is characteristically associated with low-attenuation lymphadenopathy. Non-Hodgkin's lymphoma is the second commonest AIDS-related neoplasm, and may cause multiple low-attenuation liver lesions, but it is not associated with skin lesions or high-attenuation lymphadenopathy.

Restrepo et al (2006).

87) a. ****
Radiolabelled white cell imaging is used for detection of infection and inflammation. Images reflect the distribution of white blood cells within the body, and also localize areas of infection or inflammation. Imaging is usually performed at 18–24 hours, by which time blood pool activity is normally no longer present, and the most intense uptake is seen in the spleen, followed by the liver and then the bone marrow. Imaging is also usually performed at 2–6 hours for investigation of suspected inflammatory bowel disease, as sloughed inflamed cells may move distally and provide misleading information as to the affected site if only imaged at 24 hours. Physiological diffuse lung uptake may be seen in the first 4 hours due to cellular activation from in vitro cell manipulation, but normally decreases after this. Thymus activity may be seen normally in children. Bowel and genitourinary activity are not normally seen, and gastrointestinal activity is always abnormal. In general, focal activity outside the normal white cell distribution, which is greater than that of the spleen, suggests the presence of an abscess. Activity equal to that of the liver indicates a significant inflammatory focus. Activity less than that of the bone marrow suggests a low-level inflammatory response.

Zeissman et al (2006), 389–94; Dähnert (2007), 1082–3.

88) a. ****
The WHO response criteria were devised in 1981 to standardize the criteria used for measuring therapeutic response in cancer patients. These criteria set out definitions of complete response, partial response, no change and progressive disease, based upon bidimensional measurements of tumour lesions in the axial plane. The product of the longest diameter multiplied by the greatest perpendicular diameter is calculated for each measurable lesion, and the sum of these products is used to determine treatment response. The RECIST criteria were introduced in 2000, and were designed to be used in clinical trials. The criteria involve classifying the disease burden into measurable and non-measurable disease, followed by selection of up to 10 representative target lesions. The sum of the long axis dimension of the target lesions in the axial plane is used to determine the final response category. Potential concerns about the use of the RECIST criteria include possible confusion arising when lymph node measurements are performed using the short axis dimension and the increased workload involved for the radiologist.

Royal College of Radiologists (2006), 11–13.

89) d. ****

T3 tumours penetrate the subserosa but do not invade adjacent structures. On CT, this may be appreciated as blurring of the tumour margin or wide reticular strands radiating from the tumour edge. Nodal staging depends on the number of regional nodes visible, with nodes larger than 8 mm being regarded as pathological. The presence of 1–6 regional nodes results in a stage of N1, with 7–15 nodes and >15 nodes representing nodal stages of N2 and N3 respectively. Non-regional nodes such as para-aortic and retropancreatic nodes are considered M1 disease.

Hricak et al (2007), 23–8.

90) c. **

The splenic and superior mesenteric veins join to form the main portal vein slightly to the right of the midline behind the neck of the pancreas at L1–2 level. The extrahepatic portal vein is about 8 cm long, and divides into the right and left portal veins at the porta hepatis. The inferior mesenteric vein most commonly drains into the splenic vein, but may drain into the splenic/superior mesenteric vein confluence in 30% of cases or the superior mesenteric vein in 30%.

Butler et al (1999), 234–5.

91) b. ***

Chemotherapeutic agents are commonly associated with fatty liver. Diffuse fat deposition (the commonest pattern) causes a generalized decrease in the attenuation value of the liver on CT, and may be diagnosed with an absolute liver attenuation value of less than 40 HU on contrast-enhanced CT. It may also be diagnosed at unenhanced CT if the liver attenuation value is at least 10 HU less than that of the spleen. Liver metastases usually present as focal, low-attenuation lesions on portal phase imaging. Hepatic venous congestion causes a diffuse decrease in attenuation but is associated with enlargement of the inferior vena cava and hepatic veins due to elevated central venous pressure. Amyloidosis can cause a generalized decrease in liver attenuation, but more commonly appears as discrete areas of low attenuation with reduced contrast enhancement. Budd–Chiari syndrome may also result in a diffuse decrease in liver attenuation, but there is usually patchy liver enhancement and poor visualization of the hepatic veins.

Eisenberg (2003), 538–41; Hamer et al (2006).

92) e. **

The prone-angled, overcouch view performed as described separates overlying loops of sigmoid colon.

Chapman & Nakielny (2001), 71.

93) a. ****
Percutaneous or endoscopic biliary stenting is usually performed to relieve jaundice in patients with malignant biliary obstruction. Metallic or plastic stents may be used. Metallic stents have a larger internal diameter and have higher long-term patency rates than plastic stents, as well as a low surface area that reduces bacterial colonization and subsequent fibrous deposition. However, metallic stents become incorporated into the bile duct mucosa and are not easily removed, which may present particular problems if the stent becomes infected. They are also prone to shortening following deployment, and a long-segment obstruction may therefore require multiple stents. In addition, the cost of metallic stents is approximately 10 times that of plastic stents.

Sutton (2002), 733–5.

94) c. ****
Endoscopic ultrasound is the most accurate method for local staging of oesophageal cancer. At endoscopic ultrasound, the oesophageal wall appears as five distinct alternating hyperechoic and hypoechoic bands that correspond to the histological layers of the oesophagus. The innermost hyperechoic layer represents the interface between the lumen and the mucosa. The hypoechoic second layer is a hypoechoic band that represents the muscularis mucosa. The third layer is a hyperechoic band that represents the submucosa. The fourth layer is a hypoechoic band that represents the muscularis propria. The fifth outermost layer is a hyperechoic band that represents the oesophageal adventitia. The fifth layer in the stomach, duodenum and rectum represents the serosa. For oesophageal cancer, T1 tumours invade the lamina propria or submucosa. T2 tumours invade the muscularis propria, T3 tumours invade the adventitia and T4 tumours invade adjacent tissue. Tis represents carcinoma *in situ*.

Wojtowycz et al (1995).

95) d. **
For a standard, single-slice, spiral CT of the abdomen and pelvis in a single breathhold, 100–150 ml of 300 mg/ml iodine intravenous contrast medium should be administered at 3–4 ml/s. For a portal phase examination, image acquisition should begin 65–70 s after commencement of the injection.

Royal College of Radiologists (2006), 14–16.

96) b. *****
The most common complication of administration of superparamagnetic iron oxide particles is acute severe back pain, which is seen in approximately 4% of patients. This is thought to be a side effect of particulate agents in general, and lasts for the duration of the infusion and slightly beyond. The risk is higher in patients with liver dysfunction, and when the infusion is administered more rapidly than over the

recommended 30 minutes. Slowing of the infusion rate or termination of the infusion with recommencement after resolution of the back pain is usually sufficient to alleviate the symptoms.

Semelka & Helmberger (2001).

97) b. ***
Impaired cricopharyngeus relaxation (or cricopharyngeal achalasia) is hypertrophy of the cricopharyngeus muscle with failure of relaxation. It is seen in up to 10% of asymptomatic adults as a normal variant, as a compensatory mechanism in gastro-oesophageal reflux, and in association with a range of neuromuscular disorders. It appears on barium swallow as a smooth, shelf-like posterior projection at the level of C5–6 that persists during a swallow. In severe cases, it may result in functional obstruction or overflow aspiration. Symptomatic patients may be treated by cricopharyngeal myotomy. Pharyngeal webs are thin, anterior, shelf-like protrusions into the cervical oesophagus. They are frequent incidental findings but occasionally cause dysphagia. There is an association with Plummer–Vinson syndrome. Anterior osteophytes may cause an indentation of the posterior oesophagus, but these are usually asymptomatic. Thyroid enlargement may cause a smooth impression on the lateral wall of the oesophagus.

Eisenberg (2003), 302–3.

98) d. ****
Caroli's disease is a rare congenital disorder characterized by multifocal segmental saccular dilatation of the intrahepatic bile ducts. It presents in childhood and early adulthood with upper abdominal pain, fever and transient jaundice. Up to 80% of patients have associated medullary sponge kidney. Typical CT findings are of multiple cystic structures with a central enhancing 'dot', representing the portal vein radicles surrounded by dilated ducts. Cholangiography is diagnostic and demonstrates saccular dilatation of the intrahepatic ducts of up to 5 cm in diameter, with frequent associated ectasia of the extrahepatic ducts. Choledochal cysts primarily cause cystic dilatation of the common bile duct, but there may be associated intrahepatic biliary dilatation. A choledochocele is a cystic dilatation of the intraduodenal portion of the common bile duct. Primary sclerosing cholangitis classically causes multifocal strictures of the intrahepatic and extrahepatic ducts, alternating with segments of dilatation. In polycystic liver disease, there is no communication of the cysts with the biliary tree.

Eisenberg (2003), 450–1.

99) a. ****
Gastrointestinal stromal tumours are the commonest mesenchymal tumours of the gastrointestinal tract. They are characterized by expression of KIT, a tyrosine kinase growth factor receptor, which distinguishes them from leiomyomas and leiomyosarcomas. They occur

most commonly in the stomach, and have the classic appearance of a submucosal mass on barium meal, forming an obtuse angle with the gastric wall in profile. Focal areas of ulceration are seen in 60%. On CT, the tumours measure up to 30 cm and are often predominantly extragastric. Typical features are of peripheral enhancement, with central low attenuation representing necrosis, haemorrhage and cyst formation. Lymphadenopathy is not a feature. Gastric carcinoma and lymphoma rarely demonstrate exophytic growth and commonly have associated lymphadenopathy. Adenomatous polyps are mucosal lesions. Gastric carcinoid is usually seen in the antrum and characteristically shows associated ulceration.

Levy et al (2003).

100) a. ***
The main arterial supply to the pancreas is from the splenic artery, which provides numerous small branches into the pancreatic substance as it runs along the superior pancreatic border, as well as several larger arteries including the dorsal pancreatic artery from its proximal end (which may alternatively arise from the coeliac artery) and the arteria pancreatica magna halfway along its length. The pancreatic head has a dual blood supply, from the superior pancreaticoduodenal artery (derived from the gastroduodenal artery) and the inferior pancreaticoduodenal artery (derived from the superior mesenteric artery). The transverse pancreatic artery also runs along the length of the pancreas beside the main duct, and there are multiple anastomoses between the various vessels, allowing multidirectional flow.

Butler et al (1999), 255–6.

MODULE 4
GENITOURINARY, ADRENAL, OBSTETRICS & GYNAECOLOGY, AND BREAST

Module 4: Genitourinary, Adrenal, Obstetrics & Gynaecology, and Breast: Questions

1) A patient who has no function in their native kidneys is found to have declining renal function 1 day after transplantation. A MAG3 renogram shows normal perfusion but diminished excretion. Which of the following processes is affecting the transplanted kidney?

   a. acute rejection
   b. chronic rejection
   c. acute tubular necrosis
   d. renal vein thrombosis
   e. ciclosporin toxicity

2) A portal venous-phase CT of the abdomen and pelvis is performed in a 60-year-old man to investigate upper abdominal and back pain, which is attributed to features of pancreatitis on the scan. An incidental finding is of a rounded, renal lesion of diameter 3 cm, with average attenuation value of 80 HU and containing no significant component with a negative attenuation value on pixel densitometry. There are no previous images for comparison. What is the most likely diagnosis of the renal lesion?

   a. angiomyolipoma
   b. renal cell carcinoma
   c. simple cyst
   d. high-density cyst
   e. infected cyst

3) A 30-year-old woman has a well-circumscribed, cystic, adnexal mass with areas of dense focal calcification, small enhancing soft-tissue elements, fluid–fluid levels and bright regions on T1W MRI that become dark on fat-saturated sequences. Which of the following pathologies is most likely?

   a. ovarian cyst with proteinaceous contents
   b. endometrioma
   c. mature cystic teratoma of the ovary
   d. ovarian cyst adenofibroma
   e. ovarian adenocarcinoma

4) A 55-year-old male has an ultrasound scan of the renal tract prompted by a single urinary tract infection. A kidney cyst of diameter 2 cm with a thin septum is seen. The septum has perceptible enhancement on CT. What is the most appropriate management from the choices below?

a. discharge with no follow-up
b. imaging follow-up
c. partial nephrectomy
d. nephrectomy
e. nephroureterectomy

5) A 78-year-old man presents with a palpable, non-tender, left breast lump. Mammography demonstrates a well-defined, high-density, lobulated mass in the retroareolar region. Ultrasound appearances are of a hypoechoic mass with an eccentric position relative to the nipple. The ipsilateral axilla appears unremarkable. What is the most likely diagnosis?

a. invasive ductal carcinoma
b. lipoma
c. breast abscess
d. gynaecomastia
e. lymphoma

6) At the 20-week fetal anomaly ultrasound scan, the cervix of a 25-year-old primagravida is measured to be 22 mm long. She is most likely to have been treated with which of the following?

a. oestrogens
b. progestogens
c. heparin
d. salbutamol
e. corticosteroids

7) A 40-year-old man has a testicular ultrasound scan, which demonstrates a multilobular mass that is homogeneous and hypoechoic with Doppler flow seen in internal hypoechoic bands. Which of the following is the most likely diagnosis?

a. teratoma
b. lymphoma
c. metastasis
d. seminoma
e. focal infarction

8) A general practitioner performs a vaginal examination prior to intended removal of an intrauterine contraceptive device. The locator device cannot be seen or palpated. What is the most appropriate initial investigation for this patient?

a. abdominal radiograph
b. pelvic ultrasound scan
c. pelvic CT
d. pelvic MRI
e. hysteroscopy

9) CT scan of the chest, abdomen and pelvis is performed to stage a renal cell carcinoma. The tumour arises in, and is confined to, the upper pole of the left kidney with a maximum dimension of 5 cm. There is tumour thrombus in the left renal vein, inferior vena cava and right atrium. There are no enlarged lymph nodes and no metastases seen. According to the TNM classification what is the stage of the tumour?

a. T4 N0 M0
b. T2 N0 M0
c. T3a N0 M0
d. T3c N0 Mx
e. T3c N0 M0

10) A 30-year-old female has continued ipsilateral loin pain following surgery for pelviureteric junction obstruction. Ultrasound scan shows the renal pelvis to be less dilated than prior to surgery. MAG3 renogram is inconclusive with regard to the question of ongoing obstruction, and a Whitaker test is performed. The maximum pressure difference between the collecting system (antegrade) needle and the urinary catheter is found to be 10 cmH$_2$O. What should the patient be advised regarding the findings of the Whitaker test?

a. this invasive test is also inconclusive
b. there is no evidence of pelviureteric junction or ureteric obstruction
c. there is ongoing pelviureteric junction obstruction
d. there is a second previously occult level of obstruction
e. the original diagnosis of pelviureteric junction obstruction is in doubt

11) A 30-year-old woman attends for a first-trimester ultrasound scan. Her last menstrual period was approximately 10 weeks prior to the scan, but she is unsure of the exact dates. What is the most accurate ultrasound measurement for dating the pregnancy at this stage?

a. biparietal diameter
b. mean gestational sac diameter
c. crown–rump length
d. femur length
e. abdominal circumference

12) A 40-year-old woman with a history of prior pelvic radiotherapy for cervical cancer has an ultrasound scan for cyclical pelvic pain. The endometrium is distended by predominantly echo-poor material, and both ovaries have moderately large cysts containing low-level echoes. On MRI, the cervix returns low T2 signal and the ovarian cysts return high signal on fat-suppressed T1W sequences. Which of the following is the most likely diagnosis?

a. recurrent cervical tumour with bilateral ovarian metastases
b. recurrent cervical tumour and synchronous bilateral ovarian teratomas
c. cervical stenosis and bilateral endometriomas
d. cervical stenosis and bilateral ovarian cystadenocarcinomas
e. new primary endometrial carcinoma with bilateral ovarian secondaries

13) A postmenopausal patient has a hysterectomy and bilateral salpingo-oophorectomy for bilateral ovarian masses. Histological examination confirms bilateral ovarian tumours and reveals concomitant endometrial adenocarcinoma. What is the most likely histological diagnosis of the ovarian lesions?

a. benign serous cystadenoma
b. benign mucinous cystadenoma
c. malignant serous cystadenocarcinoma
d. malignant mucinous cystadenocarcinoma
e. endometrioid tumour

14) A 60-year-old male, treated long term for hypertension with hydralazine, develops bilateral hydronephrosis. On CT KUB, the ureters are deviated medially and obstructed by a large, plaque-like, para-aortic, soft-tissue density. The aorta appears 'taped-down' to the vertebral column rather than elevated by the para-aortic tissue. Which of the following is the most likely diagnosis?

a. enlarged retroperitoneal lymph nodes due to Hodgkin's disease
b. enlarged retroperitoneal lymph nodes due to non-Hodgkin's lymphoma
c. retroperitoneal fibrosis
d. bilateral ureteral transitional cell carcinoma
e. metastatic lymph node enlargement from testicular embryonal cell carcinoma

15) An 80-year-old male has an IVU for unilateral loin pain. On the control film, the renal outline on the side of the pain is indistinct and enlarged. The same kidney has a staghorn calculus and shows no evidence of function following contrast injection. Which of the following is the most likely diagnosis?

a. xanthogranulomatous pyelonephritis
b. renal tuberculosis
c. hyperparathyroidism
d. hydatid cyst
e. carcinoma

16) On CT performed for staging purposes, a primary bladder tumour involves bladder muscle without perivesical extension. Malignant enlarged lymph nodes of 4 cm greatest dimension in the ipsilateral internal iliac and 1.5 cm greatest dimension in the common iliac lymph node groups are present. Which of the following is the most accurate TNM stage?

a. TI NI M0
b. T2 NI M0
c. T2 N2 M0
d. T2 NI MI
e. T3 NI M0

17) A 30-year-old male is investigated by renal tract ultrasound scan for renal impairment. Both kidneys are smooth in outline but enlarged. Which of the following diagnoses typically produces this pattern of renal enlargement?

a. autosomal dominant polycystic kidney disease
b. von Hippel–Lindau disease
c. sickle cell disease
d. metastases
e. nephroblastomatosis

18) A 55-year-old, hepatitis B-positive male under investigation for painless haematuria is admitted as an emergency with unilateral loin pain and hypotension. A renal arteriogram shows multiple, bilateral, small, renal artery branch aneurysms. Which of the following antibody titres is most likely to be positive?

a. anti-double-stranded DNA
b. anti-basement membrane
c. anti-Ro
d. anti-immunoglobulin G
e. perinuclear anti-neutrophil cytoplasmic

19) A 20-year-old man has radical orchidectomy for a non-seminomatous germ cell tumour. A CT of the thorax, abdomen and pelvis shortly after surgery shows no lymphadenopathy or metastasis. Which of the following is the most appropriate follow-up regimen?

a. repeat CT of the chest, abdomen and pelvis only in response to symptoms suggesting recurrence
b. repeat CT of the chest, abdomen and pelvis only when serum tumour markers rise
c. serial serum tumour marker measurement with yearly CT of the chest, abdomen and pelvis
d. serial serum tumour marker measurement with 3-monthly CT of the chest, abdomen and pelvis for 1 year followed by 6-monthly CT of the chest, abdomen and pelvis for 1 year
e. 3-monthly whole-body PET/CT

20) On ultrasound scan, a 30-year-old man is found to have bilateral testicular microlithiasis and unilateral testicular atrophy. There is a history of orchidopexy of the atrophic testicle. Which of the following is the most appropriate management?

a. discharge
b. self-examination only
c. follow-up clinical examination and surveillance sonography
d. further investigation with MRI
e. testicular biopsy

21) A patient is found to have a renal pelvis transitional cell carcinoma. The cancer invades adjacent renal parenchyma and extends into perinephric fat. No significantly enlarged lymph nodes and no metastases are seen on CT of the chest, abdomen and pelvis. Which of the following is the overall stage for this patient's disease?

a. I
b. II
c. III
d. IV
e. V

22) A 50-year-old man complains to his general practitioner of painful sexual intercourse. An ultrasound examination of the penis is performed, which identifies dense, shadow-casting abnormalities of the periphery of both corpora cavernosa. What is the likely diagnosis?

a. priapism
b. Zoon's balanitis
c. penile squamous cell carcinoma
d. Peyronie's disease
e. balanitis xerotica obliterans

23) A 16-year-old male with a history of recurrent sudden severe testicular pain at night has a surgical scrotal exploration, which establishes that one testicle has a high insertion of the tunica vaginalis on the spermatic cord. What proportion of patients with this condition will have bilateral disease?

a. none
b. 10%
c. 25%
d. 65%
e. all

24) On an axial MRI of the penis, three tubular masses of tissue, occupying much of the cross-sectional area of the penis, are entirely surrounded by a T1- and T2-hypointense layer. Breach of this layer upstages a penile cancer from T1 to T2. From the following choices, name this structure or structures.

a. corpora cavernosa
b. corpora spongiosa
c. cavernosal arteries
d. urethra
e. tunica albuginea

25) A 65-year-old female with biopsy-proven ovarian cancer has a staging CT scan. It reveals a left basal pleural effusion that after aspiration contains no malignant cytology. There is a large, complex, abdominopelvic mass, with ascites and peritoneal deposits outside the pelvis measuring over 2 cm in diameter. Pelvic and para-aortic lymph nodes are enlarged. There are liver surface and parenchymal deposits. Which of the described features results in a classification of stage IV disease?

a. ascites
b. pleural effusion
c. liver surface deposits
d. liver parenchymal deposits
e. 2 cm deposits outside the pelvis

26) A 35-year-old female has investigations for episodic right loin pain. Ultrasound scan of the renal tract is unremarkable. A DMSA scan is performed with the patient sitting, and shows only 30% contribution to the total tracer activity from the right kidney. When the counts are repeated supine, the contribution from the right kidney is 50%. What is the most likely abnormality of the right kidney?

a. nutcracker kidney
b. nephroptosis
c. pelviureteric junction obstruction
d. ureteric calculus
e. vesicoureteric reflux

27) An 80-year-old male with a history of nephrectomy for renal cell carcinoma is found at follow-up to have a heterogeneously enhancing 25 mm lesion confined to his remaining kidney. No enlarged nodes or metastases are present. The lesion is biopsied and found to be an adenocarcinoma. The patient decides upon radiofrequency ablation as treatment. A CT scan 1 month after the ablation quantifies the average post-contrast enhancement of the tumour as 8 HU. Which of the following best represents the degree of success of the radiofrequency ablation?

   a. failed
   b. residual enhancing tumour requiring repeat ablation
   c. residual enhancing tumour but no value in repeat ablation
   d. successful
   e. indeterminate

28) An imaging request is received with the clinical information, 'biopsy-proven adenocarcinoma of the cervix, for local staging'. Which of the following is the most appropriate technique?

   a. transvaginal ultrasound scan
   b. endoanal ultrasound scan
   c. CT abdomen and pelvis with intravenous and oral contrast
   d. MRI with pelvic phased-array coil
   e. ^{18}FDG PET

29) Endoanal ultrasound scan is performed on a 20-week pregnant patient who sustained perineal damage during a previous vaginal delivery, to guide the method of delivery. Scarring is seen involving more than 50% of the external sphincter, but the internal anal sphincter is intact. Which of the following best represents the degree of perineal injury?

   a. first
   b. second
   c. third (3a)
   d. third (3b)
   e. third (3c)

30) A 65-year-old male being investigated for microscopic haematuria has an ultrasound scan, which suggests a 20 mm tumour in the cortex of the interpolar region of the left kidney. CT scan confirms an enhancing mass in the same location. On DMSA SPECT, this abnormality has good uptake. Which of the following is the most appropriate management?

   a. no further action
   b. biopsy
   c. nephrectomy
   d. image-guided drainage
   e. chemotherapy

31) A 50-year-old man has surgery to remove a tumour confined to the adrenal gland. Histology reveals a phaeochromocytoma. Subsequently, he develops hypertension and urinary vanillylmandelic acid is found to be elevated. An MIBG scan is performed. Activity in which of the following organs is most likely to be a metastasis?

   a. lung
   b. bladder
   c. thyroid
   d. colon
   e. spleen

32) A 23-year-old nulliparous woman is examined for dyspareunia. Biopsy confirms a clinically small but malignant-looking cervical lesion to be adenosquamous carcinoma. In such cases, local imaging staging must indicate which of the following?

   a. tumour size and distance from the internal os plus the cervix length
   b. tumour size and distance from the external os plus the uterine length
   c. tumour size and distance from the vaginal introitus plus length of the vagina
   d. tumour size and vascularity
   e. ovarian position

33) A patient has a squamous cell carcinoma of the vulva. An MRI is performed for locoregional staging. There are significantly enlarged inguinal lymph nodes ipsilateral to the primary tumour, but none contralaterally. A short axis, ipsilateral, 1.2 cm external iliac node is also identified that has signal characteristics identical to the primary tumour throughout. Which of the following is the most accurate nodal staging?

   a. Nx
   b. N0
   c. N1
   d. N2
   e. N3

34) A 35-year-old male with autosomal dominant polycystic kidney disease has been shown on CT to have, among the innumerable renal cysts, several high-density cysts. Which of the following MRI sequences would be most useful in detecting a renal cell carcinoma among haemorrhagic or proteinaceous cysts?

   a. T1W
   b. T2W
   c. T1W post-gadolinium
   d. T1W fat-suppressed post-gadolinium
   e. T1W post-gadolinium with pre-contrast T1W signal subtracted

35) A patient with endometrial cancer previously treated with surgery has an ^{18}FDG PET scan to look for recurrence. A false-negative result could be caused by which of the following scenarios?

a. peritoneal deposits smaller than 1 cm
b. bladder diverticulum
c. post-surgical inflammation
d. abscess
e. bowel avidity

36) A 70-year-old man with biopsy-proven prostate carcinoma has an MRI of the prostate to assess suitability for radical prostatectomy. There is bilateral, multifocal, peripheral-zone, low-signal change on small FOV T2W images in locations corresponding on more than one scan plane. These changes are confined within the prostatic capsule. However, enlarged lymph nodes are seen in the left internal and common iliac groups. No other disease is seen, including on a CT of the abdomen and pelvis and a radioisotope bone scan. What is the TNM stage of this patient's cancer?

a. T2b N1 M0
b. T2c N1 M0
c. T2c N1 M1
d. T3 N1 M0
e. T3 N1 M1

37) A man is found to have a single adrenal mass of diameter 35 mm. On an unenhanced CT scan, the average attenuation value is 30 HU. On a CT timed at 60 seconds after iodinated contrast medium injection, the attenuation value of the mass is 90 HU. By 15 minutes after contrast, the attenuation value is 50 HU. Which of the following is the most likely diagnosis?

a. lipid-rich adenoma
b. lipid-poor adenoma
c. metastasis
d. adrenal cortical cancer
e. adrenal haemorrhage

38) An adult male patient who has been taking over-the-counter analgesics regularly for years has an IVU for ureteric colic. No radio-opaque calculi are seen on the control film. With contrast in the renal calyces, they are noted to be club shaped on the side of the pain. On the same image, there is a triangular filling defect in the renal pelvis. The colic is most likely to be caused by which of the following?

a. radio-opaque stone
b. radiolucent stone
c. sloughed papilla
d. blood clot
e. transitional cell carcinoma

39) A 55-year-old man has biopsy-proven penis cancer. An MRI is performed. Which of the following is the best reason for performing this examination?

a. to confirm the diagnosis
b. to refute the diagnosis
c. to perform local staging
d. to assess metastatic spread
e. to assess regional lymph node involvement

40) A 38-year-old man presents with a classic history of ureteric colic. Plain abdominal film is unremarkable, and CT KUB shows ureteric dilatation and periureteric stranding down to the vesicoureteric junction on the side of the pain. No radio-opaque calculi are seen on the CT scan. Ultrasound examination shows a tiny, densely echogenic focus within the bladder wall, at the same vesicoureteric junction. For which of the following conditions is the patient most likely to be receiving treatment?

a. diabetes mellitus
b. asthma
c. HIV
d. gastro-oesophageal reflux
e. headaches

41) A patient with a lower ureteric transitional cell carcinoma has an MRI for locoregional staging purposes and a CT of the abdomen and pelvis for lymph node involvement and metastases. An 8 mm short axis node is recorded. In which of the following abdominopelvic groups would this be significant by size criteria?

a. inguinal
b. common iliac
c. external iliac
d. internal iliac
e. retroperitoneal

42) A 23-year-old woman is found on a 10-week dating ultrasound scan to have a twin pregnancy. A repeat examination prompted by blood spotting per vaginum, later attributed to a cervical erosion, shows a singleton pregnancy and no evidence of the twin. What should this be termed?

a. foetus papyraceus
b. vanishing twin
c. fetal death *in utero*
d. immune fetal hydrops
e. non-immune fetal hydrops

43) A 45-year-old female has imaging to stage a cervical carcinoma. The primary tumour is 5 cm in longest dimension, is seen to involve the uterine corpus, and has small-volume parametrial spread that does not reach the pelvic side wall. Parametrial lymph nodes are significantly enlarged. There is no hydronephrosis. Vaginal involvement is also seen, with the caudal extent of the tumour being below the level of the urethral orifice into the bladder base. Which of the described features causes the local stage to be T3a?

a. size over 4 cm
b. uterine corpus invasion
c. parametrial spread
d. vaginal invasion
e. parametrial nodal involvement

44) A 14-year-old boy slides off his saddle while cycling, injuring his testicles. On ultrasound scan, one testicle has a paratesticular complex cystic mass, loss of testicular outline and several avascular planes within the testicle. Which of the following is the most appropriate management?

a. discharge with analgesia
b. admission for analgesia
c. admission for elective surgery
d. admission for surgery the following day
e. immediate surgical intervention

45) A 50-year-old female with a breast carcinoma that clinically involves the skin is to be staged by CT. Other than those related to the primary tumour, there are no specific symptoms. Which of these CT protocols should be used?

a. post-contrast brain
b. non-contrast brain, neck, chest, abdomen and pelvis
c. non-contrast brain, neck and chest, post-contrast abdomen and pelvis
d. post-contrast brain, neck, chest, abdomen and pelvis
e. post-contrast neck, chest, abdomen and pelvis

46) A 35-year-old male is prompted to see his general practitioner by his wife, who has noticed blood in the man's semen. An ultrasound scan of the scrotum is performed. What is the most common appearance that would accompany this symptom?

a. normal appearances
b. enlarged spermatic cord, epididymis and testicle with decreased echogenicity
c. testicular enlargement showing a hypoechoic lesion with a fluid–fluid level
d. paratesticular 'bag of worms' appearance
e. scrotal skin thickening

47) A postmenopausal patient is investigated for ascites. Cytology from the ascites reveals cells in keeping with an epithelial ovarian malignancy. Which of the following is the most appropriate staging investigation?

a. CT of the abdomen and pelvis with oral and intravenous contrast
b. CT of the chest, abdomen and pelvis with oral and intravenous contrast
c. MRI of the pelvis
d. ^{18}FDG PET
e. PET/CT

48) A CT KUB is performed on a 55-year-old South African man with unilateral loin pain. This demonstrates moderate ipsilateral hydroureteronephrosis with a stricture in the distal ureter. There is also widespread bladder calcification and bilateral distal ureter calcification. The responsible organism is most likely to be which of the following?

a. *Escherichia coli*
b. *Schistosoma mansoni*
c. *Schistosoma haematobium*
d. *Schistosoma japonicum*
e. *Mycobacterium tuberculosis*

49) Into which of the following lymph node groups does lymph from the scrotum initially drain?

a. para-aortic at the L1–2 level
b. superficial inguinal
c. obturator
d. internal iliac
e. presacral

50) A 60-year-old male has an ultrasound scan of the renal tract for renal colic. There is an echo-free, thin-walled structure in the renal sinus with posterior acoustic enhancement and dilatation of the major calyces. A CT KUB (unenhanced) does not add to this appearance, but a 10-minute delayed, contrast-enhanced CT shows that the calyces are obstructed while the renal pelvis is not dilated but stretched over the non-enhancing sinus abnormality. What is the most likely diagnosis?

a. sinus lipomatosis
b. parapelvic cyst
c. pelviureteric junction obstruction
d. transitional call carcinoma
e. renal cell carcinoma

51) A 40-year-old man has a right-sided intratesticular mass of indeterminate ultrasound appearance. A CT scan of the chest, abdomen and pelvis reveals an enlarged, round, cystic, right paracaval lymph node just caudal to the right renal vein. Other enlarged cystic lymph nodes are demonstrated in the mediastinum. No enlarged suprarenal or retrocrural nodes are seen. Considering these findings, which tumour type is most likely to be found in the orchidectomy specimen?

a. epidermoid tumour
b. malignant teratoma
c. seminoma
d. metastatic lung squamous cell carcinoma
e. adenomatoid tumour

52) On the 20-week fetal anomaly scan, it is noticed that there is less than 1 mm of hypoechoic myometrium between placenta and echo-bright uterine serosa. An MRI is performed. On T2W images, the placenta is heterogeneous and bright, and causes junctional zone interruption and marked focal myometrial thinning. The serosa looks intact. These findings describe which of the following?

a. placenta accreta
b. placenta increta
c. placenta percreta
d. placenta praevia
e. placental abruption

53) An 80-year-old man undergoes cystoscopy for macroscopic haematuria. He is found to have a 6 cm bladder tumour, biopsy of which confirms small-cell bladder cancer. He is considered suitable for radical treatment. Which of the following is the most appropriate staging strategy?

a. whole-body PET/CT
b. MRI of the bladder
c. MRI of the bladder plus CT of the abdomen and pelvis with intravenous contrast
d. MRI of the bladder plus CT of the chest, abdomen and pelvis with intravenous contrast
e. MRI of the bladder plus CT of the brain, chest, abdomen and pelvis with intravenous contrast

54) During a 20-week fetal anomaly scan, it is noticed that the umbilical cord has only two vessels. Which of the following conditions is most frequently associated with this finding?

a. triploidy
b. Turner's syndrome
c. trisomy 18
d. trisomy 13
e. Down's syndrome

55) Lymphatic drainage from the lower third of the vagina is normally first to which of the following lymph node groups?

a. obturator
b. internal iliac
c. external iliac
d. inguinal
e. retroperitoneal

56) During the third trimester of pregnancy, a multiparous, 48-year-old woman who is a smoker experiences bleeding per vaginum. Ultrasound scan shows the edge of the placenta to cover the whole of the internal cervical os. It is decided that delivery will be by caesarean section, for which of the following reasons?

a. placental separation
b. low-lying placenta
c. marginal placenta praevia
d. complete placenta praevia
e. placental abruption

57) Cystoscopy is attempted on a 65-year-old female for persistent microscopic haematuria, but the scope cannot be advanced along the urethra. A biopsy is taken and MRI is performed. Axial T2W images show a mass of high signal intensity disrupting the normal, target-like, zonal anatomy of the urethra. Which of the following cell types is the most likely histology from the biopsy?

a. squamous cell
b. transitional cell
c. adenocarcinoma
d. clear cell
e. mastocyte

58) A 28-week pregnant patient known to have uterine fibroids reports abdominal pain for the preceding 4 weeks. On questioning she admits to small amounts of brown/red vaginal loss. Ultrasound scan shows a complex but predominantly hypoechoic collection between the uterine wall and placenta. Which of the following is the most likely explanation for the imaging findings?

a. acute placental abruption
b. placental abruption 1 week previously
c. placental abruption 4 weeks previously
d. placenta membranacea
e. ectopic pregnancy

59) A 25-year-old female undergoes ultrasound scan of the pelvis for low abdominal pain. A gas reflection is seen within the uterine cavity. Which of the following is the likely cause of the pain?

a. endometriosis
b. adenomyosis
c. endometritis
d. endometrial carcinoma
e. tubo-ovarian abscess

60) MRI is performed for locoregional staging of vaginal cancer. Which of the following descriptions is the most likely appearance on a T2W sequence, given a small primary tumour confined to the vagina?

a. central high signal within the vagina; focal homogeneous, low-signal mass not breaching the surrounding ring of intermediate-signal vaginal wall
b. central high signal within the vagina; focal homogeneous, high-signal mass not breaching the surrounding low-signal vaginal wall
c. central high signal within the vagina; focal homogeneous, intermediate-signal mass breaching the surrounding low-signal vaginal wall
d. central high signal within the vagina; focal homogeneous, intermediate-signal mass not breaching the surrounding low-signal vaginal wall
e. central intermediate signal; focal homogeneous, high-signal mass contained by low-signal vaginal wall

61) A 30-year-old, nulliparous woman with Stein–Leventhal syndrome is being treated for subfertility with clomiphene. She develops abdominal pain, distension, nausea and vomiting. Ultrasound examination of the abdomen reveals both ovaries to be larger than 7 cm in length and packed with large follicles, and also reveals an ovarian cyst 12 cm in diameter. Ascites and a pleural effusion are also seen. What is the most likely diagnosis?

a. endometriosis
b. ovarian cyst torsion
c. ovarian hyperstimulation syndrome
d. ovarian serous cystadenoma
e. corpus luteum of menstruation

62) A patient with a raised PSA has MRI of the prostate. There is diffuse, low-signal change throughout the peripheral zone on T2W images. At the right base, there is focal high signal on T1W images. At the left base there is restricted diffusion. In the right mid-gland, spectroscopic analysis reveals a choline plus creatine/citrate ratio of considerably less than 0.8. In the left mid-gland, there is a diminished contrast wash-in rate. At the apex, the relative peak enhancement is less than in other regions of the prostate. Which is the most likely site of focal prostate carcinoma?

a. left base
b. right base
c. left mid-gland
d. right mid-gland
e. apex

63) On transvaginal ultrasound scan, an ovary measures $5 \times 3 \times 2$ cm. Regarding the volume of this ovary, which of the following statements is most accurate?

a. it is large for pre- and postmenopausal ovaries
b. it is normal for pre- and postmenopausal ovaries
c. it is normal for a premenopausal ovary but large for a postmenopausal ovary
d. it is normal for a postmenopausal ovary but large for a premenopausal ovary
e. not enough information is given to assess the volume

64) Calcification is seen on a screening mammogram. Which of the following patterns is the most likely to be associated with a carcinoma?

a. tortuous tramline calcification
b. thick, linear, rod-like calcifications, some with a lucent centre
c. eggshell, curvilinear calcification
d. popcorn calcification
e. a cluster of 10 calcific particles, all less than 0.5 mm

65) A transvaginal ultrasound scan is performed on a premenopausal woman on day 21 of the menstrual cycle. Given that her endometrium is normal, which of the following measurements of endometrial thickness is most likely?

a. 2 mm
b. 2–4 mm
c. 4–8 mm
d. 7–14 mm
e. greater than 14 mm

66) In antenatal ultrasound scanning, which of the following is a major marker associated with trisomy 21?

a. echogenic bowel before 20 weeks
b. echogenic intracardiac focus
c. brachycephaly
d. small cerebellum
e. hydrothorax

67) In a twin pregnancy, entanglement of the umbilical cords is discovered. Which of the following best describes the genetic and anatomical relationship of the twins?

a. dizygotic; both intrauterine
b. monozygotic; dichorionic diamniotic
c. monozygotic; monochorionic diamniotic
d. monozygotic; monochorionic monoamniotic
e. dizygotic; one ectopic

68) Which of the following unusual benign breast tumours is most likely to be locally infiltrating, aggressive and proliferative, and consist of only well-differentiated fibroblasts?

a. neurofibroma
b. granular cell tumour
c. fibromatosis
d. lipoma
e. areolar leiomyoma

69) A 68-year-old female patient has a pelvic ultrasound scan for a palpable mass. Arising within the left ovary is a 15 cm cyst with an irregular thick wall, frond-like solid elements, multiple septations over 2 mm thick and a pulsatility index of 0.5. These sonographic appearances are most in keeping with which of the following ovarian cystic structures?

a. corpus luteum cyst
b. follicular cyst
c. polycystic ovaries
d. benign ovarian neoplasm
e. malignant ovarian neoplasm

70) A 17-year-old female with primary amenorrhoea is found on clinical examination to have a hypoplastic upper/middle vagina. MRI shows an absent uterus but normal tubes and ovaries. Which of the following is the most likely diagnosis?

a. uterus didelphys
b. unicornuate uterus
c. Mayer–Rokitansky–Küster–Hauser syndrome
d. uterine agenesis
e. septate uterus

71) A 60-year-old female who has declined intervention for a renal angiomyolipoma of diameter 6 cm presents with flank pain, hypotension and tachycardia. In this scenario, which of the following is most likely to account for the presentation?

a. torsion of the angiomyolipoma
b. haemorrhage from the angiomyolipoma
c. rupture of the angiomyolipoma
d. leak from the non-aneurysmal abdominal aorta
e. nephroptosis

72) A postmenopausal woman is found on MRI to have a multicystic adnexal mass that contains fluid–fluid levels and does not show any fat suppression. In addition, her uterus shows a widened junctional zone containing small bright foci on T2W images. For which of the following diseases is she most likely to be receiving oral treatment that can account for these findings?

a. urinary tract infection
b. deep venous thrombosis
c. endometrial cancer
d. breast cancer
e. bipolar disorder

73) An 80-year-old female is found incidentally to have a unilateral, unilocular, echo-free, thin-walled ovarian cyst of diameter 4 cm. There are no papillary projections or solid parts, and the CA-125 is less than 30 U/ml. Which of the following is the most appropriate management?

a. pelvic exenteration
b. total abdominal hysterectomy and bilateral salpingo-oophorectomy
c. bilateral oophorectomy
d. laparoscopic staging
e. repeat transvaginal ultrasound scan in 4 months

74) A female has a cancer detected at the prevalent round of the NHS Breast Screening Programme. Which of the following ages is she most likely to be?

a. 45 years
b. 50 years
c. 55 years
d. 60 years
e. 65 years

75) A 70 year old, who is a lifelong smoker, is investigated for weight loss. Among other findings, an adrenal nodule of 3 cm short axis diameter is found on post-contrast CT, with an average attenuation value of 60 HU. On in-phase T1W images, the adrenal nodule is isointense to spleen; on out-of-phase T1W images, the whole of the nodule returns significantly lower signal than the spleen. Of the following, which is the most likely diagnosis for this adrenal nodule?

a. lung cancer metastasis
b. collision tumour
c. adrenal adenoma
d. phaeochromocytoma
e. hyperfunctioning adrenal cortical neoplasm

76) A 70-year-old woman is known to have uterine fibroids. There has been a clinically apparent increase in the uterine size. Transvaginal ultrasound appearances are in keeping with a large myometrial fibroid. Which of the following diagnoses must be considered in this patient?

a. lipoleiomyoma
b. endometrial hyperplasia
c. adenomyoma
d. leiomyosarcoma
e. Bartholin's gland tumour

77) On an antenatal ultrasound scan, unilateral fetal ureteric dilatation is identified. Follow-up imaging after birth reveals persistent dilatation of a non-tortuous ureter that is aperistaltic in its distal segment. There are no other associated urogenital anomalies. Which of the following is the most appropriate diagnosis?

a. prune-belly syndrome
b. primary vesicoureteric reflux
c. primary megaureter
d. neuropathic bladder
e. ureterocele

78) A 28-year-old female has a hysterosalpingogram for infertility. Both fallopian tubes distend progressively with contrast injection but without peritoneal spill of contrast. A delayed plain abdominal radiograph shows continued distension of both tubes by dense collections of contrast and no peritoneal spill. Given these findings, which of the following is the most likely predisposition to infertility for this patient?

a. tuberculosis
b. endometriosis
c. pelvic inflammatory disease
d. submucosal uterine fibroids
e. Asherman's syndrome

79) An IVU is performed on a teenager. On a 15-minute, full-length radiograph, the right ureter and collecting system appear normal, while the left collecting system is displaced laterally and inferiorly, giving a 'drooping flower' appearance. What is the most likely congenital anomaly?

a. bilateral ureteral duplication
b. left ureteral duplication
c. left ureteral diverticulum
d. recently passed left ureteric stone
e. crossed fused ectopia

80) A 25-year-old woman with pelvic inflammatory disease has a raised serum β-hCG level. Ultrasound scan reveals an empty uterine cavity and an extrauterine amniotic sac. MRI some weeks later shows circumferential bowel involvement by the placenta, which appears to be continuous with the bowel wall muscle. Which of the following is the most compelling reason for a further follow-up MRI?

a. to check that the placenta has been fully removed by surgery
b. to check for response to chemotherapy
c. to ensure that the placenta involutes following delivery and no abscess has developed
d. to stage the gestational trophoblastic neoplasia
e. to date the pregnancy

81) A 70-year-old man with previously diagnosed, bilateral renal calculi is seen with fever, rigors and left loin pain. Ultrasound scan shows a dilated left renal collecting system. Which of the following is the most appropriate management?

a. oral antibiotics with outpatient follow-up
b. urinary catheter, intravenous antibiotics and admission to hospital
c. left nephrostomy and antibiotics
d. bilateral nephrostomy
e. intramuscular anti-spasmodics

82) A 20-year-old man presents with a 4-week history of a scrotal mass. There has been no trauma and no pain. Ultrasound scan confirms an intratesticular, partly cystic, heterogeneous mass. Which of the following tumour markers is most likely to be elevated?

a. CA-125 and AFP
b. CA-15-3 and CEA
c. PSA
d. CA-19-9
e. AFP and β-hCG

83) A 28-year-old female is investigated for infertility. She has raised androgen levels and a higher than normal luteinizing hormone: follicle-stimulating hormone ratio. Pelvic ultrasound scan demonstrates bilaterally large ovaries with multiple small follicles. Which of the following is the most likely reason for the patient's infertility?

a. cervical fibroids
b. hostile cervical mucus
c. ovarian torsion
d. polycystic ovarian disease
e. bilateral ovarian endometriosis implants

84) A 60-year-old man has a 4 cm rounded mass arising within the right kidney. It has heterogeneous, strong post-contrast enhancement. Calcification is also evident within the tumour. Which of the following features of this renal mass would favour the diagnosis of renal cell carcinoma over angiomyolipoma?

a. marked vascularity
b. calcification
c. fat within the tumour
d. round morphology
e. hyperechogenic on ultrasound scan

85) A 75-year-old female is investigated for a slowly enlarging breast mass. There are no involved lymph nodes clinically. Following biopsy, clumps of tumour cells floating in pools of extracellular mucin and without a capsule are seen on histology. The 10-year survival rate for this tumour is in the region of 70–90%. Which of the following is the most likely type of breast tumour?

a. mixed mucinous carcinoma
b. pure mucinous carcinoma
c. phyllodes tumour
d. inflammatory carcinoma
e. melanoma metastasis

86) A 79-year-old female has a 6-month history of vaginal bleeding. Transvaginal ultrasound scan demonstrates an ill-defined endometrium measuring 20 mm in thickness. Outpatient clinic endometrial biopsy confirms endometrial adenocarcinoma. MRI stage is T4. Which of the following MRI features supports this stage?

a. disease limited to the endometrium
b. cancer invasion evident into the outer half of the myometrium
c. vaginal involvement
d. rectal serosal involvement
e. bladder mucosal involvement

87) A well-circumscribed, round, 15 mm mass is identified in the breast on first-round screening mammography. It has no associated calcification. From the following, choose the most appropriate management:

a. repeat mammography at the normal screening interval
b. repeat mammography in 6 months
c. MRI of the breast
d. wide local excision of the lesion
e. ultrasound examination of the mass

88) On MRI of the penis, a squamous cell carcinoma is typically seen as hypointense to the corpora on T1W and T2W images. What is the most likely appearance of this cancer on T1W images following intravenous contrast administration?

a. no change in signal compared with that on the pre-contrast T1W sequence
b. post-contrast enhancement greater than that of the corpus spongiosum but less than that of the corpora cavernosa
c. post-contrast enhancement less than that of all corpora
d. post-contrast enhancement greater than that of all corpora
e. post-contrast enhancement greater than that of the corpora cavernosa but less than that of the corpus spongiosum

89) On a midline sagittal T2W MR image of the uterus of a 25-year-old female, the endometrium, junctional zone and outer myometrium of the corpus are clearly identified. From innermost to outermost, which of the following signal intensities best describes the normal uterus?

a. high, intermediate, low
b. high, low, intermediate
c. intermediate, high, low
d. intermediate, low, high
e. low, intermediate, high

90) A 60-year-old female with urinary retention and pelvic pain is investigated with MRI of the pelvis. On sagittal T2W images, the bladder is seen to be 2 cm below the pubococcygeal line. What is the likely cause of the patient's symptoms?

a. anterior rectocele
b. enterocele
c. cystocele
d. rectal prolapse
e. bladder intussusception

91) Regarding normal pelvic floor anatomy, which of the following is contained within the middle compartment of the female pelvic floor?

a. bladder
b. urethra
c. vagina
d. rectum
e. anus

92) At a breast cancer multidisciplinary team meeting, the case of a 60-year-old female patient is discussed. Following clinical examination, she is thought to have multifocal breast cancer, but this is not supported by the ultrasound and mammography findings. Which of the following is the most appropriate next investigation?

a. repeat ultrasound scan
b. repeat mammography with additional views
c. MRI
d. CT
e. ^{18}FDG PET

93) A 45 year old who is assumed to be pregnant presents with a uterus large for dates and hyperemesis gravidarum. The β-hCG levels are raised. Transvaginal ultrasound scan shows hyperechoic soft tissue with cysts filling the uterine cavity and a septated large left ovarian cyst. Which of the following additional features favours the diagnosis of complete hydatidiform mole as opposed to any other gestational trophoblastic disease?

a. no fetal parts
b. dysmorphic fetus
c. associated prominent vessels
d. pelvic lymph node involvement
e. lung metastases

94) A diabetic patient with long-standing mild renal impairment requires an angiogram, and it is decided that iodinated contrast will be used. Which of the following is most likely to prevent the patient from developing contrast-induced nephropathy?

   a. prior administration of acetylcysteine
   b. thorough hydration of the patient
   c. oral fluid restriction
   d. concurrent diuretic administration
   e. use of high-osmolar contrast medium

95) A portal venous phase abdominal CT scan of a 65-year-old man demonstrates an ill-defined, rounded area 4 cm in diameter within a kidney. It is heterogeneous but predominantly of attenuation value above 70 HU. It contains small dense calcific foci. Which additional feature suggests that the lesion is more likely to be a renal cell carcinoma than a transitional cell carcinoma of the collecting system?

   a. thickened indurated pelvicalyceal wall
   b. central location of the tumour with centrifugal expansion that compresses renal sinus fat
   c. renal parenchymal invasion with renal contour preservation
   d. renal vein thrombus
   e. further mass arising from the urinary bladder wall

96) An adult male is initially investigated for abnormal liver function tests. Eventually, the diagnosis of Stauffer's syndrome is pronounced. What are the likely CT findings?

   a. liver mass in keeping with hepatocellular carcinoma with renal metastases
   b. renal mass in keeping with renal cell carcinoma with liver metastases
   c. renal mass in keeping with renal cell carcinoma and hepatosplenomegaly without focal hepatic or splenic lesions
   d. hepatosplenomegaly and bilateral renal enlargement without focal lesions in any of these organs
   e. renal mass in keeping with renal cell carcinoma with a pancreatic head metastasis

97) A clinical trial of a novel chemotherapy agent for renal cell carcinoma is being undertaken. The response of the primary tumour and nodal and distant metastases will be assessed according to the RECIST criteria. On axial imaging, the long axis of every lesion present on the pre-treatment scan has decreased on the post-treatment CT. However, the patient has progressive disease. Which additional feature from the list below would explain this?

a. the improvement in the summed long axes of five lesions is not more than 30%
b. a new site of disease is identified
c. the lesions have not all disappeared
d. sustained improvement was not proven by a repeat CT at 4 weeks
e. the improvement in the summed products of bidimensional measurements is not more than 50%

98) A plain abdominal radiograph is acquired for left-sided abdominal pain. The lumbar spine is osteoporotic with intervertebral disc space narrowing, vacuum phenomenon and calcification. Marginal osteophytes and endplate sclerosis are also present. In addition to nephrocalcinosis, a radio-opaque calculus is noted along the path of the left ureter. Which of the following is the most likely pattern of inheritance?

a. autosomal recessive
b. autosomal dominant
c. autosomal dominant with partial penetrance
d. mitochondrial
e. X-linked

99) Which of the following is the strongest indication for a PET/CT scan?

a. cervical cancer staging
b. endometrial cancer staging
c. ovarian cancer staging
d. prostate cancer staging
e. bladder transitional cell carcinoma staging

100) On the third day postpartum, a 25-year-old female develops right-sided lower abdominal pain and breathlessness. CT pulmonary angiogram confirms a pulmonary embolus. Bilateral leg Doppler scan is normal. Which of the following diagnoses requires the most serious consideration?

a. appendicitis
b. right ovarian vein thrombosis
c. torsion of ovarian cyst
d. broad ligament haematoma
e. pelvic abscess

Module 4: Genitourinary, Adrenal, Obstetrics & Gynaecology, and Breast: Answers

1) c. ****
Acute tubular necrosis is the commonest acute reversible cause of renal failure in the transplanted kidney and usually occurs within 24 hours. Of the complications of a transplanted kidney causing renal impairment, normal perfusion is seen in acute tubular necrosis, whereas renal vein thrombosis and transplant rejection have reduced perfusion accompanying the diminished excretion. Ciclosporin can cause a similar pattern of renal impairment but would be expected to occur 1 month after transplantation. Functional assessment of a transplanted kidney involves perfusion and excretion assessment with a MAG3 or DTPA renogram, MAG3 being the better test in transplant recipients with renal impairment. Doppler ultrasound resistive index measurement is also used, with a value of <0.7 regarded as normal.

Weissleder et al (2007), 307–10.

2) b. ***
A single portal venous phase CT is not the optimum image set to characterize renal parenchymal lesions. However, renal cell carcinoma is more commonly encountered than high-density cysts. Furthermore, carcinoma is most frequently found in men (2:1) aged over 50 years. Kidney neoplasms tend to have densities above 30 HU on an unenhanced CT and rise by more than 10–20 HU post-contrast, usually being above 70 HU in the portal phase.

Dähnert (2007), 690–1.

3) c. ***
The main differentials for an ovarian mature cystic teratoma (dermoid cyst) are endometriomas and proteinaceous ovarian cysts, which can also have fluid–fluid levels. Fat is frequently demonstrated in a dermoid cyst, but not in these differentials. Fat can be proven by a significant negative attenuation value on CT, or on MRI with chemical shift artefact in the frequency-encoding direction, a gradient echo sequence in which fat and water are in opposite phase or frequency-selective fat saturation sequences. Mature cystic teratoma contains mature tissues of germ cell (pleuripotent) origin. At least two of the three germlines should be represented. Mean patient age is 30 years, younger than for epithelial ovarian neoplasms, and it is the commonest ovarian mass in children.

Usually asymptomatic, they can cause abdominal pain or other non-specific symptoms. They are bilateral in 10% of cases.

Outwater et al (2001).

4) b. **
An incidental, mildly complicated renal cyst has been uncovered. The Bosniak classification is a useful tool for evaluating cystic renal lesions, and guiding management. Simple cysts (Bosniak grade I) are thin walled, are of water density and have no enhancement. Minimally complicated cysts (grade II) may be clustered or septated, and have small curvilinear calcifications, a minimally irregular wall or high-density contents. Follow-up lesions (grade IIF) have perceptible enhancement of otherwise thin septations or are above 3 cm in diameter with high-density contents. Surgical lesions (grade III) have thicker septa or walls, measurable enhancement, coarse irregular calcification and irregular margin, are multiloculated or can be a non-enhancing nodular mass. Clearly malignant lesions (grade IV) can have necrotic components, irregular wall thickening and enhancing solid elements.

Dähnert (2007), 961.

5) a. ***
Most symptomatic male breast lesions are benign, with gynaecomastia representing the commonest benign entity. Characteristic mammographic features are of a central, retroareolar, flame-shaped density. Male breast cancers are usually invasive ductal carcinomas, which typically appear as a discrete, high-density, well-defined mass with lobulated or spiculated margins at mammography. Microcalcification is seen less commonly than in females, but secondary signs, such as nipple retraction and skin thickening, occur earlier than in females due to smaller breast size. Ultrasound scan is particularly helpful in assessing the relationship of the mass to the nipple. An eccentric position is highly suspicious for breast cancer. Axillary lymphadenopathy is seen in approximately 50% of patients.

Chen et al (2006).

6) a. ****
Uterine cervix length can be measured transabdominally or transvaginally. With the former approach, the measurement can be 10% greater than the corresponding transvaginal measurement, because, while the full urinary bladder is a desirable acoustic window, it increases the cervical length. Transvaginally, the normal cervical length is 40 ± 8 mm in the first 14 weeks of pregnancy, 42 ± 10 mm in the second trimester and 32 ± 12 mm from 28 weeks on. An incompetent cervix usually develops during the second or early third trimester. Incidence is

increased after cervical trauma, *in utero* diethylstilbestrol exposure (cervical hypoplasia), and oestrogen treatment. On imaging, dilatation of the cervical canal is seen to begin at the internal os and extend out. It produces a beaking or funnelling appearance and shortens the cervical canal to less than 25 mm. Clinically, the membranes or even fetal parts may be seen through the external os.

Dähnert (2007), 1047.

7) d. ***
Ninety-five per cent of testicular tumours are germ cell tumours. Others include sex-cord and stromal tumours such as Leydig cell and Sertoli cell tumours. Primary lymphoma and metastases can also occur in the testicle. Non-seminomatous germ cell tumours include teratoma, embryonal carcinoma and choriocarcinoma, but these affect a younger population of 20–30 years. Ultrasound scan is the investigation of choice for detection of a testicular tumour and for assessing normality of the contralateral testicle. Seminomas present with mass or pain, and are generally lobulated masses on ultrasound scan with hypoechoic fibrovascular septations in which colour flow can be visible. T2W MRI demonstrates uniform intermediate signal with band-like low-signal septa. There is contrast enhancement, especially of the septations. They rarely calcify, but, if they do, the calcification is speckled or stippled.

Ueno et al (2004).

8) b. **
The device should be seen within the endometrial cavity on ultrasound scan as an echo-bright structure casting an acoustic shadow. If it is not identified in the uterus on ultrasound scan, then a plain abdominal film is indicated to exclude perforation and migration.

Dähnert (2007), 1048.

9) e. ***
T1 and T2 renal cell carcinomas are limited to the kidney, and measure ≤7 cm and >7 cm respectively. T3 tumour extends beyond the kidney, into either the adrenal gland or perinephric tissues (T3a), the renal vein or vena cava below the diaphragm (T3b) or the vena cava above the diaphragm, or it invades the wall of the vena cava (T3c). T4 tumour invades beyond Gerota's fascia. N1 or N2 nodal disease refers to involvement of a single regional node, or more than one regional node, respectively. Overall, T3c N0 M0 disease represents stage III disease.

Hricak et al (2007), 122–9.

10) b. ***

The Whitaker test is a pressure–flow study to evaluate ureteral obstruction or resistance in dilated non-refluxing upper tracts. Being invasive and time-consuming, it is usually performed only when excretory renograms are equivocal. A pressure difference of greater than 15 cmH$_2$O is abnormal.

Weissleder et al (2007), 305.

11) c. **

Estimation of gestational age is most accurate in the first trimester. The crown–rump length is used, which has a range of $\pm$ 0.7 weeks. Beyond about 13 weeks, the measurement becomes less reliable as the fetus becomes increasingly flexed. In the very early first trimester, the mean gestational sac diameter can be used to estimate gestation age with similar accuracy, but this measurement should not be used once the embryo can be seen. Biparietal diameter (or alternatively head circumference) becomes the most reliable measurement in the second trimester with an accuracy of $\pm$ 1.2 weeks up to 20 weeks. Femur length is less precise. Abdominal circumference is the least accurate measurement, and is generally used only to assess fetal growth and proportionality. Estimation of gestational age becomes considerably less reliable with advancing pregnancy; beyond about 22 weeks, fetal growth becomes the main determinant of fetal size.

Middleton et al (2004), 307–8, 310–15.

12) c. ***

Cervical stenosis can be congenital or acquired. When it is acquired, causes include cervical (after the menopause) or endometrial (before the menopause) carcinoma. Radiation and curettage can also produce cervical stenosis. On imaging, the endometrial cavity is distended by secretions and blood products. Reflux endometriosis can complicate cervical stenosis.

Dähnert (2007), 1014.

13) e. ****

Benign serous cystadenoma is bilateral in 20% of cases, benign mucinous cystadenoma in 5%, malignant serous cystadenocarcinoma in 50% and malignant mucinous cystadenocarcinoma in 25%. However, not only are endometrioid ovarian tumours frequently bilateral (30–50%) but they are also often (30%) found with concomitant endometrial adenocarcinoma.

Weissleder et al (2007), 352–4.

14) c. *

Retroperitoneal fibrosis can cause extrinsic compression of both ureters and retroperitoneal vascular structures such as the aorta, inferior vena cava and iliac vessels. It can be idiopathic or secondary to inflammatory aortic aneurysm, retroperitoneal metastases, haemorrhage, abscess, urinoma, diverticulitis, appendicitis, Crohn's disease, and drugs such as ergot alkaloids and hydralazine. Malignant retroperitoneal lymphadenopathy causing ureteric obstruction tends to encircle the aorta, elevating it off the vertebral column. In contrast, retroperitoneal fibrosis rarely extends between the aorta and the vertebrae, and therefore appears to tape the aorta down to the spine.

Sutton (2002), 981.

15) a. *

On the IVU, the features of xanthogranulomatous pyelonephritis are unilateral reniform enlargement, ipsilateral renal hypofunction and nephrolithiasis. The condition is probably produced by chronic low-grade obstruction and chronic bacteriuria. Renal parenchyma is replaced by lipid-laden histiocytes causing renal expansion. This expansion can cause 'stone fracture' with obvious separation of the fracture fragments on plain film. Renal tuberculosis causes dystrophic calcification that can be nodular, curvilinear or amorphous. The calcification is typically multifocal, involving other sites of the urinary tract, and there may be kidney scarring. Hyperparathyroidism causes medullary calcification. Six per cent of renal carcinomas have amorphous, irregular or occasionally curvilinear calcification, while hydatid cysts exhibit curvilinear or heterogeneous calcification.

Zagoria (2004), 139–41.

16) c. **

Bladder cancer achieves the T3 status by perivesical involvement. The N status is determined by the greatest dimension of the regional nodes. When the greatest dimension is less than or equal to 2 cm, the nodal status is N1. N2 is for regional nodes measuring 2–5 cm. N3 is achieved when the greatest dimension of the largest regional node is more than 5 cm. Inguinal and retroperitoneal nodes are staged as metastases.

Hricak et al (2007), 141–6.

17) c. **

Causes of bilateral smooth renal enlargement include diabetic nephropathy, acute glomerulonephritis, collagen vascular disease, vasculitis, AIDS nephropathy, leukaemia, lymphoma, autosomal recessive polycystic renal disease, acute interstitial nephritis, sickle cell disease, thalassaemia, acromegaly, amyloidosis, myeloma and acute urate nephropathy. When the bilateral renal enlargement is caused by masses, the differential diagnosis includes autosomal dominant polycystic disease, acquired renal cystic disease, lymphoma, metastases, Wilms' tumours, tuberous sclerosis, von Hippel–Lindau syndrome, multiple oncocytomas and nephroblastomatosis.

Zagoria (2004), 144–5.

18) e. ****
While several forms of arteritis can cause multiple small renal aneurysms, it is polyarteritis nodosa that does so most commonly, affecting men more than women with a mean age of 55 years, the range being 18–81 years. It is associated with HIV and hepatitis B infection, and pANCA is usually positive. Systemic lupus erythematosus is associated with anti-double-stranded DNA antibodies, Goodpasture's disease with anti-basement membrane antibodies, Sjögren's syndrome with anti-Ro and anti-La antibodies and rheumatoid arthritis with anti-immunoglobulin G (anti-IgG), also known as rheumatoid factor.

Dähnert (2007), 649–50.

19) d. ***
Stage I, non-seminomatous, germ cell tumour patients should enter a surveillance programme of this type following orchidectomy. Such programmes are rarely used for seminoma, particularly when retroperitoneal radiation treatment is used. Rising tumour markers between surveillance scans or thereafter should provoke CT of the chest, abdomen and pelvis plus ultrasound scan of the remaining testicle. If no new disease is identified, MRI of the brain is indicated.

Royal College of Radiologists (2006), 90–2.

20) c. ***
Atrophic maldescended testes are at higher risk of developing malignancy, particularly seminoma, even after orchidopexy. The increased risk applies to the contralateral testicle also. Microlithiasis is also associated with testicular cancer. In combination, these features require clinical and sonographic follow-up.

Zagoria (2004), 325.

21) d. ***
In the TNM staging of urothelial malignancies, T1 refers to invasion of the subepithelial connective tissue, whereas a T2 tumour invades the muscularis. T3 tumours in the renal pelvis invade the peripelvic fat or renal parenchyma, whereas those in the ureter invade the periureteric fat. T4 tumours invade adjacent organs or perinephric fat, as in this case. For renal and ureteric transitional cell carcinoma, the group stages I–III are determined by the T status, all these stages having no involved nodes

and no metastases. T4 primaries or any involved nodes or metastases give stage IV disease. There is no stage V.

Hricak et al (2007), 131–6.

22) d. ***
The cause of Peyronie's disease is unknown, but the result is fibrous thickening of Buck's fascia and the septum between the corpora cavernosa. Calcified plaques are also seen. The fibrous areas do not engorge with blood, causing the penis at erection to be bent; this can make intercourse painful or impossible. Priapism is persistent painful erection of the penis but is not associated with penile calcification. Zoon's balanitis is an idiopathic lymphocytic inflammatory condition of the penis, which may respond to topical steroid but is also treated by circumcision. Balanitis xerotica obliterans is the severe form of penile lichen sclerosus, which is an uncommon inflammatory dermatosis. It can cause phimosis and urinary retention.

Weissleder et al (2007), 337–8.

23) d. ***
A bell-clapper deformity is described. This is bilateral in 50–80% of cases. High insertion of the tunica vaginalis on the spermatic cord means that this tunic completely surrounds the testis, epididymis and distal spermatic cord, allowing intravaginal torsion. Extravaginal torsion is rare and occurs when the testis and tunic twist at the external ring.

Dähnert (2007), 974–5.

24) e. ***
Invasion of the corpora cavernosa or corpora spongiosa by a penile cancer is via the tunica albuginea, making the local stage T2. If the urethra, found centrally within the corpora spongiosa, is involved, it becomes T3. Each corpus cavernosum contains a central artery. Having rapidly flowing blood, this will also be hypointense on both T1W and T2W images because of flow void.

Singh et al (2005).

25) d. ***
Liver capsule deposits are stage T3/III. The pleural effusion cannot be regarded as M1/IV, because it requires positive cytology for this. Any involved regional nodes give stage IIIc and include obturator, common, internal and external iliac, laterosacral, inguinal and para-aortic.

Hricak et al (2007), 84–9.

26) b. ****

Ptosis of the mobile kidney when erect can cause symptoms and underestimation of parenchymal DMSA uptake. Since the differential function may be a factor in considering removal of a kidney, the technique should account for the possibility of nephroptosis influencing the counts. A nutcracker kidney is a rare cause of left-sided loin pain and haematuria; it is caused by compression of the left renal vein between the aorta and superior mesenteric artery.

Plas et al (2001).

27) d. ****

The practice of radiofrequency ablation of renal tumours is emerging. Currently, CT 1 month after the procedure is used to assess treatment success. If enhancing prior to ablation, the tumour is regarded as ablated if there is < 10 HU rise in attenuation following contrast administration. Bulky persistent irregular peripheral enhancement is the commonest appearance of an incompletely treated lesion.

Lui et al (2003).

28) d. **

MRI is the technique of choice for local staging of cancer of the uterine cervix. CT is less useful for staging of the primary tumour but has value in detecting involved lymph nodes and distant metastases. [18]FDG PET may be useful in some cases for detection of distant metastases or the identification of recurrent disease. Its value will vary with the histological diagnosis on account of varying radiotracer avidity, with squamous cell carcinomas typically being avid.

Hricak et al (2007), 90–6.

29) d. ****

First-degree perineal tear involves skin only. Perineal muscle is torn in a second-degree tear and so includes episiotomy. Anal sphincter damage defines third-degree injury, this being subdivided into types 3a, involving less than 50% of external sphincter, 3b, more than 50% of external sphincter, and 3c, when the internal sphincter is torn. A tear extending into the anal epithelium is a fourth-degree tear.

Baker (2006), 257.

30) a. **

The abnormality described is prominent or hypertrophic cortex since it takes up DMSA, which in the kidneys is a parenchymal tracer. Renal cell carcinoma, cysts, abscess, haematoma, scar and infarct would be seen as photopenic areas on DMSA SPECT, if large enough.

Dähnert (2007), 1123.

31) a. **

Normal MIBG uptake is seen in myocardium, liver, spleen, bladder, adrenal glands, salivary glands, nasopharynx, thyroid and colon. Abnormal MIBG activity is seen in phaeochromocytoma (paraganglioma when extra-adrenal), neuroblastoma, carcinoid tumour, medullary thyroid carcinoma and ganglioneuroma. Ten per cent of phaeochromocytomas are familial, 10% bilateral or multiple, 10% extra-adrenal and 10% malignant. Metastatic spread is to bone, lymph nodes, liver and lung.

Chapman & Nakielny (2003), 311.

32) a. ***

Trachelectomy may be considered to conserve the uterus and preserve fertility in young women with small tumours. Tumour size, distance from the internal os, cervix length and size of the uterus are required from the imaging. Surgery, radiation and chemotherapy are treatment options for cervical cancer dependent on stage. From 85% to 90% of cervical carcinomas have squamous cell histology, the remainder being mostly adenocarcinoma or adenosquamous.

Royal College of Radiologists (2006), 96.

33) c. **

NX is used when regional nodes cannot be assessed, and N0 when there are no involved regional nodes. N1 denotes ipsilateral involved femoral or inguinal lymph nodes. N2 signifies bilateral regional nodal involvement. All intrapelvic nodes are regarded as metastases and therefore do not influence the N stage. There is no N3 for vulval cancer.

Hricak et al (2007), 104–8.

34) e. ****

The cornerstone of diagnosis here is the post-contrast enhancement of renal cell carcinoma. To identify this among the high T1 signal of haemorrhage or protein within cysts, it is ideal to subtract the pre-contrast T1 signal. Fat suppression will not remove the distracting high signal from mildly complicated cysts. Risk of renal cell carcinoma is increased in adult polycystic renal disease when in renal failure. Hence, caution may be required since at certain levels of renal impairment the use of MRI contrast is not advised.

Weissleder et al (2007), 291.

35) a. ****

False positives can occur with PET because [18]FDG is a metabolic tracer, and activity is seen in normal bowel, ovaries (cyclical), endometrium (cyclical), blood vessels, bone marrow and skeletal muscle. [18]FDG is renally excreted; hence, focal accumulation can be seen in ureters,

bladder diverticula, pelvic kidneys and urinary diversions. Benign processes can also take up this tracer, including abscesses, uterine fibroids, endometriosis, post-surgical inflammation, post-radiotherapy inflammation and sacral fractures. Fusion of the PET with a CT scan can reduce these common pitfalls. However, using CT for attenuation correction can introduce other artefacts, such as apparently increased activity around metal prostheses. The PET acquisition is considerably longer than the CT one, allowing movement of bowel or bladder wall (with distension over time) and hence misregistration of PET activity on the anatomical CT data. False-negative PET scans can be caused by small tumour deposits close to the urinary bladder, where they cannot be resolved from each other.

Subhas et al (2005).

36) c. ****
Being bilateral prostate-confined disease, this cancer is T2c. Internal iliac, obturator, external iliac and sacral are the regional nodal groups. Common iliac, para-aortic and inguinal involved lymph nodes are regarded as metastases.

Hricak et al (2007), 152–8.

37) b. ****
An unenhanced CT attenuation value of less than 10 HU is in keeping with a lipid-rich adenoma. With a threshold of 60% or higher for absolute contrast-enhancement washout, a sensitivity of 98% and specificity of 92% can be achieved in differentiating adenomas from non-adenomas. Percentage of enhancement washout = ([attenuation at 60 s − attenuation at 15 min] / [attenuation at 60 s − attenuation on plain CT]) × 100. Applying this to the figures quoted in the question gives an absolute washout of around 66.6%.

Caoili et al (2002).

38) c. **
Predisposing factors to papillary necrosis include diabetes mellitus, analgesic nephropathy/abuse, sickle cell disease, pyelonephritis, obstructive uropathy, tuberculosis, trauma, cirrhosis, coagulopathy and renal vein thrombosis. None of the other options easily explains the club-shaped calyx. Blood clots from renal or tumour haemorrhage do cause ureteric colic but tend to elongate along the pelvis and ureter.

Zagoria (2004), 194.

39) c. **
MRI offers good soft-tissue contrast that is of value in local staging of the primary tumour. Local extent is used to guide the type of treatment, which includes partial penile amputation, total penectomy and radiation

therapy. MRI will also show enlarged regional lymph nodes, but the principal purpose of MRI is local staging. CT can also be used for nodal spread and metastatic disease.

Hricak et al (2007), 166–70.

40) c. **

While around 10% of renal and ureteric stones are radiolucent on plain film, almost all are opaque on CT. One exception is the tiny radiolucent calculi formed in patients on protease inhibitors such as indinavir used in the treatment of HIV/AIDS.

Sutton (2002), 965–7.

41) d. ****

A short axis measurement of 7 mm or greater represents significant enlargement of internal iliac nodes. Regarding other nodal regions, significant enlargement for inguinal nodes is 10 mm, for common iliac 9 mm, for external iliac 10 mm, for obturator 8 mm and for retroperitoneal nodes between renal arteries and the aortic bifurcation 12 mm. In addition to size, there may be morphological clues to nodal involvement by cancer. Clustering of nodes, round nodes, nodes with irregular capsules, and nodes sharing CT or MRI characteristics of the primary tumour (attenuation, signal, cystic or necrotic changes, and contrast-enhancement pattern) are features suggesting lymph node involvement.

Royal College of Radiologists (2006), 27.

42) b. ***

'Vanishing twin' occurs at less than 13 weeks when one twin is completely resorbed with no residuum evident on ultrasound scan. In foetus papyraceus, one twin is compressed and seen plastered to the adjacent membranes. Fetal death *in utero* or intrauterine death is signalled by absent heart and somatic movement in the second and third trimesters. Hydrops is excess total body water manifested as extracellular liquid accumulation in tissues and serous cavities. In hydrops of immune orgin, antibodies to red blood cells are present.

Dähnert (2007), 1042–3.

43) d. ***

The urethra is used as a landmark for the lower third of the vagina. Cervical cancer involvement of the upper two-thirds of the vagina is T2a. When the lower third is involved, it becomes T3a. T3b disease denotes disease that reaches the pelvic side wall or has caused hydronephrosis. Extension of disease into bladder or rectal mucosa is T4, as is disease extending out of the true pelvis. Extension into the corpus only is disregarded. T1b1 disease and T1b2 disease differ in being less or greater than 4 cm respectively. Parametrial lymph nodes are regional nodes and represent N1 disease; they do not influence the T stage.

Hricak et al (2007), 90–6.

44) e. **

Testicular rupture is described; it is an indication for immediate surgical intervention to salvage the testicle and prevent anti-sperm antibody development (testicles are immune-privileged sites). Other consequences of testicular trauma are fracture, haematoma and haematocele. Associated torsion may occur, due to trauma-stimulated, forceful, cremasteric muscle contraction.

Weissleder et al (2007), 336.

45) e. ***

A T4 stage primary is described. Lower-stage breast cancers (T1/T2, less than 5 cm) are not usually staged by CT, as there is a less than 2% incidence of metastases at the time of diagnosis. Incidence of metastases at diagnosis for higher-stage cancers (T3/T4) is 15–20%. When staged with CT, a suitable protocol would be 100–150 ml of iodinated intravenous contrast agent used, with the neck and chest scanned 20–25 seconds after injection, and the abdomen and pelvis scanned 70–80 seconds after injection.

Royal College of Radiologists (2006), 124–6.

46) a. ***

Investigation in most cases of haemospermia is not fruitful. In patients under 40 years, the causes are usually idiopathic or inflammatory (prostatitis, epididymo-orchitis, urethritis and urethral warts). The same causes apply in those over 40 years, but further possible causes include prostate cancer, benign prostatic hypertrophy, prostatic or seminal vesicle calculi, hypertension and carcinoma of the seminal vesicles.

Weissleder et al (2007), 335.

47) a. **

Plain chest radiograph may be added to this as a routine, but chest CT would be requested only with an additional reason to do so. MRI of the ovaries can be helpful in characterizing ovarian masses where ultrasound scan and CA-125 are equivocal. There may be a role for PET/CT in defining disease extent, but cystic tumour deposits, particularly when they may be on or close to bowel or associated with ascites, present a challenge for this technique.

Royal College of Radiologists (2006), 93–5.

48) c. ****

Schistosomiasis (bilharzia) is a parasitic infection that, worldwide, is the commonest cause of bladder wall calcification. *Schistosoma japonicum* and *S. mansoni* cause gastrointestinal tract infection, while *S. haematobium* affects the genitourinary tract. Schistosomiasis is endemic in South Africa, Egypt, Nigeria, Tanzania, Zimbabwe and Puerto Rico. The calcification spreads proximally up the ureters. In contrast, tuberculosis begins in the kidneys and spreads distally. Transitional cell carcinoma and cyclophosphamide-induced cystitis also cause bladder wall calcification. Causes of calcification within the urinary bladder lumen include stones and encrusted foreign bodies such as catheter balloons.

Chapman & Nakielny (2003), 350.

49) b. **

Testes drain to the para-aortic nodes at the L1–2 level. The penile body drains to superficial inguinal nodes, while the proximal penis lymph drainage is to deep inguinal nodes. Appreciation of these patterns of lymph drainage is of vital importance when staging testicular, penile and other scrotal malignancies.

Butler et al (1999), 292–4.

50) b. **

The main differential diagnosis for a parapelvic or renal sinus cyst is hydronephrosis. Such cysts may present with pain due to obstructive caliectasis, but rarely cause hydronephrosis. They are found in 1.5% of autopsies and represent 4–6% of all renal cysts. A distinction is made in this question between renal and ureteric colic, the former symptom located to the loin and the latter more typically being loin to groin.

Dähnert (2007), 961.

51) b. ***

Seminoma tends to spread to contiguous nodes with the primary sites being, for a right-sided testicular tumour, right paracaval and interaortocaval nodes just below the junction of the right renal vein and inferior vena cava. Left-sided testicular tumours usually spread first to nodes just caudal to the left renal vein. Teratoma and other malignant, non-seminomatous, germ cell tumours of the testes can occupy mediastinal nodes without such direct cranial extension along the nodal groups. Nodes involved by seminoma tend to be soft-tissue density while nodes inhabited by non-seminomatous, germ cell tumours are frequently cystic. Metastases to the testicle are rare on account of the testicle being an immunologically privileged site with a blood–testicular barrier. Adenomatoid tumour is a benign epididymal lesion. Epidermoid tumour is also benign, appearing as an intratesticular, hypoechoic lesion, characteristically with an echogenic capsule. Classically, it assumes an 'onion-skin' appearance of concentric echogenic layers. Internal shadowing can be produced by calcification.

Hricak et al (2007), 159.

52) b. ****
The normal decidua forms a barrier between chorionic villi and uterus, preventing deep invasion of placental material. An underdeveloped or absent decidua permits direct contact of chorionic villi with the myometrium, known as placenta accreta. When the villi invade the myometrium, it becomes placenta increta; if the serosa is penetrated, it is placenta percreta. Diagnosis is difficult on ultrasound scan, but MRI can help. Risk factors are previous caesarean section and myomectomy, multiparity and increasing maternal age. Complications include maternal haemorrhage, premature delivery, intrauterine growth retardation and 5% chance of perinatal death. To protect the mother, balloon catheters can be placed over the internal iliac arteries prior to caesarean delivery.

Dähnert (2007), 1060.

53) d. **
MRI is indicated for local (in fact locoregional) staging. CT of the chest is required in addition to the abdomen and pelvis because of the histological tumour type. ^{18}FDG PET is not useful for staging urothelial tumours because of the urinary excretion of this radiotracer.

Royal College of Radiologists (2006), 81–5.

54) c. ****
In 67% of cases of single umbilical artery, there are chromosomal abnormalities. Trisomy 18 has a stronger association than trisomy 13, Turner's syndrome or triploidy. Down's syndrome is not associated.

Dähnert (2007), 1063.

55) d. **
The upper two-thirds of the vagina drain to the pelvic nodes, which is of relevance when imaging vaginal cancer. This cancer is uncommon, representing 1–2% of gynaecological malignancy. Eighty-five per cent of cases of vaginal cancer are squamous and 15% are adenocarcinoma. Clear-cell carcinoma is a rare form of adenocarcinoma found in young patients with *in utero* diethylstilbestrol exposure. Even less common are melanoma, sarcoma and adenosquamous carcinoma occurring as vaginal primaries. The two commonest cell types have different natural histories. Adenocarcinoma tends to involve pelvic and is more likely to involve supraclavicular lymph nodes, while squamous carcinomas are

more likely to give rise to liver metastases. They are equally likely to metastasize to the lungs.

Hricak et al (2007), 110–15.

56) d. **
This occurs in 1 in 200 pregnancies, and the incidence rises with increasing maternal age, multiparity, smoking and previous caesarean section. Delivery is by caesarean section. Third-trimester bleeding occurs in 90% of cases of placenta praevia, with premature delivery and perinatal and maternal death as other complications. A low-lying placenta is one within 2 cm of the internal cervical os. Marginal placenta praevia describes a placental edge up to the os. Partial praevia covers some of the os. From 60% to 90% of patients with placenta praevia in the second trimester have a normal placenta by term because of differential growth of the lower uterine segment.

Weissleder et al (2007), 806.

57) a. ****
Urethral tumour is rare and occurs more in women than in men. Squamous cell carcinoma is the most common histological type followed by transitional cell carcinoma and then adenocarcinoma. MRI is the technique of choice for local staging.

Hricak et al (2007), 147–51.

58) b. ***
Abruption can be regarded as premature separation of the placenta from the uterine wall secondary to maternal haemorrhage after 20 weeks' gestation. Manifestations include vaginal bleeding, pain and disseminated intravascular coagulation. Risk factors include hypertension (pre-eclampsia), previous abruption, smoking, cocaine, leiomyoma, idiopathic factors, fetal malformation and trauma. Placental abruption is responsible for 15–25% of perinatal deaths. On ultrasound scan, acute haemorrhage appears hyperechoic or isoechoic, and may be difficult to distinguish from the adjacent placenta. The haematoma forms a complex hypoechoic collection within 1 week of abruption, and usually appears as an anechoic collection within 2 weeks. Placenta membranacea refers to the presence of placental villi in the peripheral membranes.

Dähnert (2007), 1059.

59) c. **
Endometritis is the commonest cause of gas in the uterus. Gas is also seen in the uterus when a submucosal fibroid becomes infected, when necrotic neoplastic tissue is metabolized by bacteria, because of fistula to the gastrointestinal tract, in pyometra secondary to cervix

obstruction by cancer, or in cases of gas gangrene due to clostridial infection following septic abortion. Ovarian gas can be seen with infection within an ovarian neoplasm. Numerous gas-filled spaces in the vaginal submucosa and exocervix can occur in pregnancy; this is termed 'vaginitis emphysematosa'.

Dähnert (2007), 1014.

60) d. ***
The vaginal epithelial layer and mucus are bright on T2W images. This is normally surrounded by low-signal (fibromuscular) vaginal wall.
Tumours are typically intermediate signal on T2W images. If gadolinium is used, cancers often have early phase enhancement. Large tumours may have central necrosis. T1 tumours do not breach the low-T2-signal vaginal wall, whereas T2 tumours do and extend into the paracolpal fat. T3 tumours reach the pelvic side wall while T4 tumours extend beyond the true pelvis or involve bladder or rectal mucosa.

Hulse & Carrington (2004), 112.

61) c. ***
Ovarian hyperstimulation syndrome is more commonly seen with human menopausal gonadotrophin therapy but can also be seen with clomiphene. Severe complications relate to volume depletion, such as hypovolaemia, oliguria, electrolyte imbalance and thromboembolic events. Intra-abdominal haemorrhage is also reported.

Dähnert (2007), 1056.

62) a. ****
In staging prostate cancer with MRI, the large-FOV T1W sequence is useful for demonstrating haemorrhage (high signal), enlarged lymph nodes and bone metastases. Small-FOV T2W images of the prostate in axial, coronal and sagittal planes show the zonal anatomy well, with normal peripheral zone returning high signal. Cancer within the peripheral zone typically returns low signal on T2W images. Other typical findings in carcinoma of the prostate are increased relative peak enhancement, increased contrast wash-in rate, reversal of the choline plus creatine/citrate ratio on spectroscopy, restricted diffusion and increase in permeability on pharmacokinetic modelling.

Choi et al (2007).

63) c. **
Normal ovarian volume is less than $18\,cm^3$ before the menopause and less than $8\,cm^3$ after. The volume can be estimated by multiplying the three diameters and dividing by two.

Weissleder et al (2007), 340.

64) e. **

Microcalcifications are those less than 0.5 mm. When there are more than five in a tissue volume of 1 cm³, particularly if segmentally distributed, 30% will be malignant. Other features also suggesting malignancy are a mixture of sizes and shapes of the calcific foci, associated soft-tissue opacity and progression on serial mammography.

Chapman & Nakielny (2003), 365–7.

65) d. **

The menstrual endometrium is under 4 mm. After menstruation and up to day 14, the proliferative endometrium is 4–8 mm. Days 14–28 are secretory with the endometrium 7–14 mm. On ultrasound scan, the endometrium is seen as an echo-bright stripe. Unless the patient is taking tamoxifen or hormones, the postmenopausal endometrium should be less than 4 mm. A cut-off of 3 mm when performing screening for endometrial cancer has a 99% negative predictive value.

Weissleder et al (2007), 339–40.

66) e. ***

Major markers for Down's syndrome include ventriculoseptal defect, cystic hygroma, omphalocele, duodenal atresia, hydrothorax, mild cerebral ventricular dilatation, corpus callosum agenesis and imperforate anus. The other options given are minor markers.

Dähnert (2007), 70–1.

67) d. *

For cord entanglement, the twins must be in the same amniotic sac. Dizygotic twins are non-identical and result from fertilization of two separate ova.

Dähnert (2007), 1021–2.

68) c. ****

In 80% of cases of fibromatosis of the breast, there is β-catenin or adenomatous polyposis coli gene mutation. Granular cell tumour is most commonly found in the upper inner quadrant corresponding to the supraclavicular nerve territory and is thought to be of Schwann cell origin. Neurofibromas of von Recklinghausen's disease are associated in an autosomal dominant fashion with a gene on chromosome 17.

Porter et al (2006).

69) e. ***

Features of an ovarian cyst that suggest malignancy are thick irregular walls and thick septations (>2 mm), large overall size, solid elements and, on Doppler scan, a high peak systolic velocity and low-impedance diastolic flow. Together, these give a resistive index (RI) of <0.4 and a pulsatility index (PI) of <1.

Weissleder et al (2007), 353.

70) c. ***

The uterus, fallopian tubes and upper vagina arise from the paired paramesonephric (müllerian) ducts. The caudal parts fuse and ultimately form the uterus and upper vagina with resorption of the midline septum. The cranial parts remain unfused and form the fallopian tubes. Congenital uterine abnormalities arise with failure of development or fusion of this duct, or failure of midline resorption following fusion. Mayer–Rokitansky–Küster–Hauser syndrome describes uterine agenesis accompanied by hypoplastic proximal/middle third of the vagina but normal tubes and ovaries. Forty per cent of patients with the syndrome have pelvic kidneys and other urinary tract anomalies are also associated. They have a normal genotype.

Scarsbrook & Moore (2003).

71) b. ***

Angiomyolipomas are benign hamartomatous tumours that can occur in the kidneys. They contain fat, smooth muscle and abnormal blood vessels. Eighty per cent are sporadic and occur most often in females aged 50–80 years. Twenty per cent of patients with angiomyolipomas have tuberous sclerosis. Retroperitoneal bleed is the most significant complication and can be catastrophic. The risk increases with size of the lesion due to increased abnormal vasculature. Haemorrhage occurs because of large tortuous vessels and aneurysms. Embolization is performed for symptomatic (flank pain) angiomyolipomas, those that have bled at any size, and prophylactically when over 4 cm.

Rimon et al (2006).

72) d. ****

The patient is receiving tamoxifen. Side effects include subendometrial cystic atrophy, endometrial hyperplasia and endometrial polyps. Less frequent side effects are endometriosis, polypoid endometriosis, adenomyosis and cervical polyps. There is an increased risk of endometrial carcinoma. On MRI, an endometrioma can appear as a multicystic adnexal mass of high T1 and both hypo- and hyperintense T2 signal, but without the fat suppression that would be expected with a mature cystic teratoma. Adenomyosis on MRI may manifest as a uterus with a thickened, low-signal, junctional zone on T2W images, containing small foci of high T2 signal.

Kraft & Hughes (2006).

73) e. ***
The Risk of Malignancy Index (RMI) is used to stratify the likelihood of an incidentally identified ovarian cyst being malignant. The RMI is the product of the ultrasound score, the CA-125 level and the score assigned according to menopausal status. Low-risk cysts can be managed conservatively. A cyst below 5 cm in diameter that is unilocular, unilateral and echo-free, and has no solid parts or papillary formations has a risk of malignancy of less than 1%, and a 50% chance of resolving spontaneously in 3 months.

Royal College of Obstetricians and Gynaecologists (2003).

74) b. ****
1988 was the year of introduction of the NHS Breast Screening Programme following the recommendation of the Forrest Report (HMSO 1986). Women aged 50–70 are currently invited for breast screening in the UK, with those over 70 encouraged to self-refer, but this age range will shortly be extended to 47–73 years. The prevalent round is the first round of screening, which aims to detect all those in the screened population at that time with the disease. It is a rolling programme, meaning that women receive their first invitation at some time in the 3-year interval from their 50th birthday, so they may in practice be aged 50–53 at their first screening appointment. The incident rounds, at 3-year intervals, aim to detect the cancers that have appeared in this interval. Two mammographic views (mediolateral oblique and craniocaudal) are currently routinely performed at both prevalent and incident rounds.

Osborn et al (2006).

75) c. ***
Signal dropout during out-of-phase T1W sequences occurs in lipid-rich adenomas by virtue of their fat content. Adrenal primaries and metastases do not share this feature. Collision tumours arise when a metastasis occurs in an adrenal gland that already contains an adenoma, in which case signal characteristics of both are seen on the T1W in- and out-of-phase sequences.

Mayo-Smith et al (2001).

76) d. ***
Uterine fibroids are oestrogen dependent and should involute following the menopause. Increase in size of a fibroid after the menopause should raise the possibility of sarcomatous degeneration. On ultrasound scan, the appearance of leiomyosarcoma may be indistinguishable from that of a benign fibroid.

Weissleder et al (2007), 344–5.

77) c. ****
The primary megaureter occurs because of developmental aperistalsis of the distal ureter. The ureter tends to be dilated but straight in a congenital primary megaureter. Primary vesicoureteric reflux and obstructive secondary megaureter tend to cause tortuous ureteric dilatation.

Berrocal et al (2002).

78) c. ***
The patient's fallopian tubes are occluded, giving bilateral hydrosalpinx. The commonest cause of proximal or distal tubal occlusion is pelvic inflammatory disease. Endometriosis, infection following birth or abortion, and tuberculosis are other causes. Indications for hysterosalpingogram include infertility, recurrent miscarriage, assessment of the tubes after surgery and assessment of the integrity of a post-caesarean uterine scar. Contraindications are pregnancy, purulent vulval or cervical discharge, pelvic inflammatory disease in the preceding 6 months and contrast sensitivity. Historical contraindications include the immediate post-menstruation phase and recent dilatation and curettage, because of the risks associated with intravasation of oily contrast media.

Sutton (2002), 1089.

79) b. ***
The 'drooping flower' appearance on IVU occurs with a duplicated system when the obstructed dilated upper pole collecting system displaces the contrast-opacified, lower collecting system laterally and inferiorly. The Weigert–Meyer rule describes the commonest relationship of insertion of the duplicated ureters into the bladder. The upper collecting system ureter inserts ectopically into the bladder inferior and medial to the orthotopic ureter, which enters the bladder near the trigone. The ectopic ureter may be stenotic or obstructed with or without ureterocele.

Weissleder et al (2007), 857.

80) c. *****
The history and imaging features are of extrauterine abdominal pregnancy, which occurs when the fertilized ovum implants directly on the peritoneal surface of the abdomen. This is more likely when the prevalence of pelvic inflammatory disease and ectopic pregnancy is higher. The diagnosis is often established with ultrasound scan. MRI can be used to identify the location and assess adherence to abdominal viscera by the placenta. MR angiography can suggest feeding arteries. MRI at this stage also has a role in detecting fetal anomalies. If the placenta is adherent to abdominal viscera, it is not removed, because this could precipitate catastrophic arterial haemorrhage. Therefore, MRI is performed later to ensure involution of the placenta and exclude

abscess formation. Placental adherence is suggested on MRI when it is contiguous with liver or spleen parenchyma, shows circumferential involvement of bowel or shows continuity with muscle of bowel wall.

Lockhat et al (2006).

81) c. ***
Pyonephrosis secondary to an obstructing calculus is the likely diagnosis. Percutaneous nephrostomy is indicated for temporary or permanent relief of an obstructed urinary system (malignant or benign obstructive uropathy), pyonephrosis, renal stones, iatrogenic ureteric injury, transplant kidney ureteric obstruction, and vesicovaginal fistula. A 'one-stab' puncture technique or Seldinger technique can be used. For any procedures where urinary infection is suspected or in stone disease, prophylactic antibiotics are mandatory – for example, 80 mg gentamicin or 750 mg cefuroxime. Clotting must also be checked and if necessary corrected. The major complication rate is around 3% while minor complications occur in around 15%. Major complications are septicaemia, blood loss requiring transfusion, pleural or abdominal viscera puncture, or transcolonic approach. Minor complications include retroperitoneal urine extravasation, clot colic from macroscopic haematuria and tube complications. Tube complications include catheter dislodgement, blockage, leaking, kinking and fracture.

Lewis & Patel (2004).

82) e. ***
The patient's age and ultrasound findings favour a non-seminomatous germ cell tumour. These are associated with elevated serum AFP and β-hCG. Together, CA-125 and AFP are associated with hepatocellular carcinoma, while CA-125 is also associated with ovarian cancer. CA-15-3 and CEA together are serum markers associated with breast cancer. PSA is associated with prostate cancer as well as several benign prostate conditions. CA-19-9 is mainly associated with malignancy of the pancreas and biliary tree.

Kulkarni et al (2008).

83) d. **
Polycystic ovarian disease is diagnosed by clinical, biochemical and ultrasound findings. Clinically, oligomenorrhoea, hirsutism and obesity are features. Luteinizing hormone is increased as is the luteinizing hormone: follicle-stimulating hormone ratio. Androgen levels are increased. Sonographic findings vary from normal-looking ovaries through hypoechoic ovaries without individual cysts to multiple, 5 mm or more, peripherally located cysts in bilaterally large ovaries.

Weissleder et al (2007), 350.

84) b. ***
Angiomyolipoma should not have calcification whereas it is seen in 10% of renal cell carcinomas. Both these tumours can be hypervascular. The cornerstone of diagnosis of an angiomyolipoma is identifying fat on CT or MRI; however, fat has been reported in renal cell carcinoma, and peripheral or renal sinus fat can become trapped in any large renal tumour.

Weissleder et al (2007), 293.

85) b. ****
Pure mucinous breast carcinoma tends to be slow-growing, rarely metastasizes and has a good prognosis. It is important to differentiate this from mixed mucinous carcinomas, which are invasive carcinomas of no specific type with a mucinous component. The prognosis of mixed mucinous carcinomas is worse than that of pure mucinous carcinoma, tumour behaviour depending on the non-mucinous part. Mixed mucinous tumours comprise around 2% of breast cancers, and 33–46% have lymph node metastases at presentation. Pure mucinous carcinoma accounts for 1–2% of breast malignancies with an average age of 65, older than the average for breast cancer in general, which is 60 years. Many features of pure mucinous tumours mean that there is significant potential for them to be misdiagnosed as benign masses.

Dhillon et al (2006).

86) e. ****
Endometrial carcinoma is the commonest gynaecological malignancy, and the fourth commonest site of female malignancy. It is very unlikely if the endometrial thickness on transvaginal ultrasound scan is less than 4 mm. Endometrial carcinoma becomes stage T4 when bladder or bowel mucosa is involved, whereas the stage remains T3 if other layers of bowel or bladder are invaded. On MRI, endometrial carcinoma has homogeneous signal intensity, isointense to myometrium on T1W images and hypointense to endometrial lining on T2W images. Endometrial cancers demonstrate slower contrast enhancement to a lower peak of enhancement than normal myometrium.

Barwick et al (2006).

87) e. ***
Ultrasound scan is useful in determining whether mass lesions seen on the mammogram are cystic or solid.

Weissleder et al (2007), 775.

88) c. ***
Most cancers of the penis (95%) are squamous cell carcinoma, but basal cell carcinoma, sarcoma, melanoma, lymphoma and urethral transitional

cell carcinoma are also possible. Typical appearances of a primary penile cancer are of an ill-defined infiltrating lesion hypointense to the corpora on both T1W and T2W images. Tumours enhance following contrast, but to a lesser degree than the normal corporal bodies. Signal characteristics of melanotic melanoma will be notably different from the other tumour types, returning a bright signal on T1W images.

Singh et al (2005b).

89) b. **

The premenopausal uterus normally has a bright endometrium within a dark junctional zone and an intermediate outer myometrium on T2W images. Cancer disrupts the zonal anatomy seen on T2W MRI. T1W sequences do not demonstrate uterine zonal anatomy. On T2W images, the uterine cervix has a distinct zonal signal pattern that is particularly well seen on sequences acquired perpendicular to the long axis of the cervix. These are especially useful for cervical cancer staging. The cervix lumen is bright, the cervical mucosa is intermediate to bright, and the fibromuscular cervical stroma is dark and surrounded by the intermediate signal outer layer of cervical stroma. With age or radiation treatment, the uterus involutes and loses this zonal appearance on T2W MRI. Notably, the outer corpus and especially the cervical muscles return a lower signal.

Hulse & Carrington (2004), 33–7.

90) c. **

Suspected pelvic floor prolapse can be investigated with MRI. Usually, there is minimal movement of pelvic organs even on maximal strain. When the pelvic floor is lax, the organs descend below the pubococcygeal line by 1–2 cm. When descent exceeds 2 cm, the prolapse may require surgical intervention. An enterocele describes small bowel descending 2 cm or more between vagina and rectum. Anterior bulging of the rectal wall is known as a rectocele, while bladder descent of more than 1 cm is a cystocele.

Weissleder et al (2007), 357–8.

91) c. **

The pelvic floor is supported by the endopelvic fascia and the levator ani muscle complex. This complex consists of three muscle groups, iliococcygeal, pubococcygeal and puborectalis. The anterior compartment of the female pelvic floor contains the bladder and urethra. The middle compartment contains the vagina and the posterior compartment the rectum.

Weissleder et al (2007), 357.

92) c. ***

Multifocal/multicentric cancer in the breast may alter treatment choice and when clinically suspected should be investigated with MRI. MRI can also be used to assess the extent of residual disease in the breast after breast conservation surgery in cases where the surgical resection margins are positive. An acceptable series of sequences for breast MRI would be: 4mm slice-thickness, transverse, spin echo T2W images of both breasts; 4-mm-thick, sagittal, spin echo T2W images of the affected breast; 4-mm-thick, sagittal, dynamic contrast-enhanced T1W gradient echo with fat saturation of the affected breast; and a delayed post-contrast sequence with the same parameters.

Royal College of Radiologists (2006), 124–6.

93) a. ***

Gestational trophoblastic disease (GTD) is abnormal proliferation of the trophoblast, which can give rise to a complete or partial hydatidiform mole, invasive mole or choriocarcinoma. Increasing age and previous GTD are risk factors. Elevation of β-hCG aids diagnosis and is of value in assessing risk of metastatic disease (hence prognosis), and can be used to assess treatment response or detect recurrence. Complete moles have a higher malignant potential than partial moles. A complete mole has no fetal parts and has a 46,XX or, less often, a 46,XY karyotype. A partial mole has fetal parts and a triploid karyotype with 69 chromosomes. Eighty per cent of hydatidiform moles resolve with evacuation, 15% are locally invasive and 5% give rise to metastatic choriocarcinoma. When GTD is staged, there are no 'regional' nodes, and any nodal spread is considered metastatic with a significant worsening of prognosis. On ultrasound, the mole is echogenic but with a vesicular appearance. Fifty per cent of cases are associated with a large, septated theca lutein cyst. On Doppler ultrasound scan, they have prominent associated vessels with low resistance and high peak systolic velocity.

Weissleder et al (2007), 808–9.

94) b. ***

A significant contribution to the evidence base used to guide practice in contrast-induced nephropathy (CIN) comes from the NEPHRIC study group. The trial was a randomized, prospective, double-blind, multicentre study performed in 17 centres in Denmark, France, Germany, Spain and Sweden, and consisted of 129 patients. CIN is acute renal impairment with an absolute increase in serum creatinine of at least 0.5mg/dl (44.2 μmol/l) or a relative increase of at least 25% from baseline. A rise of 1 mg/dl is less frequently used as the definition. CIN usually peaks on day 2 or 3 following iodinated contrast injection, with a return to baseline within 2 weeks. Return to baseline is not always seen. Low-osmolar iodinated contrast media have a low rate of CIN in the general population – less than 2%. In patients with increased risk of CIN due to diabetes mellitus or pre-existing renal impairment, this rate rises significantly. It has also been shown that low-osmolar contrast causes less CIN than high-osmolar (order of 1800 mosmol/kg water) contrast in high-risk patient groups. No difference in CIN rate is observed in low-risk groups when iso-osmolar is compared with low-osmolar contrast agents. The NEPHRIC study group shows that in people with diabetes or those with renal impairment having iliofemoral or coronary angiography there is a reduced rate of CIN when using iso-osmolar iodinated contrast as opposed to low-osmolar contrast medium. Osmotic diuresis causing increased sodium load to the distal nephron, with consequent increased medullary work, possible hypoxia and volume depletion giving rise to activation of vasoregulatory hormone systems, is suggested as the reason for the findings. Vigorous hydration is encouraged as perhaps the most important measure to try to avoid CIN. There is evidence both supporting and rejecting the nephroprotective effect of the free radical scavenger acetylcysteine when given before the iodinated contrast media.

Aspelin et al (2003).

95) d. ***
Differentiation of renal cell from transitional cell carcinoma is helpful for planning surgical treatment since transitional cell carcinoma of the renal collecting system requires the more extensive surgical procedure of nephroureterectomy. Renal vein thrombus is seen with renal cell carcinoma while all other options given are features of transitional cell carcinoma of the kidney. Delayed contrast CT offers a pyelographic phase on which collecting system, ureter and bladder filling defects are clearly demonstrated. A urothelial field effect can occur, resulting in multiple transitional cell carcinomas throughout the renal tract. Renal cell carcinoma, as it expands, tends to distort the renal outline and is more likely to be peripheral and exophytic.

Dähnert (2007), 958, 979.

96) c. *****
Stauffer described a syndrome of nephrogenic hepatopathy in which a renal cancer without liver metastases causes hepatosplenomegaly and abnormal liver function. Renal cell carcinoma paraneoplastic phenomena include erythrocytosis and hypercalcaemia.

Dähnert (2007), 959.

97) b. ****
Two criteria are commonly used for assessing cancer response to treatment: WHO and RECIST. The latter stands for Response Evaluation Criteria in Solid Tumours, and it is this tool that is usually used in treatment trials. The WHO criteria compare a summed area product (longest axial dimension multiplied by the longest axial dimension perpendicular to this). RECIST sums the longest axial dimension and compares this across scans. Complete response for both

criteria is disappearance of disease, confirmed at 4 weeks. A partial response according to the WHO is 50% or more reduction in the summed area product following treatment and confirmed at 4 weeks. RECIST requires a 30% or greater decrease in the summed longest diameters, confirmed at 4 weeks. Progressive disease is defined as a 25% increase in summed area product for the WHO criteria and a 20% increase in summed longest diameter according to RECIST. Progressive disease also results from the appearance of any new site of disease. Stable disease reflects changes of magnitude that do not achieve partial response or progressive disease.

Therasse et al (2000).

98) a. ****
Alkaptonuria is the unifying diagnosis and is usually autosomal recessive. In this condition the absence of homogentisic acid oxidase causes accumulation of homogentisic acid, which is excreted in urine and sweat. Ochronotic deposition in the cardiovascular system causes atherosclerosis, aortic and mitral valve calcification, and myocardial infarction.

Chapman & Nakielny (2003), 533.

99) a. ****
In the pelvis, ^{18}FDG PET/CT is recommended for use in staging colorectal cancer, cervical cancer and non-Hodgkin's lymphoma. It is also indicated for detecting recurrence of colorectal, cervical, endometrial and ovarian cancers. It is not recommended for primary urothelial malignancy or prostate cancer. Usefulness is limited in the renal tract by urinary excretion of FDG. It is less than satisfactory in prostate cancer because of the poor sensitivity for osseous metastases.

Subhas et al (2005).

100) b. **
The puerperium is a hypercoagulable state, and puerperal endometritis can seed bacteria along the ovarian vein. Eighty per cent of thromboses are on the right and 14% are bilateral. Incidence is between 1 in 600 and 1 in 2000 deliveries. On contrast-enhanced CT, a tubular structure with low-density centre and peripheral enhancement is seen. Complications include inferior vena caval thrombosis, pulmonary embolus (25%), septicaemia, metastatic abscess formation and death (5%).

Dähnert (2007), 1056–7.

MODULE 5

PAEDIATRICS

1) A finding of bilateral meningiomas in a child suggests a diagnosis of which of the following phakomatoses?

   a. neurofibromatosis type 1
   b. neurofibromatosis type 2
   c. von Hippel−Lindau disease
   d. Sturge−Weber syndrome
   e. tuberous sclerosis

2) A 14-year-old boy who is a keen gymnast and fast bowler gives a history of several months of central low back pain that suddenly worsened during a game of cricket when he also developed bilateral shooting pains in his legs. There is no overt deformity on clinical examination, but lower back tenderness with generally restricted movement is noted. He undergoes radiographic, CT and MR imaging. What is the most likely radiological finding to explain the patient's current symptoms?

   a. herniated intervertebral disc
   b. discitis
   c. Scheuermann's disease
   d. spondylolysis
   e. spondylolisthesis

3) A 2-day-old, full-term baby boy is found to have a palpable abdominal mass during a routine examination. He is otherwise well. A plain abdominal radiograph demonstrates a well-defined, dense mass containing multiple calcifications in the right lower quadrant. What is the most likely diagnosis?

   a. neuroblastoma
   b. duplication cyst
   c. meconium peritonitis
   d. meconium ileus
   e. Hirschsprung's disease

4) A 3-year-old child with aniridia is found to have a palpable abdominal mass. The mass is shown to arise from a kidney and to contain cystic elements on ultrasound scan. No calcification is seen in the tumour on CT. Which of the following diagnoses is the most likely?

   a. renal cell carcinoma
   b. neuroblastoma
   c. angiomyolipoma
   d. Wilms' tumour
   e. ossifying renal tumour of infancy

5) A 6-month-old infant presents with irritability, joint swelling and flattened occiput. Radiographs of the limbs show bowing of the long bones, widened growth plates with cupped metaphyses and generalized osteopenia with coarse trabeculation seen throughout. A diagnosis of rickets is made. Which additional finding is likely to suggest hypophosphatasia as the underlying cause rather than primary vitamin D deficiency?

a. irregular poorly mineralized epiphyses
b. sclerotic rim to the epiphyses
c. lucent extensions into the metaphyses
d. fraying of the metaphyses
e. relatively normal mineralization

6) A 6-year-old boy presents with learning disability, seizures and a facial rash. MRI of the brain shows several cortical lesions with low signal on T1W and high signal on T2W images. They show no enhancement with administration of intravenous gadolinium. Low-signal subependymal nodules are identified on all sequences. Subsequent renal ultrasound scan demonstrates multiple, bilateral hyperechogenic lesions. What is the most likely diagnosis?

a. neurofibromatosis type I
b. Sturge–Weber syndrome
c. von Hippel–Lindau disease
d. tuberous sclerosis
e. metachromatic leukodystrophy

7) A neonate in neonatal intensive care has an abdominal film showing an umbilical arterial catheter (UAC) and an umbilical venous catheter (UVC), both in good position. Which of the following features would help to determine which catheter is which?

a. UAC is smaller in calibre
b. tip of the UAC lies at T8 level
c. UAC courses down into pelvis before approaching thorax
d. UVC is longer than UAC
e. UAC tip always lies to the left of tip of the UVC

8) A 5-year-old, previously well girl is found to have a palpable abdominal mass. Ultrasound scan demonstrates a 5 cm cystic lesion in the right upper quadrant. The wall of the lesion has an outer hypoechoic layer and an inner echogenic layer. The remainder of the abdomen appears normal. What is the most likely diagnosis?

a. Wilms' tumour
b. ovarian cyst
c. pancreatic pseudocyst
d. duplication cyst
e. choledochal cyst

9) A baby boy is investigated for renal failure. The imaging findings are of bladder distension and a posterior urethral valve, ureters measuring 10 mm in diameter bilaterally, undescended testes and widely separated abdominal rectus muscles. What is the most likely diagnosis?

a. prune-belly syndrome
b. primary vesicoureteric reflux
c. developmental aperistalsis of the distal ureter
d. neuropathic bladder
e. ureterocele

10) A 12-year-old boy with known Langerhans' cell histiocytosis presents with tachypnoea, cough and dyspnoea. A chest radiograph and then high-resolution CT are performed. What are the most likely findings?

a. bilateral, symmetrical consolidation
b. bronchiectasis
c. reticulonodular changes in mid-zones
d. bronchial wall thickening
e. bilateral hilar lymphadenopathy

11) A 2-year-old girl presents with respiratory distress following recent treatment for a chest infection that has been slow to resolve. A chest radiograph shows a large, well-defined mass in the lower right thorax. This comprises multiple cysts, with apparent hypoplasia of the ipsilateral lung, and is causing contralateral mediastinal shift. What is the most likely diagnosis?

a. bronchopulmonary sequestration
b. hypogenetic lung syndrome
c. congenital lobar emphysema
d. bronchogenic cyst
e. type I cystic adenomatoid malformation

12) A 2-year-old boy presents to his general practitioner with decreased visual acuity and pain in the left eye. Examination reveals a white light reflex (leukocoria) in the affected eye. Subsequent CT shows a retrolental, solid, lobulated, hyperdense mass with punctate calcification. The vitreous humour is abnormally dense. What is the most likely diagnosis?

a. orbital pseudoglioma
b. retrolental fibroplasia
c. retinoblastoma
d. Coats' disease
e. persistent hyperplastic primary vitreous

13) A newborn baby presents with coughing and choking during feeding. On examination, the baby is noted to drool excessively. Attempted passage of a feeding tube into the stomach is unsuccessful, and a chest radiograph shows the coiled feeding tube in the proximal oesophagus. An abdominal radiograph demonstrates gas within the stomach. What is the most likely diagnosis?

a. oesophageal atresia alone
b. oesophageal atresia and proximal tracheo-oesophageal fistula
c. oesophageal atresia and distal tracheo-oesophageal fistula
d. oesophageal atresia with proximal and distal tracheo-oesophageal fistulae
e. tracheo-oesophageal fistula without oesophageal atresia

14) A 3-day-old boy presents with respiratory distress without cyanosis. Clinically, there is reduced air entry in the right hemithorax with dull percussion note. A chest radiograph shows an opaque right hemithorax with mediastinal shift to the left. Ultrasound scan shows a large effusion, which aspiration demonstrates to be milky. What is the most likely cause?

a. idiopathic
b. birth trauma
c. lymphangioleiomyomatosis
d. thoracic duct atresia
e. lymphangiectasia

15) Of the following findings on a cervical spine radiograph in a 10-year-old child, which is abnormal in the context of a traumatic injury?

a. anterior wedging of the C3 vertebral body
b. anterolisthesis in flexion at C2–3
c. prevertebral soft-tissue thickness of 15 mm at C6
d. predental space of 6 mm in flexion
e. predental space of 3 mm in neutral

16) A newborn is found to have reduced air entry and breath sounds in the right hemithorax, but is otherwise well. A chest radiograph shows an opaque right hemithorax with ipsilateral mediastinal shift. Which feature on ventilation–perfusion scintigraphy would make the diagnosis of pulmonary hypoplasia more likely than complete collapse due to bronchial obstruction?

a. matched marked reduction in ventilation and perfusion
b. more marked reduction in perfusion than ventilation
c. more marked reduction in ventilation than perfusion
d. normal ventilation with reduced perfusion
e. normal perfusion with reduced ventilation

17) A 6-year-old girl is investigated for abdominal pain, jaundice and a palpable right upper quadrant mass. Ultrasound scan of the abdomen demonstrates a 5 cm cystic structure at the porta hepatis, which is separate from the normal gallbladder, and communicates with normal intrahepatic ducts. What is the most likely diagnosis?

a. biliary atresia
b. choledochal cyst
c. pancreatic pseudocyst
d. duodenal duplication cyst
e. pericholecystic abscess

18) A 3-year-old boy presents with fever, skin rash and abdominal pain. On examination, he has a maculopapular rash on the extensor surfaces, erythema of the oral mucosa, palms and soles, and multiple enlarged cervical lymph nodes. He is tender in the right upper quadrant. Abdominal ultrasound scan demonstrates a markedly enlarged gallbladder with a thin wall and a positive sonographic Murphy's sign is elicited. No gallstones are seen. What is the most likely diagnosis?

a. acute acalculous cholecystitis
b. acute gallbladder hydrops
c. choledochal cyst
d. acute calculous cholecystitis
e. emphysematous cholecystitis

19) A 7-year-old boy who has recently arrived in the country from south-east Asia presents with colicky abdominal pain. Blood tests show eosinophilia. He undergoes small bowel follow-through examination, which reveals multiple tubular filling defects in the small bowel averaging 20 cm in length, some of which contain a central, barium-filled canal. What is the most likely diagnosis?

a. ancylostomiasis (hookworm)
b. ascariasis (roundworm)
c. strongyloides infection
d. anisakiasis (herring worm disease)
e. taeniasis (tapeworm)

20) A 7-year-old boy presents with a 1-week history of a cough productive of green sputum. He is pyrexial with a mildly raised white cell count. Which feature on the chest radiograph would be more suggestive of bacterial pneumonia than viral pneumonia?

a. pleural effusion
b. peribronchial cuffing
c. atelectasis
d. airspace opacification
e. cavitation

21) A 10 year old presents with increasing dyspnoea on exertion. A chest radiograph shows dilatation of the left pulmonary artery with mural calcification. The right pulmonary artery and lungs are normal. An ECG shows right ventricular hypertrophy. What is the most likely diagnosis?

a. aneurysm of pulmonary artery
b. patent ductus arteriosus
c. right pulmonary atresia
d. pulmonary stenosis
e. Swyer–James syndrome

22) A 4-year-old boy is investigated for abnormal gait, with swelling and deformity of the right lower leg. Radiographs reveal epiphyseal irregularity and multiple abnormal ossifications around the medial portions of the distal femoral, and proximal and distal tibial epiphyses of the affected leg, with normal appearances of the lateral epiphyses and the whole of the contralateral lower limb. MRI demonstrates that the ossifications lie within the epiphyseal cartilage. What is the described condition?

a. hereditary multiple exostoses
b. Trevor's disease
c. Ollier's disease
d. Morquio's syndrome
e. warfarin embryopathy

23) MRI of the brain in a premature baby reveals ischaemic lesions adjacent to the trigone of the lateral ventricle. What is the most likely insult to have caused these appearances?

a. prolonged partial asphyxia
b. acute profound asphyxia
c. germinal matrix haemorrhage
d. rupture of a choroid plexus cyst
e. venous sinus thrombosis

24) Abdominal ultrasound is performed on a neonate on the high-dependency unit to investigate a palpable mass. A heterogeneous avascular suprarenal mass is identified. Cystic change and a peripheral hyperechoic rim develop over a series of scans. Which of the following is the most likely cause of the abdominal mass?

a. nephroblastoma
b. neuroblastoma
c. adrenal haematoma
d. phaeochromocytoma
e. myolipoma

25) A 6-year-old boy attends accident and emergency following an injury to his elbow. Radiographs show apparent ossification in the regions of the capitellum, radial head and trochlea, and there is marked soft-tissue swelling and a joint effusion. Which of the following is the most likely underlying injury?

  a. avulsed medial epicondyle
  b. avulsed lateral epicondyle
  c. avulsed olecranon
  d. supracondylar fracture
  e. fractured radial head

26) A 7-year-old boy presents with a painless, 2 cm midline mass in the neck just below the hyoid bone. This moves superiorly on protrusion of the tongue. Ultrasound scan shows a cystic lesion. What is the most likely diagnosis?

  a. branchial cleft cyst
  b. ectopic thyroid
  c. thyroglossal duct cyst
  d. obstructed laryngocele
  e. necrotic lymphadenopathy

27) What is the normal position of the duodenojejunal junction on frontal views during an upper gastrointestinal contrast examination?

  a. to the left of the left pedicles of the vertebral body at the level of the duodenal bulb
  b. to the left of the left pedicles below the level of the duodenal bulb
  c. overlying the vertebral body at the level of the duodenal bulb
  d. to the right of the right pedicles below the level of the duodenal bulb
  e. to the right of the right pedicles above the level of the duodenal bulb

28) A 5-year-old boy has recurrent urinary tract infection. A micturating cystourethrogram is performed, during which contrast from the bladder enters both ureters and reaches the pelvis and calyces bilaterally without any urinary tract dilatation. Of what grade is this vesicoureteric reflux?

  a. I
  b. II
  c. III
  d. IV
  e. V

29) In hyaline membrane disease, which is the first feature usually seen on a chest radiograph in the initial stages?

a. reduced lung volumes
b. bilateral consolidation
c. granularity in both lungs
d. pleural effusions
e. white-out of lungs

30) An 8-year-old boy has sudden-onset, severe, unilateral, testicular pain. What is the most likely cause?

a. torsion of appendix testis
b. torsion of appendix epididymis
c. torsion of testis
d. epididymitis
e. orchitis

31) Regarding reduction of intussusception in children, which of these is a feature of hydrostatic reduction using barium, rather than pneumatic reduction using air?

a. lower intracolonic pressures
b. faster reduction
c. higher successful reduction rate
d. less contamination of the peritoneal cavity
e. lower radiation dose

32) Of the choices below, which best describes the pattern of normal myelination of the brain in the first 9 months of life?

a. cranial to caudal, posterior to anterior, deep to superficial
b. cranial to caudal, anterior to posterior, deep to superficial
c. cranial to caudal, posterior to anterior, superficial to deep
d. caudal to cranial, posterior to anterior, deep to superficial
e. caudal to cranial, anterior to posterior, superficial to deep

33) A 4-year-old boy presents with a mixed endocrine syndrome of precocious puberty and cushingoid features. CT reveals a 10 cm mass replacing the left adrenal gland with cystic areas in keeping with haemorrhage and necrosis. The mass is continuous with the upper pole of the left kidney, which is expanded and has acquired the same CT appearance as the adrenal mass. No enlarged nodes or distant metastases are identified. Choose from the following the correct stage grouping:

a. I
b. II
c. III
d. IV
e. V

34) Ultrasound scan of the abdomen of a newborn girl reveals an abdominopelvic cyst. It is thin walled and anechoic, and has a 'daughter cyst'. Of the following which is the most likely diagnosis?

    a. Wilms' tumour
    b. ovarian cyst
    c. cystic lymphatic malformation
    d. choledochal cyst
    e. cystic teratoma

35) In a review of a paediatric skull radiograph that shows a generalized increase in bone density, which additional feature would suggest a diagnosis of pyknodysostosis rather than the more common osteopetrosis?

    a. premature closure of the anterior fontanelle
    b. multiple wormian bones
    c. insufficiency fractures
    d. sparing of the calvarium
    e. narrowing of the medulla

36) A 1-month-old girl has liquid discharge from the umbilicus. Which of the following provides a suitable explanation?

    a. vesicourachal diverticulum
    b. urachal cyst
    c. patent urachus
    d. bladder exstrophy–epispadias complex
    e. cloacal exstrophy

37) A female neonate develops respiratory distress. A radiograph of the chest shows a narrow chest with very short ribs that do not extend beyond the anterior axillary line, platyspondyly with curved vertebral bodies and short curved humeri. What is the described dysplasia?

    a. thanatophoric dysplasia
    b. asphyxiating thoracic dysplasia
    c. camptomelic dysplasia
    d. achondroplasia
    e. Ellis–van Creveld syndrome

38) Immature skeletons often break with a pattern that differs from the mature skeleton, with incomplete fractures and plastic bowing. What is the most important factor in the paediatric skeleton that accounts for this?

a. malleable bones
b. thick periosteum
c. loosely tethered periosteum
d. decreased bone mineral density
e. partially mineralized osteoid

39) A neonate with Down's syndrome presents with persistent bilious vomiting within a few hours of birth. An abdominal radiograph demonstrates a dilated, gas-filled stomach and duodenal bulb, with a total absence of gas in the small and large bowel. What is the most likely diagnosis?

a. Hirschsprung's disease
b. hypertrophic pyloric stenosis
c. duodenal atresia
d. duodenal duplication cyst
e. annular pancreas

40) At 6 months old, an infant with a cardiac murmur, learning disability, physical handicap, and abnormal facies is investigated after a urinary tract infection. Ultrasound scan reveals unilateral ureteric obstruction by an echo-bright focus in the bladder wall at the vesico-ureteric junction. On the same examination, a bladder diverticulum is also noticed. Choose the most likely unifying diagnosis.

a. Marfan's syndrome
b. Maffucci's syndrome
c. Morquio's syndrome
d. Williams' syndrome
e. Mikity–Wilson syndrome

41) At a 20-week, antenatal ultrasound scan, a fetus has a renal pelvis diameter measured at 7 mm unilaterally. When the scan is repeated at 35 weeks, the renal pelvis measures 12 mm. Which of the following is the most appropriate follow-up for the neonate?

a. discharge
b. ultrasound scan at 6 weeks
c. ultrasound scan within 24 hours of birth
d. micturating cystourethrogram soon after birth
e. ^{99m}Tc-labelled DMSA scan soon after birth

42) Which of the following findings on ultrasound examination of the hips in an 8-week-old child suggests the diagnosis of a concentrically located but unstable joint?

a. multiple epiphyseal ossification centres
b. alpha angle of 48°
c. beta angle of 55°
d. acetabular coverage of 50%
e. inverted acetabular labrum

43) A 10-year-old girl being treated for acute lymphoblastic leukaemia presents with a sudden onset of weakness. The leukocyte count is well below 100 000/mm^3, and the platelet count is well below 10 000/mm^3. Unenhanced CT brain is normal. Which of the following imaging techniques is most likely to demonstrate the cause of the signs?

a. post-contrast CT brain
b. CT venogram
c. MR venogram
d. DWI
e. gradient echo MRI

44) An 18-month-old girl has a cough. A chest radiograph shows consolidation in the right upper lobe. This is treated and a follow-up chest radiograph is performed, which shows a triangular-shaped mass arising from the mediastinum projecting over the right upper lobe. This has a rippled border. What is the most appropriate next investigation?

a. CT of chest
b. blood film
c. MR of chest
d. denatured red blood cell scintigraphy
e. no further investigation

45) What is the commonest chest radiograph finding seen in tetralogy of Fallot?

a. pulmonary plethora
b. bulging right heart border
c. concavity at the level of the pulmonary trunk
d. elevated cardiac apex
e. bulging of the superior left heart border

46) A 5-week-old boy presents with projectile vomiting. Examination of the abdomen is normal. He undergoes ultrasound scan of the abdomen, during which the following measurements are obtained: pyloric canal length of 18 mm, transverse pyloric diameter of 12 mm and pyloric muscle wall thickness of 3 mm. What is the most appropriate next step in management?

a. 24-hour pH probe monitoring
b. symptomatic management
c. pyloromyotomy
d. repeat ultrasound scan in 2–3 days
e. upper GI contrast examination

47) A 2-day-old, full-term, male neonate presents with failure to pass meconium. A water-soluble contrast enema demonstrates a dilated sigmoid colon with a narrowed, poorly distensible rectum and a persistent corrugated appearance to the rectal mucosa. What is the most likely diagnosis?

a. colonic atresia
b. meconium ileus
c. imperforate anus
d. Hirschsprung's disease
e. meconium plug syndrome

48) A 17-year-old girl presents with abdominal pain and rectal bleeding. She undergoes colonoscopy, which demonstrates multiple polypoid lesions in the colon. Which feature would favour a diagnosis of juvenile polyposis rather than familial adenomatous polyposis?

a. a total of 10 polyps in the colon
b. a histological diagnosis of tubulovillous polyps
c. involvement of the rectum
d. mucocutaneous pigmentation
e. a first-degree relative with multiple colonic polyps

49) A 7 year old presents with back pain, mild fever and leukocytosis. A plain film shows collapse of a lower thoracic vertebra with increased density. There is no kyphosis and disc spaces are preserved. The remaining bones are normal. What is the most likely diagnosis?

a. osteomyelitis
b. Ewing's sarcoma
c. eosinophilic granuloma
d. steroid usage
e. osteogenesis imperfecta

50) A 14-year-old girl is admitted following trauma and undergoes CT of the abdomen and pelvis. The large bowel is incidentally noted to lie on the left side of the abdomen, with the small intestine on the right. The superior mesenteric artery lies to the right of the superior mesenteric vein. What is the most likely diagnosis?

a. normal appearances
b. non-rotation
c. malrotation
d. reversed rotation
e. midgut volvulus

51) A 12-year-old girl presents with altered sensation in the upper and lower limbs. Clinical assessment demonstrates weakness of the lower limbs with reduced pain and temperature sensation. MRI shows syringohydromyelia and tonsillar ectopia of 7 mm with the fourth ventricle in normal position. No myelomeningocele is seen. What is the most likely diagnosis?

a. Chiari I malformation
b. Chiari II (Arnold–Chiari) malformation
c. Chiari III malformation
d. Dandy–Walker syndrome
e. diastematomyelia

52) Antenatal ultrasound scan performed at 31 weeks' gestational age shows hydrops, for which there is no identifiable immunological cause. The scan also demonstrates cardiac enlargement and hydrocephalus. Which of the following is the most likely associated ultrasound finding?

a. unilateral megalencephaly
b. renal cysts
c. aberrant right subclavian artery
d. cerebral median tubular cystic space with high-velocity, colour Doppler flow
e. retinal tumour

53) At 18 months old, a child is seen in the accident and emergency department for a first seizure. On examination, there are cutaneous bruises and burns. Radiographs reveal posterior rib and long bone fractures of varying ages. Which of the following is the most likely finding on CT of the brain?

a. epidural haematoma
b. subdural haematoma
c. subarachnoid haemorrhage
d. acute cerebral contusion
e. cortical tubers

54) A 12-year-old boy is investigated for abdominal pain. On ultrasound scan, there are large, echo-free, septated, cystic collections around both kidneys causing scalloping of the renal outline. On CT, these collections are close to water density. Which of the following is the most likely diagnosis?

a. renal lymphangiectasia
b. bilateral Wilms' tumours
c. bilateral adrenal neuroblastoma
d. bilateral hydronephrosis
e. medullary sponge kidney

55) A 15-year-old female, whose father had progressive renal failure, presents with anaemia, polyuria and haematuria. On ultrasound scan, her kidneys are small and smooth. Which associated finding is most likely?

a. pancreatic cysts
b. posterior fossa haemangioblastoma
c. cystocele
d. nerve deafness
e. hypertension

56) A neonate presents with respiratory distress shortly after birth. A chest radiograph shows hazy opacification in the left upper zone, which improves over the next 7 days, and the chest radiograph becomes normal. Two months later, the baby re-presents with respiratory distress, and a chest radiograph shows hyperlucency in the left upper zone with contralateral mediastinal shift and compression of the adjacent left lower lobe. What is the likely diagnosis?

a. congenital lobar emphysema
b. Macleod's syndrome
c. bronchiolitis obliterans
d. foreign body
e. carcinoid

57) A 6-year-old boy presents with lower gastrointestinal bleeding. He undergoes a [^{99m}Tc]-pertechnetate study, which demonstrates a small focal area of increased activity in the right lower quadrant 5 minutes after tracer injection, which increases in intensity with time paralleling the activity of the stomach. What is the most likely diagnosis?

a. Meckel's diverticulum
b. appendicitis
c. duodenal duplication cyst
d. intussusception
e. peptic ulcer disease

58) A full-term baby boy born to a diabetic mother presents during the first day of life with abdominal distension and failure to pass meconium. Plain abdominal radiograph demonstrates a dilated, meconium-filled, proximal colon to the level of the splenic flexure, with an empty descending colon, sigmoid and rectum. Administration of a water-soluble enema results in passage of meconium, and the baby is discharged well 2 days later. What is the most likely diagnosis?

a. intussusception
b. Hirschsprung's disease
c. meconium plug syndrome
d. meconium ileus
e. ileal atresia

59) A 3-year-old boy presents with a cough of 1 week's duration. There is no relevant preceding history. A chest radiograph shows lucency in the right lower zone, and an expiratory film demonstrates air trapping in the same region as well as mediastinal shift to the left. No masses are seen. What is the likely diagnosis?

a. foreign body aspiration
b. congenital lobar emphysema
c. congenital cystic adenomatoid malformation type I
d. bronchiolitis obliterans
e. bronchogenic cyst

60) A 2-year-old girl is admitted with abdominal pain and vomiting. No history of trauma is provided. On examination, she is tachycardic and has upper abdominal tenderness. Ultrasound scan of the abdomen demonstrates an echogenic intramural mass in the duodenum in keeping with an intramural haematoma. There is mild proximal dilatation of the duodenum and a small amount of free fluid within the abdomen. What is the most likely underlying cause?

a. duodenal diverticulum
b. haemophilia
c. pancreatitis
d. Henoch–Schönlein purpura
e. non-accidental injury

61) A 7-year-old boy is admitted with colicky abdominal pain and rectal bleeding. He is noted to have a purpuric skin rash on the extensor surfaces of his arms and legs. What are the most likely findings on CT of the abdomen?

a. multifocal bowel wall thickening
b. multiple small polyps in the colon
c. focal outpouching of the distal ileum
d. inflammatory changes at the terminal ileum
e. dilatation of the small bowel

62) A 10-year-old boy is brought to accident and emergency after falling on his bike and sustaining a blunt abdominal injury by impacting the handlebars. CT shows free intraperitoneal fluid with a more focal collection of fluid at the mesenteric root. Additional findings of mesenteric stranding and focal bowel wall thickening are seen. There is diffuse homogeneous hyperattenuation of the pancreas, kidneys and bowel wall. What is the most likely underlying injury?

a. mesenteric rupture
b. bowel perforation
c. splenic rupture
d. renal contusion
e. pancreatic contusion

63) A 12-year-old presents with increasing back pain over 2 weeks associated with malaise. He has mild pyrexia. Plain films of the lumbar spine show reduced disc space between the second and third lumbar vertebrae with loss of clarity of the endplates. What investigation would be most likely to help make the diagnosis?

a. CT
b. MRI
c. bone scan
d. labelled white cell scan
e. gallium scan

64) A 10 month old presents with recurrent chest infections, the most recent caused by *Pseudomonas aeruginosa*. The chest radiograph shows patchy infiltrates in the right base. Which feature on high-resolution CT would make the diagnosis of cystic fibrosis more likely than Williams–Campbell syndrome?

a. cystic bronchiectasis
b. emphysematous bullae
c. mucus plugging
d. lower lobe involvement
e. pleural effusions

65) A frontal radiograph of the pelvis in a child demonstrates flaring of the iliac wings with flattening of the acetabular roof and decreased acetabular and iliac angles giving an abnormal iliac index. There is associated elongation and tapering of the ischia. These are pelvic features of which condition?

   a. achondroplasia
   b. osteodysplasty
   c. Down's syndrome
   d. mucopolysaccharidosis
   e. fibrous dysplasia

66) During a routine new-baby check, a unilateral, firm, tense, non-pitting, parietal mass is noticed. Ultrasound scan demonstrates a crescent-shaped lesion adjacent to the outer table of the skull. The mass is most likely to be which of the following?

   a. caput succedaneum
   b. cephalocele
   c. cephalhaematoma
   d. leptomeningeal cyst
   e. fibrous dysplasia

67) Hyperechoic lesions are seen within the brain of a preterm neonate during a cranial ultrasound scan. Of the following, which most strongly suggests that the appearances are due to germinal matrix haemorrhage rather than periventricular leukomalacia?

   a. the baby is premature
   b. the hyperechoic changes are anterior to the caudothalamic groove
   c. the hyperechoic changes are adjacent to the trigone of the lateral ventricle
   d. cystic changes follow the acute phase in the affected brain
   e. there was no birth trauma

68) On plain radiographs of paediatric long bones, osteomalacia may manifest as all but which of the following?

   a. Looser's zones
   b. bowing
   c. insufficiency fracture
   d. generalized osteopenia
   e. increased trabeculae

69) Which of the following conditions is the most common underlying aetiology for intussusception in childhood?

   a. viral gastroenteritis
   b. Meckel's diverticulum
   c. Henoch–Schönlein purpura
   d. duplication cyst
   e. small bowel polyp

70) A 15-year-old girl with a history of multiple febrile convulsions as an infant presents to the neurologist with complex partial seizures. The episodes start with special and somatosensory aura followed by a wide-eyed stare with behavioural arrest, before finally proceeding to a generalized tonic-clonic seizure. MR imaging is requested. Which sequence is best to evaluate the temporal lobes for signs of mesial temporal sclerosis?

   a. axial T1W
   b. axial T2W
   c. axial FLAIR
   d. coronal T1W
   e. coronal T2W

71) A 14-year-old, overweight boy is seen in orthopaedic clinic with a 3-week history of left hip pain and reduced range of movement. Radiographs show mild proximal femoral osteopaenia, an ill-defined area of increased opacity in the proximal metaphysis, widening of the growth plate, and a small epiphysis. What is the most likely diagnosis?

   a. irritable hip
   b. Perthes' disease
   c. slipped upper femoral epiphysis
   d. septic arthritis
   e. insufficiency fracture

72) An asymptomatic, 15-month-old girl is brought to the emergency department following witnessed ingestion of a hearing aid battery. A junior casualty officer asks for your advice about whether the patient requires imaging. What is the most appropriate imaging strategy?

   a. reassurance that imaging is not indicated
   b. patient to return for imaging if battery not passed within 48 hours
   c. abdominal radiograph (and chest radiograph if abdominal radiograph negative)
   d. ultrasound scan of the abdomen
   e. patient to be referred straight for endoscopic removal

73) An incidental finding made in a 13-year-old girl is of unilateral ovarian atrophy. The atrophic ovary has stippled calcification. Given these features, which is the most likely explanation?

   a. ovarian teratoma
   b. amputated ovary
   c. follicular ovarian cyst
   d. ovarian leiomyoma
   e. ovarian vein thrombosis

74) A neonate is delivered following an uncomplicated pregnancy and presents with respiratory distress but no cyanosis. No resuscitation or ventilation is required. A chest radiograph shows a pneumothorax, which is treated by aspiration. What investigation should be considered?

   a. cranial ultrasound scan
   b. renal ultrasound scan
   c. abdominal radiograph
   d. barium swallow
   e. ascending urethrogram

75) Which of the following features on ultrasound scan is most suggestive of a horseshoe kidney?

   a. unilateral upper pole calyx dilatation
   b. unilateral lower pole calyx dilatation
   c. bilateral upper pole calyx dilatation
   d. laterally oriented renal long axis
   e. medially oriented renal long axis

76) What type of fracture is the most commonly seen in the presentation of non-accidental injury in a child?

   a. diaphyseal transverse
   b. metaphyseal corner
   c. posterior ribs
   d. skull vault
   e. vertebral body wedge

77) A 30-week premature baby is delivered normally and shortly after birth develops tachypnoea and expiratory grunting. What feature on the chest radiograph would make respiratory distress syndrome of the newborn more likely than meconium aspiration syndrome?

   a. bilateral consolidation
   b. pneumothorax
   c. pleural effusion
   d. air bronchograms
   e. hyperinflation with air trapping

78) Germinal matrix haemorrhage is identified on a cranial ultrasound scan of a neonate. Which of the following imaging features confers the worst prognosis?

   a. subependymal haemorrhage
   b. intraventricular haemorrhage
   c. intraventricular haemorrhage with ventricular dilatation
   d. intraparenchymal haemorrhage
   e. choroid plexus pulsation

79) On antenatal ultrasound scan, oligohydramnios, non-visualization of the urinary bladder and bilateral enlarged hyperechoic kidneys are recorded. Renal failure ensues within the first month of life. An older sibling aged 5 years has established portal hypertension. The parents are phenotypically normal. What are the odds of further offspring of the same parents having the same disease?

   a. zero
   b. I in 5
   c. I in 4
   d. I in 2
   e. unity

80) A 3-week-old baby boy born at full term presents with persistent jaundice. Clinical examination demonstrates hepatomegaly, and blood tests confirm hyperbilirubinaemia. He undergoes pheno-barbital-augmented ^{99m}Tc-labelled IDA (iminodiacetic acid) cho-lescintigraphy, which demonstrates good hepatic activity within 5 minutes but no biliary clearance into the bowel on delayed images at 24 hours. What is the most likely diagnosis?

   a. biliary atresia
   b. neonatal hepatitis
   c. cystic fibrosis
   d. choledochal cyst
   e. physiological jaundice

81) Which of the following sites is not typical of an avulsion fracture in a child?

   a. anterior inferior iliac spine
   b. ischial tuberosity
   c. tibial spine
   d. medial epicondyle
   e. radial head

82) A 13-year-old male presents with recurrent epistaxis. CT shows a highly vascular mass in the nasopharynx, with widening of the pterygopalatine fossa and invasion of the sphenoid sinus. Which arterial branch is the feeding vessel likely to be arising from?

   a. ascending pharyngeal
   b. facial artery
   c. superficial temporal artery
   d. internal maxillary artery
   e. internal carotid artery

83) A term neonate whose birth per vaginum was notably protracted has an MRI of the brain at age 4 days. There are changes in keeping with hypoxic ischaemic encephalopathy. Affected areas are marked by T1 shortening without T2 signal change. Which of the following is the most likely explanation for this pattern of abnormal signal?

   a. high T2 signal is masked by a high degree of myelination
   b. high T2 signal is masked by a low degree of myelination
   c. high T1 signal is accentuated by a high degree of myelination
   d. high T1 signal is accentuated by a low degree of myelination
   e. low T1 signal is masked by a high degree of myelination

84) Radiographs of the lower limbs in a child show bilateral bowing of the femora and tibiae with genu varum. Additional findings of generalized osteopenia, deficient trabeculation, multiple fractures and cortical thinning suggest which underlying cause?

   a. rickets
   b. Blount's disease
   c. osteogenesis imperfecta
   d. neurofibromatosis
   e. yaws

85) Craniosynostosis of the sagittal suture of the skull results in which skull vault shape abnormality?

   a. brachycephaly
   b. scaphocephaly
   c. trigonocephaly
   d. oxycephaly
   e. plagiocephaly

86) A 2-year-old boy presents with jaundice, abdominal pain and precocious puberty. Ultrasound scan of the abdomen reveals a heterogeneous, hyperechoic, 10 cm mass with areas of coarse calcification in the right lobe of the liver. What is the most likely diagnosis?

    a. hepatocellular carcinoma
    b. hepatoblastoma
    c. haemangioma
    d. pyogenic abscess
    e. choledochal cyst

87) Which of the following would be regarded as abnormal during ultrasound scan of the kidneys in a neonate?

    a. echogenicity of the renal cortex similar to that of liver
    b. large hyperechoic medullary pyramids
    c. paucity of renal sinus fat
    d. lobulated renal contour
    e. echogenic septum at anterosuperior margin of the kidney

88) From the following renal and adrenal findings, choose that which favours a diagnosis of neurofibromatosis type 1 above von Hippel–Lindau syndrome or tuberous sclerosis.

    a. renal cysts
    b. renal cell carcinoma
    c. phaeochromocytoma
    d. renal artery aneurysm
    e. angiomyolipoma

89) A 12 year old presents with a painless swelling in the right side of his neck, at the angle of the mandible. Ultrasound scan shows a cystic lesion with internal debris. CT confirms a cystic lesion with a beak of tissue pointing between the internal and external carotid arteries. What is the most likely diagnosis?

    a. cystic hygroma
    b. abscess
    c. branchial cleft cyst
    d. carotid body tumour
    e. lymphadenopathy

90) An 8-year-old boy with a 3-month history of increasing chest wall pain presents with a tender lump on the chest wall. Imaging of the chest shows a large inhomogeneous mass arising from a rib with a large intrathoracic component and preservation of tissue planes. There is associated rib destruction and a lamellated periosteal reaction is seen. What is the most likely diagnosis?

a. Ewing's sarcoma
b. neuroblastoma
c. Hodgkin's disease
d. osteomyelitis
e. hamartoma of chest wall

91) Which of the following injuries is one that is not suggestive of non-accidental injury in a 2-year-old boy?

a. metaphyseal corner fracture
b. lateral rib fractures
c. posterior rib fracture
d. spiral tibial fracture
e. depressed occipital fracture

92) An 8-year-old girl presents with back pain. Clinically, there is a double-curve scoliosis convex to the left in the thoracic region and to the right in the lumbar region. There is no focal neurology. MRI shows the conus behind the L3 vertebral body, and the filum terminale is 3 mm in thickness at the L5–S1 level. A high-signal lesion is seen on T1W and T2W images in the canal behind the L5 and S1 vertebral bodies. What is the most likely diagnosis?

a. diastematomyelia
b. meningocele
c. syringomyelia
d. tethered cord
e. developmental scoliosis

93) A 3-week-old girl presents with congestive cardiac failure and is found to have hepatomegaly on examination. Ultrasound scan of the abdomen shows an ill-defined, complex, heterogeneous, 5 cm mass in the right lobe of the liver containing multiple vascular channels on Doppler ultrasound scan. What is the most likely diagnosis?

a. infantile haemangioendothelioma
b. hepatoblastoma
c. cavernous haemangioma
d. mesenchymal hamartoma
e. hepatocellular carcinoma

94) A 15-year-old boy presents to accident and emergency with signs of meningitis but no pyrexia. CT and MRI show a retroclival midline cystic tumour with localized mass effect. Which feature would support the diagnosis of a dermoid rather than an epidermoid cyst?

a. restricted diffusion on DWI
b. no enhancement with intravenous gadolinium on MRI
c. multiple septations on either modality
d. focal low attenuation on CT
e. well-defined calcifications on CT

95) An 11-year-old boy presents with fever, vomiting and right lower quadrant pain. Ultrasound scan of the right lower quadrant demonstrates a blind-ending, compressible, fluid-filled, tubular structure measuring 4 mm in diameter, as well as enlarged mesenteric lymph nodes and several thickened loops of small bowel. What is the most likely diagnosis?

a. acute appendicitis
b. mesenteric lymphadenitis
c. Crohn's disease
d. Meckel's diverticulum
e. enteric duplication cyst

96) A 16-year-old female with a history of imperforate anus corrected soon after birth is investigated for primary amenorrhoea. Ultrasound scan shows the uterus and upper vagina distended by moderately echogenic material. Which of the following is the most likely cause of the amenorrhoea?

a. longitudinal vaginal septum
b. transverse vaginal septum
c. cervical dysgenesis
d. obstructed uterine horn
e. endometritis

97) An 11-year-old boy falls at school and lands on his outstretched arm. He complains of elbow pain and is taken to accident and emergency, where radiographs show no fracture but elevation of the anterior humeral fat pad and a visible posterior fat pad. What is the most likely occult injury?

a. supracondylar fracture
b. radial head fracture
c. medial epicondyle avulsion
d. lateral epicondyle avulsion
e. articular chondral fracture

98) A 4-month-old boy presents with cyanosis. Examination reveals right ventricular heave and systolic murmur. A chest radiograph shows a bulging right heart border and widening of the superior mediastinum, creating a 'snowman' appearance. What is the most likely diagnosis?

a. Fallot's tetralogy
b. total anomalous pulmonary venous return
c. partial anomalous pulmonary venous return
d. transposition of the great vessels
e. coarctation of the aorta

99) A 9-year-old boy with leukaemia and severe neutropenia presents with right lower quadrant abdominal pain and bloody diarrhoea. CT of the abdomen demonstrates circumferential thickening of the caecum with decreased bowel wall attenuation and pericolonic inflammatory changes. What is the most likely diagnosis?

a. appendicitis
b. typhlitis
c. leukaemic infiltration of the bowel
d. diverticulitis
e. Crohn's disease

100) A preterm male infant develops abdominal distension and blood-stained stools 2 days after birth. Plain abdominal radiograph shows distended and thickened bowel loops with curvilinear gas collections within the bowel wall. What is the most likely diagnosis?

a. necrotizing enterocolitis
b. Hirschsprung's disease
c. meconium ileus
d. imperforate anus
e. viral gastroenteritis

Module 5: Paediatrics: Answers

1) b. ***

The phakomatoses are neuroectodermal disorders with skin and central nervous system manifestations. Neurofibromatosis type 2 (central neurofibromatosis) accounts for only 10% of cases, type 1 accounting for 90%. Although the hallmark finding of type 2 is bilateral acoustic schwannomas, multiple meningiomas, particularly in a child, should bring the diagnosis to mind. A mnemonic for remembering the associations is MISME (multiple inherited schwannomas, meningiomas and ependymomas), and tumours may be seen in the brain or spinal cord. In the spine, multiple nerve sheath tumours are often located in the cauda equina. Skin manifestations are seen relatively infrequently, unlike in the more common type 1.

Dähnert (2007), 319.

2) e. ***

Back pain in adults is common and most frequently non-specific. In contrast, back pain in children is less common and often caused by a serious underlying condition. Spondylolysis is a defect in the pars interarticularis, the weakest part of the vertebra, and is an acquired condition even in childhood, where it is usually due to repetitive microtrauma in athletically active children. In isolation, it does not cause neurological symptoms, but bilateral defects can allow slippage of one vertebra over another, creating an abnormality of alignment, a spondylolisthesis. Disc herniation in children is rare and occurs as a result of a traumatic event rather than degeneration. It is usually lateral. Scheuermann's disease is associated with a kyphotic deformity.

Afshani & Kuhn (1991).

3) c. ****

Meconium peritonitis is a chemical peritonitis that occurs *in utero* following perforation of bowel as a result of bowel obstruction or ischaemia. Most commonly, the perforation seals off *in utero*, but the extruded meconium may be palpable as an abdominal mass, or may become calcified and therefore visible on plain film as a dense calcified mass or as calcific plaques throughout the peritoneal cavity. It may also be identified on ultrasound scan as echogenic material between bowel loops with a 'snowstorm' appearance. In other cases, active perforation is still present at birth, and the baby presents with clinical peritonitis. Meconium ileus may result in abdominal calcifications in the neonate, but these are intramural in location. Hirschsprung's disease and other causes of intestinal obstruction may be associated with intraluminal calcifications in the neonate. Neuroblastoma is frequently associated with calcification, but is suprarenal in location and usually symptomatic. Duplication cysts are not usually associated with calcification.

Chapman & Nakielny (2003), 221; Dähnert (2007), 856.

4) d. ***
Wilms' tumour is the commonest renal tumour of childhood. Seventy-five per cent occur in children under 5 years, 5–10% are bilateral and 10% are multifocal. Calcification is seen in less than 15%. Nephroblastomatosis is a precursor, and the disease is associated with the *WT1* and *WT2* genes of chromosome 11. The *WT1* abnormal gene is found in the WAGR syndrome of Wilms' tumour, aniridia, genitourinary abnormalities and learning disability. It is also found in the DRASH syndrome of male pseudohermaphroditism and progressive glomerulonephritis. The abnormal *WT2* gene is found with the Beckwith–Wiedemann syndrome and hemihypertrophy.

Weissleder et al (2007), 865–6.

5) c. *****
Rickets is osteomalacia occurring in an immature skeleton, resulting in poorly mineralized osteoid and bone softening. The fundamental deficiency is of the active form of vitamin D (1,25-dihydroxycholecalciferol), which is required for normal osteoid mineralization. Dietary vitamin D (7-dehydrocholesterol) is converted in the skin to cholecalciferol (vitamin D$_3$) by sunlight. In the liver, cholecalciferol is hydroxylated to 25-hydroxycholecalciferol by the enzyme 25-hydroxylase; this is then further converted into the active form of vitamin D in the kidney. Abnormality anywhere in this pathway can lead to rickets, and its causes include dietary deficiency (most common), lack of sunlight, and renal or liver disease. Phosphate has a significant influence in the regulation of vitamin D metabolism, and hypophosphataemia is noted in many cases of vitamin D-refractory rickets. Hypophosphatasia is a rare inherited metabolic disorder of decreased tissue non-specific alkaline phosphatase causing defective bone mineralization, which is refractory to vitamin D treatment. It resembles rickets radiologically, with irregular, poorly mineralized epiphyses with a sclerotic rim and metaphyseal fraying. However, in hypophosphatasia, associated irregular lucent extensions into the metaphyses representing uncalcified bone matrix are characteristic, allowing differentiation from rickets.

Resnick & Kransdorf (2005), 569.

6) d. ***
Tuberous sclerosis is a member of the phakomatoses, a group of neuroectodermal disorders characterized by coexistence of skin and central nervous system tumours. The classic clinical triad of seizures, learning disability and adenoma sebaceum (a facial rash) is seen in approximately half of presenting patients. Imaging findings seen on MRI

and sometimes CT are periventricular nodules, which often calcify, and 'cortical tubers', which represent brain parenchymal hamartomas. These lesions are low signal on T1 and high signal on T2W images, and typically do not enhance. Enhancement of a lesion suggests associated giant cell astrocytoma, which is most commonly seen at the foramen of Monro, where it may obstruct, causing hydrocephalus. Common associations are renal angiomyolipoma, bone abnormalities and spontaneous pneumothorax.

Altman et al (1988).

7) c. ****
The UAC passes along the umbilical artery to the internal iliac artery, from which it arises. It then passes up the common iliac artery into the aorta. The UVC passes up the umbilical vein to the left portal vein, through the ductus venosus, into the middle or left hepatic vein and into the inferior vena cava. The tips of the catheters may vary in position, but ideal placement of the UVC is around the T8–9 level, with high placement of the UAC being at the T7–9 level. The tip of the UVC may lie on either side of the UAC depending on whether it reaches the inferior vena cava or remains in the left lobe of the liver. The UAC and UVC are usually of the same diameter. Their length is determined by their course, and is not a reliable predictor in identifying whether the catheter is arterial or venous.

Hogan (1999).

8) d. ***
Gastrointestinal duplication cysts account for 15% of paediatric abdominal masses. They most commonly arise from the small bowel and colon and, although usually asymptomatic, those that contain ectopic gastric or pancreatic tissue may present with ulceration or haemorrhage. Contrast studies are not useful for diagnosis, as most cysts do not communicate with the bowel lumen. Ultrasound scan is the most appropriate technique and demonstrates a simple anechoic cyst with a characteristic two-layered wall, representing the inner echogenic mucosa and the outer hypoechoic muscle. These appearances are characteristic of bowel wall, and help to distinguish a duplication cyst from other cystic lesions such as ovarian cyst, which are typically thin walled. Pancreatic pseudocyst is unlikely in the absence of previous episodes of pancreatitis.

Brant & Helms (2007), 321.

9) a. ***
(a) to (e) are all causes of a megaureter – that is, a ureter over 7 mm in diameter. The hallmark of prune-belly syndrome is a distended bladder, and it is associated with posterior urethral valves. Bladder distension causes the triad of widely spaced abdominal rectus muscles,

hydroureteronephrosis and cryptorchidism. The last occurs because the large bladder interferes with testicular descent.

Berrocal et al (2002).

10) c. ****

Langerhans' cell histiocytosis presents with features similar to adults in children over 10 years. Typically, there are reticular/reticulonodular changes that progress to cysts and honeycombing. These predominate in the upper zones and mid-zones with sparing of the costophrenic angles. The diagnosis is made by the characteristic radiographic and clinical findings. Bronchoalveolar lavage or biopsy may be necessary if the diagnosis is in doubt.

Kilborn et al (2003).

11) e. ***

Cystic adenomatoid malformation (CAM) is a congenital cystic abnormality of the lung. There are three types: I – single/multiple large cysts of >20 mm; II – multiple cysts of 5–12 mm; III – solitary mass with microcysts. If undetected *in utero*, they usually present in the first year with respiratory distress and cyanosis, but can present later with recurrent infections. In type I CAM, the chest radiograph shows an expansile mass with multiple air- or fluid-filled cysts, with compression or hypoplasia of ipsilateral lung and contralateral mediastinal shift. Extra-lobar bronchopulmonary sequestration produces a wedge-shaped mass, usually posteromedially in either lung. Bronchogenic cysts are usually well-defined soft-tissue masses arising from the mediastinum and often present later in life. Hypogenetic lung syndrome produces a small hemithorax with reduced vascularity rather than a mass. Congenital lobar emphysema produces overinflation of one, or occasionally two, lobes, with hyperlucency. This may be mass like at birth due to delayed clearance of fluid.

Dähnert (2007), 487–8.

12) c. ***

Retinoblastoma is a highly malignant primary ocular tumour of childhood occurring in sporadic and heritable form and arising from primitive photoreceptor cells of the retina (in the group of primitive neuroectodermal tumours). It is the most serious intraocular process in a child, and calcification in a paediatric orbit must be considered to represent retinoblastoma until proved otherwise. Once tumour extends beyond the orbit, mortality rate is virtually 100%. Heritable forms are often multifocal in a single orbit or bilateral. Trilateral retinoblastoma is bilateral orbital tumours and associated pineoblastoma.

Hopper et al (1992).

13) c. ****

Oesophageal atresia is suspected when a newborn baby presents with drooling, and is confirmed on a chest radiograph by the presence of a gas-distended, proximal oesophageal pouch, or a coiled feeding tube within the pouch. Absence of gas in the abdomen on an abdominal radiograph implies oesophageal atresia either alone or with a proximal fistula. However, gas within the abdomen implies the presence of a distal tracheo-oesophageal fistula. Occasionally, there may be both proximal and distal tracheo-oesophageal fistulae, but this situation is rare, accounting for only 1% of patients, as opposed to around 80% with distal fistula alone. Oesophageal atresia and tracheo-oesophageal fistula may be part of the VACTERL association, which includes vertebral, anorectal, cardiovascular, tracheo-oesophageal fistula, renal and limb anomalies.

Dähnert (2007), 816–18.

14) a. ****

Chylothoraces in neonates are usually right sided, and in most cases no obvious cause is found. Treatment is conservative with special formula and intermittent aspiration. All of the listed conditions are causes of chylothorax, but lymphangioleiomyomatosis presents in adult females and not in the neonatal period.

Alford & McIlhenny (1999).

15) d. **

The maximum predental space is 2.5–3 mm in an adult and 5 mm in a child. Any widening suggests injury to the alar ligamentous complex in the context of trauma. Other causes of widening are Down's syndrome, rheumatoid arthritis, neurofibromatosis and osteogenesis imperfecta. Anterior wedging of C3 and pseudosubluxation at C2–3 and C3–4 are within normal limits in children. Additionally, prevertebral soft tissues can be greater than in the adult, certainly up to 100% of the anteroposterior dimension of the vertebral body at the C6 level.

Lustrin et al (2003).

16) a. ***

Pulmonary hypoplasia is the presence of a completely formed but congenitally small bronchus with rudimentary parenchyma and vessels. This produces a matched marked reduction in ventilation and perfusion or, in severe cases, complete absence of both ventilation and perfusion. In total lung collapse, the ventilation would be reduced or absent with often reduced, but better, perfusion.

Dähnert (2007), 501.

17) b. ***

Choledochal cyst is a congenital condition characterized by aneurysmal dilatation of the common bile duct, which in the majority of cases is associated with an anomalous junction of the common bile duct and pancreatic duct, allowing reflux of pancreatic enzymes into the common bile duct and resulting in weakening of the wall. The most common type (type I) is a localized dilatation of the common bile duct below the cystic duct. Communication with the common hepatic or intrahepatic ducts is demonstrated, and intrahepatic ducts are usually not dilated. Biliary atresia presents in the neonatal period with jaundice. Typical findings include an echogenic triangular structure at the porta, representing the atretic biliary plate, and a small or non-visualized gallbladder. Pancreatic pseudocyst and duodenal duplication cyst do not communicate with the biliary tree. A pericholecystic abscess would be unlikely in the presence of a normal gallbladder.

Dähnert (2007), 703–4.

18) b. ****

Kawasaki's syndrome is an acute multisystem vasculitis with a predilection for the coronary arteries, generally affecting children under 5 years of age. As well as skin, joint and cardiovascular manifestations, patients may develop acute hydrops of the gallbladder, probably caused by transient obstruction of the cystic duct. Ultrasound scan demonstrates a markedly enlarged and tender gallbladder with a thin wall. Acute acalculous cholecystitis may be seen in children in the high dependency or intensive care setting, especially with septicaemia and trauma, but it usually results in gallbladder wall thickening and less marked gallbladder dilatation. Choledochal cyst (aneurysmal dilatation of the common bile duct) is seen as a fusiform cyst beneath the porta hepatis separate from the gallbladder. Acute calculous cholecystitis is associated with gallstones within a thickened gallbladder wall. Emphysematous cholecystitis usually occurs in adults over 50, and gas is seen as arc-like, high-level echoes outlining the gallbladder wall.

Brant & Helms (2007), 1316.

19) b. ****

Ascariasis is the most common parasitic infection worldwide, predominantly affecting children aged 1–10 years. Worms mature in the small bowel and may be identified on plain films as tubular soft-tissue densities or on barium studies as linear or coiled filling defects of 15–35 cm in length. Barium ingested by the worms causes opacification of their central linear enteric canals. Patients may present with abdominal pain, appendicitis and haematemesis; occasionally, a bolus of worms may cause small bowel obstruction. Tapeworms may also appear as linear filling defects, but are usually much longer, reaching many feet in length. In addition, tapeworms have no alimentary canal and do not ingest barium. Hookworms measure 8–13 mm and cannot be visualized on barium studies. Anisakiasis of the small intestine usually appears radiologically as bowel wall thickening and luminal narrowing. Strongyloides infection may manifest as fold thickening and effacement, with a pipestem appearance of the jejunum in advanced cases.

Herlinger et al (1999), 291–5; Dähnert (2007), 805.

20) e. ***
Bacterial pneumonia is a combination of airway and alveolar disease, whereas viral pneumonia tends to affect airways and peribronchial tissues. Bacterial pneumonia produces two patterns of disease: lobar (consolidation, no volume loss, usually in one lobe, may cavitate) or bronchopneumonic (patchy airspace change which enlarges and coalesces, and volume loss due to mucus plugging). Viral pneumonia tends to produce peribronchial linear densities and an interstitial pattern, though airspace change may be seen in up to 50% of cases. Hilar adenopathy is not often seen, but effusions are present in 20% of cases. Pneumatoceles, pneumothorax and cavitation do not occur. Viral pneumonia may sometimes be complicated by bacterial pneumonia.

Sutton (2002), 131–3, 136; Dähnert (2007), 411–12.

21) d. *****
Pulmonary stenosis is often asymptomatic, but it presents when there is a high gradient across the pulmonary valve. There is dilatation of the pulmonary trunk and left pulmonary artery (post-stenotic dilatation), but the right pulmonary artery is unaffected, as the jet preferentially enters the left pulmonary artery. Calcification of the pulmonary arterial wall is highly suggestive. Pulmonary atresia is associated with a small hemithorax and mediastinal shift towards the affected side. Swyer–James syndrome presents with a hyperlucent lung with reduced vascularity and a small hilum. Neither of these conditions is associated with dilatation of the pulmonary arteries.

Sutton (2002), 378–80; Dähnert (2007), 652–3.

22) b. ***
Trevor's disease (also called dysplasia epiphysealis hemimelica) is a rare developmental bone dysplasia. It primarily occurs in children aged 2–4 years and affects boys more commonly than girls. It shows a preponderance for the lower limbs, most commonly affecting the knee and ankle, and demonstrates single or multiple osteocartilaginous tumours arising from epiphyses. The lesion is characteristically hemimelic, involving either the medial (two-thirds of cases) or lateral aspect of the ossification centres. Cases can be classified as localized, classic or generalized.

Araujo et al (2006).

23) a. ****
There are three patterns of hypoxic ischaemic encephalopathy. Periventricular leukomalacia occurs in watershed areas of arterial

distribution. It is caused by prolonged partial asphyxia in preterm or term babies. Acute profound asphyxia causes lesions in the deep grey matter, hippocampus and dorsal brain stem. Lastly, there is multicystic encephalomalacia that follows devastating encephalopathy and generalized brain oedema.

Khong et al (2003).

24) c. ***

Adrenal haemorrhage is not only the commonest cause of neonatal adrenal mass, but is also more likely to be seen in neonates in a high-dependency unit because it is associated with perinatal stress, hypoxia, septicaemia and hypotension. It can be unilateral or bilateral, but, even when bilateral, it does not usually cause adrenal insufficiency. Initially, the haematoma appears as an avascular heterogeneous mass on ultrasound scan that becomes cystic and smaller over a period of weeks. A hyperechoic rim can form, representing peripheral calcification. Haematomas can become infected, resulting in an abscess. Neuroblastoma is the main differential diagnosis; on ultrasound scan, it appears as a hyperechoic mass that can have internal flecks of calcification. Repeat ultrasound scan at 1 week will not show the changes that haematoma undergoes.

Sutton (2002), 876–7.

25) a. **

There are six ossification centres around the elbow. The absolute age at which they appear varies slightly, but the order of appearance does not. The order in which they appear is capitellum, radial head, internal (medial) epicondyle, trochlea, olecranon and external (lateral) epicondyle. This can be remembered as 'CRITOE', with typical ages in boys of 1, 5, 7, 10, 10 and 11 years, being up to 2 years earlier in girls. The importance of the order is in recognizing medial epicondyle avulsion injuries, which are relatively common due to the powerful forearm flexors. The medial epicondyle epiphyseal fragment is pulled medially into the joint to lie in the region of the trochlea. This gives the appearance of the 'C', 'R' and 'T' but no 'I', and therefore can be identified as pathological.

Weissleder et al (2007), 872.

26) c. **

Thyroglossal duct cyst is the commonest congenital neck mass. It presents as a painless midline neck lump, which moves superiorly on protruding the tongue. Imaging shows a smooth cystic lesion, which may take up pertechnetate on nuclear medicine studies due to the presence of functioning thyroid tissue. Ectopic thyroid is an important differential diagnosis, as this may be the only functioning thyroid tissue present and therefore should not be excised. Laryngoceles and branchial cleft cysts present with masses to the side of the neck rather than in the midline.

Lymphadenopathy will usually present as solitary or multiple solid lumps in either side of the neck, but may be 'cystic' when necrotic.

Dähnert (2007), 399–400.

27) a. ***
Intestinal malrotation is defined as a congenital abnormal position of the bowel within the peritoneal cavity, occurring as a result of disruption of the normal embryological process of gut rotation and fixation. It is associated with abnormal bowel fixation by mesenteric bands or lack of fixation of parts of the bowel, which may result in obstruction, volvulus and bowel necrosis. The position of the duodenojejunal junction (and by implication the ligament of Treitz) can help to identify the presence of malrotation and its type, and should be determined on every paediatric upper gastrointestinal contrast examination. The duodenojejunal junction normally lies to the left of the left-sided pedicles of the vertebral body, at the level of the duodenal bulb on frontal views. Malrotation is associated with medial and inferior displacement of the duodenojejunal junction. Occasionally, the normal duodenojejunal junction may be displaced inferiorly by a distended stomach or dilated adjacent bowel segment, due to laxity of the peritoneal ligaments, which may mimic malrotation.

Applegate et al (2006).

28) b. **
The international grading system for vesicoureteric reflux divides reflux into five classes. Grade I describes reflux into the ureter only, with grade II referring to reflux into the pelvicalyceal system without calyceal dilatation or blunting. Grade III reflux is associated with mild pelvicalyceal and ureteric dilatation, though forniceal angles remain distinct. Grade IV is associated with a tortuous ureter and moderate dilatation of the pelvicalyceal system, with blunting of the forniceal angles. Grade V reflux describes grossly dilated tortuous ureters with marked pelvicalyceal dilatation and obliteration of the forniceal angles.

Dähnert (2007), 992; Weissleder et al (2007), 864.

29) c. ***
Hyaline membrane disease is due to deficiency of pulmonary surfactant, which causes alveolar collapse. Prematurity, caesarean section and perinatal asphyxia are predisposing factors. In the mild form, granularity is seen throughout the lungs as the first sign. As the condition progresses, air bronchograms appear with eventual complete opacification of the lungs. Changes are usually symmetrical if the condition is uncomplicated.

Sutton (2002), 256–7.

30) c. **

Torsion of the testicle is the commonest acute problem in the prepubertal age group. Including all ages below 20 years, epididymitis occurs in a ratio of 3:2 with torsion. This ratio is 9:1 above 20 years. Torsion of the testicular appendages accounts for around 5% of scrotal pathology overall, with the appendix testis being affected far more commonly than the appendix epididymis.

Dähnert (2007), 901.

31) a. ****

Compared with use of barium, pneumatic reduction of intussusception using air allows generation of higher intracolonic pressures, which is associated with faster and more effective reduction (70–90% success rate), and therefore less fluoroscopic time and lower radiation dose. If perforation does occur (around 1% of cases), the use of air results in smaller tears and less contamination of the peritoneal cavity. A potential complication of the pneumatic method is tension pneumoperitoneum, which may result in respiratory and haemodynamic compromise, requiring prompt needle puncture of the peritoneal cavity. Overall, pneumatic reduction is considered the optimal technique, and has replaced the use of barium in most centres. However, hydrostatic reduction with water-soluble contrast remains a viable alternative, but the contrast column needs to be elevated to a height of 150 cm to generate similar pressures.

Sutton (2002), 872–3; Dähnert (2007), 846–7.

32) d. ****

Myelination is an important feature of the maturation of the normal central nervous system. It is a dynamic process that begins *in utero* and continues after birth in a predetermined manner. It is well demonstrated on MRI, where initially white and grey matter show the reverse signal characteristics to those seen in the adult brain, with the white matter appearing of lower signal on T1 and higher signal on T2 than grey matter. As myelination occurs, the white matter gains fat content and so becomes of higher signal on T1 and lower signal on T2 than grey matter, with completion at around 9 months. The process progresses caudal to cranial, posterior to anterior, and deep to superficial, beginning with the brain stem and cerebellum, then the basal ganglia, with the final areas to mature being the peripheral cortical white matter.

Ballesteros et al (1993).

33) d. ****

The clinical and radiological findings are of adrenal cortical carcinoma, which is a disease with two age peaks, the first in early childhood (two-thirds of affected children being younger than 5 years) and the second in the fourth and fifth decades. Preliminary staging is performed with CT, though MR may be useful in evaluation of vascular or local invasion. T1 and T2 tumours are ≤5 cm and >5 cm, respectively, with no evidence of invasion. T3 tumours extend outside the adrenal into fat, and T4 tumours invade adjacent organs. Stage IV disease includes any 'T' or 'N' staging with metastases, T3 N1 and T4 disease. There is no stage V.

Hricak et al (2007), 137–40.

34) b. ***
Ovarian cysts in the newborn are more common than enteric duplication cysts, giant meconium pseudocysts, cystic lymphatic malformations or choledochal cysts. Other rarer causes of intra-abdominal cystic structures in the newborn include cystic teratomas, gastric teratomas, cystic granulosa cell tumour of the ovary, ovarian teratomas and cystadenomas. Ovarian cysts may become echogenic due to the haemorrhage that can occur if they tort (twist). These cysts also have associated normal ovarian tissue, and the daughter cyst represents a follicle along the wall. Wilms' tumours are solid and occur later in life. A giant meconium pseudocyst has a thick echogenic wall, and viscous echogenic contents. It is formed by meconium leak following fetal bowel perforation due to intestinal obstruction in meconium ileus, ileal atresia or volvulus. Twenty-five per cent show peritoneal or cyst calcification, which is pathognomonic for meconium pseudocyst. Bowel obstruction may be present also. Cystic lymphatic malformations appear as large, well-circumscribed, cystic, thin-walled structures with multiple thin septa. Internally, the fluid can be echo free or echoic because of haemorrhage, debris, chyle or infection. Mesenteric, omental or retroperitoneal cysts are seen. Choledochal cysts are subhepatic or in the porta hepatis. They are seen separate from the gallbladder and are round, tubular or teardrop shaped, and connected to the biliary tree.

Khong et al (2003).

35) b. ****
Causes of a generalized increase in bone density in childhood include osteopetrosis, pyknodysostosis and craniodiaphyseal dysplasia (in order of increasing rarity). Features of pyknodysostosis that allow differentiation from the other conditions are thick calvaria (spared in osteopetrosis), multiple wormian bones, and widened lambdoid sutures and fontanelles. Other manifestations include short limbs, mandibular hypoplasia, poor pneumatization of the paranasal sinuses, non-segmentation of C1−2 and L5−S1, and clavicular dysplasia. This final feature has led to speculation that it is a variant of cleidocranial dysostosis. Insufficiency fractures may be seen in both conditions. Cortical expansion resulting in narrowing of the medulla is a feature of fluorosis.

Glass et al (2004).

36) c. **

Embryologically, the cloaca is divided by the urorectal septum into a dorsal part that develops into the rectum and a ventral part that gives rise to the allantois, bladder and urogenital sinus. The wolffian and müllerian ducts drain into the ventral cloaca. The allantois becomes the urachus, which is the umbilical attachment of the bladder. Ordinarily, this atrophies to become the umbilical ligament. If it remains patent throughout its entire length, urine can drain via the umbilicus. A urachal sinus and a vesicourachal diverticulum describe patent portions of the urachus at the umbilical and bladder ends respectively.

Weissleder et al (2007), 855.

37) a. *****

Thanatophoric dysplasia is transmitted by a dominant gene mutation, and is the commonest lethal neonatal skeletal dysplasia after osteogenesis imperfecta type II. Infants with this condition are frequently stillborn or die shortly after birth from respiratory failure. The appearances on the chest radiograph are pathognomonic, with short ribs that characteristically do not extend beyond the anterior axillary line. The vertebral bodies are curved into an H or U shape (best seen on a lateral radiograph), and the humeri are curved and short. Other skeletal abnormalities such as polydactyly may be present. Dysplasias associated with short ribs often present early in life with respiratory distress due to a critically small chest diameter.

Glass et al (2002).

38) b. ****

Paediatric fractures are commonly classified into five types: plastic deformation, buckle fracture, greenstick fracture, complete fracture and physeal injuries. The most important anatomical characteristics in the paediatric skeleton that result in these fracture patterns are the presence of growth plates and the thick periosteum, which in children contributes immensely to rapid fracture healing and helps in the reduction and the maintenance of reduction. It also decreases the likelihood that fractures will involve the entire circumference of the bone, creating torus and greenstick patterns, with the intact periosteum on one cortex preventing displacement of that cortex and acting as a hinge (particularly in greenstick patterns). This allows for accurate reduction with manipulation and retention with a cast, avoiding open reduction and internal fixation.

Rodríguez-Merchán (2005).

39) c. ***

Duodenal atresia is the commonest cause of congenital duodenal obstruction, and is often associated with Down's syndrome and other congenital anomalies. Patients present soon after birth with persistent vomiting. The site of obstruction is usually distal to the ampulla of Vater, and a 'double-bubble' sign is seen on plain abdominal radiograph, representing gas within the duodenal bulb and stomach, but no gas is seen distally. Annular pancreas is also associated with Down's syndrome, and may present neonatally with vomiting and the double-bubble sign, but obstruction is incomplete, with gas seen in the bowel distal to the stenosis. Hypertrophic pyloric stenosis usually presents with vomiting around 4–6 weeks of life, and a dilated duodenal bulb is not a feature. Duodenal duplication cyst may cause compression or displacement of the first and second parts of the duodenum, but rarely causes high-grade stenosis. The double-bubble sign is not a feature of Hirschsprung's disease.

Eisenberg (2003), 360–1.

40) d. ***
The features of idiopathic hypercalcaemia of infancy (Williams' syndrome) include elfin-like facies, neonatal hypercalcaemia that can form renal stones, learning disability, physical retardation, colonic and bladder diverticula, aortic and pulmonary valve stenosis, cardiac septal defects, osteosclerosis and metastatic calcification. Marfan's syndrome is an autosomal dominant, connective tissue disorder that, in addition to skeletal manifestations, may involve the cardiovascular system, particularly the mitral valve and ascending aorta. Morquio's syndrome is the commonest of the mucopolysaccharidoses, with multiple skeletal manifestations occurring within the first 18 months of life. Wilson–Mikity syndrome is similar to bronchopulmonary dysplasia, occurring in normal preterm infants breathing room air, but is seldom seen now due to the use of mechanical ventilation. Maffucci's syndrome is a dysplasia characterized by enchondromatosis and multiple soft-tissue haemangiomas. Learning disability and urinary tract abnormalities are not features of any of these conditions.

Dähnert (2007), 175.

41) c. ****
Pyelectasis can be regarded as a renal pelvis diameter greater than 4–5 mm at 20 weeks' gestation or 7 mm at 33 weeks, or above 10 mm at birth. Local protocol varies as to which fetuses to follow up and how. Some centres perform an ultrasound scan on all neonates who have had a renal pelvis diameter of above 5 mm at any point; others may only investigate if there is a renal pelvis above 10 mm persisting to birth. Ultrasound scan soon after birth, however, is the best way of detecting severe obstructive pathology, such as posterior urethral valves, that may warrant rapid surgical intervention. On this scan, if there is persisting dilatation above 10 mm, antibiotic prophylaxis and micturating cystourethrogram (MCUG) are appropriate. If reflux is seen on the MCUG, DMSA and repeat ultrasound scan at 6 weeks are appropriate. DMSA is used to assess parenchyma for scarring. If no reflux is seen,

MAG3 scan within 6 weeks is suggested to look for obstruction. If the renal pelvis diameter is less than 10 mm within 24 hours of birth, follow-up ultrasound scan 6 weeks later is suggested.

Duncan (2007).

42) b. ****

In performing hip ultrasound scan, the views should be taken in the coronal plane with the leg in internal rotation. The alpha angle refers to the angle between the iliac bone and the acetabular margin, and 60° or greater represents normal acetabular development. The femoral head should sit so that half of it lies within the acetabulum (equator sign). In poorly developed sockets seen in developmental dysplasia, the shallow acetabulum shows a reduced alpha angle of less than 49°, which is suggestive of potential instability regardless of concentric or eccentric location of the head. The beta angle allows for sub-categorization of the hip sonographically, less than 55° being normal and over 70° suggestive of instability. An inverted labrum is seen in severe cases only.

Dähnert (2007), 67.

43) e. ****

In children with cancer, acute neurological symptoms may be caused directly by the cancer or by its treatment. Paediatric tumours commonly metastasizing to the brain include neuroblastoma, osteosarcoma and Ewing's sarcoma. Rarer causes are melanoma, Wilms' tumour and rhabdomyosarcoma. Of these, the sarcomas are most commonly associated with intratumoral bleeding. Spontaneous bleeding is seen in thrombocytopenia (platelets $< 10\ 000/mm^3$) and disseminated intravascular coagulation. Large areas of haemorrhage will be evident on CT, but petechial haemorrhage is best seen on gradient echo MR. Ischaemia or infarction can be caused by non-bacterial thrombotic endocarditis, disseminated intravascular coagulation, septic infarction, tumour embolism, venous occlusion and radiation-induced vasculopathy. Radiation-induced vasculopathy can be acute (1–6 weeks) or early delayed (3 weeks to several months), and both are caused by oedema and transient myelin injury. All radiation injury is confined to the field of treatment. Late delayed reaction (several months to years) is accelerated atherosclerosis and white matter infarction consequent on this. Extensive demyelination, white matter necrosis and subsequent astrogliosis can also occur. With ischaemic damage, hyperintense signal may be seen on DWI as early as 1 hour. Hyperleukocytosis (leukocyte count $>100\ 000/mm^3$) causes vascular thrombosis, into which there can be secondary haemorrhage. CT or MR venography can be used to look for venous occlusion, particularly venous sinus thrombosis.

Chu et al (2003).

44) e. **

The appearance is of a normal thymus, which is visible in 50% of children up to 2 years of age. It is usually seen as a triangular density arising from the superior border of the mediastinum ('sail sign'), which has a rippled border due to indentation by the ribs ('wave sign'). The shape may change with position and respiration.

Dähnert (2003), 458.

45) d. ****

Tetralogy of Fallot accounts for 8% of congenital heart disease and consists of ventricular septal defect, overriding aorta, right ventricular hypertrophy and right ventricular outflow obstruction. On the chest radiograph, the most common finding is elevation of the cardiac apex due to right ventricular enlargement. This, with concavity at the level of the pulmonary trunk due to reduced pulmonary blood flow, produces the classic boot-shaped heart. A slight bulge in the upper left heart border may be seen due to the right ventricular infundibulum. Other associated features sometimes seen are aortic enlargement and right-sided aortic arch.

Ferguson et al (2007).

46) c. ***

Hypertrophic pyloric stenosis (HPS) is an idiopathic condition in which the circular muscle fibres of the pylorus undergo hypertrophy and hyperplasia, resulting in elongation and narrowing of the pyloric canal. Infants, often firstborn males, usually present at 4–6 weeks with projectile vomiting. If an experienced clinician can palpate an olive-shaped mass, no imaging is required. Otherwise, ultrasound scan is the imaging method of choice for diagnosis. Ultrasound findings include increased gastric peristalsis, failure of the pyloric canal to open, and elongated pylorus with thickened muscle. Pyloric canal length of >16 mm, transverse pyloric diameter of >11 mm and muscle wall thickness of >2.5 mm are indicative of HPS. The definitive treatment is pyloromyotomy.

Adam et al (2007), 1505.

47) d. ***

Hirschsprung's disease is caused by an absence of parasympathetic ganglia in the muscle and submucosal layers of the distal colon, resulting in abnormal peristalsis and impaired evacuation of the colon. The rectum is virtually always involved, but the proximal extent of disease varies. Presentation is usually with failure to pass meconium by 48 hours. Characteristic features on contrast enema in the neonate include inversion of the rectosigmoid index (the normal neonatal rectum is of greater calibre than the sigmoid colon), tortuosity and corrugation of the narrowed aganglionic segment, and difficulty in obtaining good rectal distension. A discrete zone of transition is more commonly seen in older infants and children. Colonic atresia causes massive distension of the colon proximal to the area of stenosis, but is relatively rare. Meconium plug syndrome typically results in a dilated right and transverse colon with a transition point at the splenic flexure. Meconium ileus causes small bowel obstruction.

Sutton (2002), 860–1; Dähnert (2007), 842.

48) a. ****
In familial adenomatous polyposis (FAP), multiple (usually around 1000) tubular or tubulovillous adenomatous polyps are seen in the GI tract, predominantly in the colon. Patients usually become symptomatic in the third to fourth decades and present with abdominal pain, weight loss and diarrhoea. Juvenile polyposis (JP) is the commonest cause of colonic polyps in children, and usually presents with rectal bleeding. The polyps are hamartomatous and may occur throughout the GI tract. They are less numerous than in FAP, and the condition may be diagnosed with five or more polyps. Both conditions are autosomal dominant, with 80% penetrance in FAP and variable penetrance in JP. The rectosigmoid is involved in 80% of cases of JP, whereas the rectum is always involved in FAP. In both conditions, patients are at increased risk of associated adenocarcinoma, seen in 15% of patients by 35 years of age in JP, but in 100% of patients by 20 years after diagnosis in FAP. Mucocutaneous pigmentation is a feature of Peutz–Jeghers syndrome.

Dähnert (2007), 832, 848.

49) c. ***
Eosinophilic granuloma is a benign variety of Langerhans' cell histiocytosis. Fifty per cent of cases involve the skull and 25% affect the axial skeleton. It is the commonest cause of vertebra plana (collapsed dense vertebra) in children. The posterior elements are rarely involved. Ewing's sarcoma may cause destruction of a vertebra, but vertebra plana is not a feature. The other conditions are all causes of vertebra plana but are less common in this age group.

Dähnert (2007), 110–11.

50) b. ****
Non-rotation is an abnormality of bowel rotation in which the midgut loop returns to the peritoneal cavity without undergoing rotation. It is usually asymptomatic and is often found incidentally in older children or adults. The small bowel is located on the right side of the abdomen and the colon on the left side, and the small and large bowel have a common mesentery. The superior mesenteric vein lies to the left of the superior mesenteric artery, the reverse of the normal situation. In malrotation, the superior mesenteric vein tends to lie anterior to the superior mesenteric artery, and there is abnormal positioning of the duodenojejunal junction to the right and inferiorly, usually also with cephalad positioning of the caecum. Reversed rotation is rare, and

results in the colon lying posterior to the superior mesenteric artery, with duodenum and jejunum in front of it. Midgut volvulus may complicate abnormalities of bowel rotation, resulting in torsion of the gut around the superior mesenteric artery due to a short mesenteric small bowel attachment. A clockwise 'whirlpool' sign may be seen on colour Doppler ultrasound scan, representing the superior mesenteric vein wrapping clockwise around the superior mesenteric artery.

Chapman & Nakielny (2003), 220; Dähnert (2007), 860–1.

51) a. ***
Chiari I malformation is characterized by tonsillar ectopia. The fourth ventricle is elongated but normal in position. It is associated with syringohydromyelia, hydrocephalus and malformations of the skull base. Chiari II (Arnold–Chiari) malformation is characterized by hindbrain abnormalities, with caudal displacement of the fourth ventricle. A lumbar myelomeningocele is seen in over 95% of cases. Chiari III malformation is rare and has a high cervical/low occipital meningomyelo-encephalocele. Survival beyond infancy is unusual. In Dandy–Walker syndrome, there is enlargement of the posterior fossa with cystic dilatation of the fourth ventricle and abnormalities of the cerebellar vermis. Diastematomyelia results in sagittal splitting of the spinal cord into two hemi-cords, and is sometimes associated with a myelomeningocele.

Dähnert (2007), 275–6.

52) d. ***
The unifying diagnosis is vein of Galen aneurysm. Three anatomical types are recognized, all of which are vascular malformations that dilate the vein of Galen, straight and transverse sinuses, and torcular herophili secondarily. Type 1 is an arteriovenous fistula, type 2 is an angiomatous malformation of the basal ganglia, thalami and midbrain, and type 3 has both features. It can be detected *in utero* or may present with a neonatal pattern of features (less than 1 month), an infantile pattern or an adult pattern (above 1 year). The *in utero* and neonatal manifestations are due to high-output cardiac failure and mass effect of the vein of Galen aneurysm, particularly on the aqueduct. It can undergo haemorrhage and cause infarction by a steal mechanism.

Dähnert (2007), 333.

53) b. **
The child has features of non-accidental injury. Subdural haematoma is the commonest CT finding and is frequently interhemispheric, although shallow posterior fossa subdural haematomas are also seen. If there is more than one subdural haematoma, varying densities can be seen,

indicating differing ages. Non-accidental injury is the commonest cause of serious intracranial injury in children less than 1 year old.

Dähnert (2007), 52–3.

54) a. ****
Renal lymphangiectasia is a very rare developmental malformation probably caused by a failure of the developing kidney lymphatics to establish communication with the extrarenal lymphatic system. Abnormal lymphatic channels dilate, resulting in cystic lesions in the parapelvic, perinephric and, less commonly, retroperitoneal regions. The lesions are of water attenuation on CT and may cause contour deformities of the renal outlines.

Upreti et al (2008).

55) d. ***
Alport's syndrome or chronic hereditary nephritis is the unifying diagnosis. It is inherited, probably in an autosomal dominant fashion. Ocular abnormalities can also occur, including congenital cataracts, nystagmus, myopia and spherophakia. Hypertension is not a feature. The renal impairment is progressive in affected males but non-progressive in females. Cerebellar and retinal haemangioblastomas occur in von Hippel–Lindau syndrome, along with renal, pancreatic and adrenal cysts.

Dähnert (2007), 929.

56) a. ****
Congenital lobar emphysema results in progressive overinflation of one or more pulmonary lobes; it presents in the first 6 months of life with respiratory distress and cyanosis. The left upper lobe is most commonly affected. Imaging features immediately after birth are of a hazy, mass-like opacity, which represents delayed clearing of lung fluid in the emphysematous lobe. After clearing of the fluid, the affected lobe becomes expanded and hyperlucent on imaging, and causes mass effect and mediastinal shift. Macleod's syndrome is a complication of bronchiolitis, usually presenting with hyperlucency of one or both lungs. Bronchiolitis obliterans usually occurs in adults, but may present in children following infection.

Schwartz et al (1999); Dähnert (2007), 485–6.

57) a. ***
Meckel's diverticulum is a true diverticulum arising from the small bowel, usually 80–90 cm from the ileocaecal valve, representing failure of closure of the omphalomesenteric duct. Heterotopic gastric mucosa

is present in 10–30% of diverticula, but is seen in 98% of those that present with bleeding. A [^{99m}Tc]-pertechnetate study demonstrates uptake in gastric mucosa within Meckel's diverticulum, seen as a focal area of uptake, usually in the right lower quadrant with activity paralleling that of the stomach. Duodenal duplication cysts may contain heterotopic gastric mucosa, which may be a cause of a false-positive scan, but they often appear as larger areas of increased activity, and would be expected to be in the upper abdomen. Tracer uptake may be seen in inflammatory, obstructive and neoplastic conditions, including intussusception, peptic ulcer disease and appendicitis, but activity does not parallel that of the stomach.

Zeissman et al (2006), 375–9.

58) c. ****
Meconium plug syndrome is also known as small left colon syndrome and functional immaturity of the colon. It occurs most commonly in large infants and infants of diabetic mothers and is believed to be due to relative immaturity of bowel innervation. Characteristic features are of a dilated proximal colon with a calibre change at the splenic flexure and an empty descending colon. The functional obstruction is transient and usually self-limiting, and contrast enema may act as a stimulus for subsequent passage of (normal) meconium. Hirschsprung's disease with a transition zone at the splenic flexure may mimic these findings, but the obstruction usually persists after contrast enema. Intussusception in this age group and at this site would be unusual. Meconium ileus and ileal atresia are causes of distal small bowel obstruction.

Sutton (2002), 861; Brant & Helms (2007), 1286.

59) a. ***
Foreign body aspiration is most common in children under 3 years of age. It presents with varying degrees of cough, and the chest radiograph usually shows overinflation, atelectasis, infiltrates and/or air trapping, which almost exclusively involve the lower lobes, with the right most commonly affected. A foreign body is seen in only about 9% of cases. Congenital lobar emphysema presents with increased lucency, usually in the upper zones, with air trapping and mediastinal shift. Cystic adenomatoid malformation type I usually presents as an expansile mass with multiple cysts. Bronchiolitis obliterans tends to present in adults, though it may present in children, usually with generalized hyperinflation and patchy air trapping.

Dähnert (2007), 467.

60) e. ****
Duodenal intramural haematoma is usually traumatic, particularly following bicycle-handlebar accidents and lap-belt injuries. However, it is also commonly seen in non-accidental injury, where the mechanism of

injury is thought to be a blunt blow to the abdomen that compresses the duodenum against the vertebral column. Trauma to the duodenum may result in duodenal rupture, intramural tear or, most commonly, intramural haematoma. Ultrasound appearances are of an echogenic intramural mass that becomes progressively hypoechoic with maturation of the haematoma. There may be associated deformity or obstruction of the duodenum. CT may demonstrate free intraperitoneal fluid, though free air and frank perforation are uncommon. Spontaneous intramural haematoma may occur in Henoch–Schönlein purpura, but other features of the condition would be expected to be present. It may occur with anticoagulant therapy and blood dyscrasia, but haemophilia in females is extremely rare. Duodenal diverticula may cause gastrointestinal bleeding, but this is usually intraluminal rather than intramural. Duodenal intramural haematoma has been described in association with pancreatitis but is very rare.

Carty (1997).

61) a. *****
Henoch–Schönlein purpura is an acute systemic vasculitis that affects the skin, gastrointestinal tract, joints and kidneys. Children aged 3–10 years are predominantly affected, and may present with a purpuric rash on the extensor surfaces of the limbs, arthralgia and crampy abdominal pain with intestinal bleeding. Imaging demonstrates multifocal areas of bowel wall thickening due to intramural haemorrhage and oedema. Gastrointestinal complications include bowel infarction and perforation, as well as intussusception.

Brant & Helms (2007), 1302; Dähnert (2007), 839.

62) a. ****
The most common mechanism for traumatic mesenteric rupture is a road traffic collision, although such an injury can occur in children following any blunt abdominal trauma, with handlebar injuries and child abuse being well-recognized causes. Use of a lap belt makes children more prone to the injury. Bowel perforation, infarction and active haemorrhage are indications for immediate surgery and can be identified on CT. Most of the remaining cases are treated conservatively. Free intraperitoneal air, extraluminal contrast or visible bowel wall defect is specific for perforation. Free fluid, haemorrhage and stranding are seen in perforation or mesenteric injury, with fluid at the root more likely to indicate the latter. Hyperattenuation of the pancreas, kidneys and bowel wall is a feature of hypoperfusion, along with small-calibre aorta and vena cava, and should not be mistaken for visceral injury.

Sivit et al (1992); Strouse et al (1999).

63) b. ***
Discitis is the commonest paediatric spinal disease. It is secondary to bacterial invasion of the disc through the endplate. Plain films typically

show reduced disc-space height and loss of clarity of the endplates in the acute phase. MRI is the best investigation, as it is the most sensitive. Reduced T1 signal is seen in the adjacent marrow due to oedema, with initially variable, then increased, T2 signal. Complications such as epidural abscess are well demonstrated. CT will show the endplate changes and any paravertebral inflammatory mass. Bone scans and white cell scans have much poorer sensitivity than MRI, though this is improved with the use of SPECT.

Dähnert (2007), 205.

64) c. ***

Cystic fibrosis usually presents in the first year of life with cough and recurrent infections or progressive respiratory insufficiency. The upper lobes are predominantly affected. High-resolution CT shows mucus plugging (tubular opacities), bronchiectasis, peribronchial thickening, bullous formation and collapse/consolidation. Williams–Campbell syndrome is a congenital deficiency of cartilage in the fourth to sixth generation bronchi. This produces cystic bronchiectatic changes beyond the third bronchial generation and bullous changes. Mucus plugging is not a feature.

Dähnert (2007), 488–9.

65) c. ***

Down's syndrome is a common genetic abnormality that results from trisomy of chromosome 21. The pelvic features in infantile Down's syndrome were first described by Caffey. The iliac index (sum of the acetabular and iliac angles) is decreased in Down's syndrome, and is particularly useful in making an early diagnosis. Flaring of the iliac wings due to their rotation into the coronal plane is a typical finding that gives them an increased prominence on frontal radiographs, with the appearance likened to Mickey Mouse or elephant ears. Down's syndrome is associated with a wide array of skeletal abnormalities, with the skull, spine and appendicular skeleton all potentially involved.

Eich et al (1992).

66) c. ***

Cephalhaematoma is seen with birth trauma, particularly following poor instrumentation and skull fracture during delivery. It is seen in 1–2% of deliveries. It can grow after birth and takes weeks or months to resolve. It does not cross sutural lines because the haematoma is beneath the outer layer of periosteum. The haematoma can calcify. Caput succedaneum is localized scalp oedema that does cross sutural lines. A cephalocele is a skull defect through which meninges, brain and cerebrospinal fluid may protrude.

Willatt & Quaghebeur (2004).

67) b. ****
Germinal matrix is highly vascular tissue seen at 24–32 weeks' gestational age, located anterior to the caudothalamic groove and inferior to the lateral ventricles. It is at risk of hypoxaemia and ischaemia. Haemorrhage here can be promoted by trauma at birth or coagulopathy including rhesus incompatibility. Germinal matrix haemorrhage less than 7 days old is hyperechoic but without shadowing. Within 2–3 weeks, the abnormal area decreases in size and the echogenicity reduces. Periventricular leukomalacia is white matter necrosis following hypoxaemia. It is seen in 5–10% of preterm babies. It occurs in arterial watershed areas and may appear acutely as a broad region of periventricular increased echogenicity. Cystic degeneration may follow after 2 weeks or more.

Weissleder et al (2007), 890–1.

68) e. ***
Osteomalacia is bone softening due to accumulation of excessive amounts of uncalcified osteoid and poor bone mineralization of that osteoid, which in children is called rickets. As there is reduced mineralization, the bones may appear of diffusely reduced density on radiographs, which should be termed 'osteopenia' rather than 'osteoporosis', as the latter term refers to a reduced quantity of normally mineralized bone. There is also a decrease in the number of trabeculae, which appear fuzzy and coarse. The softening of the bone leads to insufficiency fractures and bowing deformities. Fractures may heal with unmineralized osteoid that gives the appearance on radiographs of persistent lucent lines called Looser's zones. The underlying abnormality is a deficiency of vitamin D, which is required for normal bone mineralization. The two commonest causes of this are dietary and secondary to renal pathology (renal osteodystrophy).

Dähnert (2007), 4–5, 152–3.

69) a. **
Most intussusceptions occur in childhood, usually between 6 months and 2 years of age. The vast majority are idiopathic or related to mucosal oedema and lymphoid hyperplasia following viral gastroenteritis. In the 5% of patients with a pathological lead point, causes include those listed above. Patients classically present with cramping abdominal pain, screaming episodes, 'redcurrant jelly stools' and a palpable abdominal mass. Most childhood intussusceptions are ileocolic. In contrast, a specific cause is identified in 80% of adult cases, and ileoileal intussceptions are more common than ileocolic.

Dähnert (2007), 845–7.

70) e. ****
Mesial temporal sclerosis is a pattern of hippocampal neuronal loss that can occur with long-standing temporal lobe epilepsy as a result of

excessive neuronal depolarization leading to cytotoxic oedema. Three patterns of loss are described, with relative sparing of the CA2 subfield often a feature. The typical findings are of asymmetrical atrophy of the hippocampus with abnormally high signal returned on T2W images. Ipsilateral findings in the limbic system include atrophy of the fornix and maxillary body. Cortical abnormalities may exist in the temporal cortex, and this is best evaluated on high-resolution T1 sequences.

Lee et al (1998).

71) c. ***
Slipped upper femoral epiphysis is the most common hip abnormality in adolescents and is a frequent cause of premature osteoarthritis, pain and disability. The most commonly affected demographic are overweight teenage boys. Radiographs are still the initial investigation of choice, and recognition of early subtle signs allows earlier diagnosis and prompt treatment, improving long-term prognosis. The femoral head often slips posteriorly prior to slipping medially, and early slippage is best seen on lateral or frog lateral views. Early signs on the AP projection include widening of the physis with local demineralization. Posterior slippage of the femoral head may then give the appearance of a small epiphysis due to rotation and narrowing of the physis, and lateral views may show the displacement. The line of Klein is a line drawn along the lateral femoral neck, which should intersect with a small portion of the lateral femoral head. If it does not, it suggests medial slippage. An ill-defined area of increased opacification (metaphyseal blanch sign) may be seen in the proximal metaphysis, which is thought to represent a healing response.

Boles & El-Khoury (1997).

72) c. ***
Generally, in the case of ingested foreign bodies, a chest radiograph (including neck) at initial presentation is indicated. An abdominal radiograph is usually considered after 6 days only if there is doubt whether the foreign body has passed. However, if a sharp or potentially poisonous foreign body has been ingested, an abdominal radiograph is indicated at the time of presentation; a chest radiograph is indicated if the abdominal film is negative. Ingestion of disc batteries (small, coin-shaped batteries found in hearing aids, watches and calculators) may be associated with serious sequelae, particularly if the battery becomes lodged in the oesophagus, as is more likely with younger children and larger batteries. In this situation, leakage of alkaline material, and sodium hydroxide generated by electrolysis at the anode, can cause ulceration and perforation within a relatively short time. Radiography is indicated to locate the battery. If it lies within the oesophagus, emergency endoscopic removal is indicated. Batteries located beyond the oesophagus rarely require endoscopic removal, unless subsequent radiographs indicate delay in transit of the battery.

Royal College of Radiologists (2007), 170–1.

73) b. ***

An amputated ovary occurs as the result of ovarian torsion and infarction. Both an ovarian teratoma and leiomyoma will enlarge the affected ovary rather than appear atrophic. A follicular cyst will usually be a simple cyst, although it may have internal echoes produced by haemorrhage.

Weissleder et al (2007), 870.

74) b. ****

Spontaneous pneumothorax may occur in babies where there are renal anomalies, and routine ultrasound scan is recommended. This is often associated with maternal oligohydramnios, but this may not necessarily be present.

Alford & McIlhenny (1999).

75) e. **

Ninety per cent of horseshoe kidneys are joined at the lower poles by a parenchymal or fibrous isthmus. The isthmus lies at the L4–5 level, where renal ascent is arrested by the inferior mesenteric artery. The pelves and ureters are anterior, and pelviureteric junction obstruction is more common. Incidence is 1–4/1000 births, making it the commonest renal fusion abnormality. Cardiovascular, skeletal, central nervous system, anorectal and genitourinary malformations are associated. There are associations with trisomy 18 and Turner's syndrome. Associated genitourinary anomalies include hypospadias, undescended testes, bicornuate uterus and ureteral duplication. The incidence of infection and stones increases in a horseshoe kidney.

Dähnert (2007), 929.

76) a. **

Non-accidental injury (NAI) is the third leading cause of death in children after sudden infant death and true accidents, and represents about 1% of all childhood trauma. The hallmark of NAI is multiple fractures at different sites and of different ages, suggesting repeated episodes of abuse. Often, as these fractures are not treated, they show exuberant callus formation. Several locations and patterns of injury have been described as being relatively specific for NAI. However, a study of over 400 fractures showed that the most common presentation was a single, simple, transverse fracture of the middle third of a long bone, which is indistinguishable from a fracture sustained in a true accident. Whole-body imaging with isotope bone scan is sensitive for identifying all sites of injury in equivocal cases.

King et al (1988).

77) d. ****

Respiratory distress syndrome of the newborn is the commonest cause of respiratory distress in premature neonates, and is due to relative immaturity of type II pneumocytes. Features seen on chest radiograph are reduced lung expansion, bilateral and symmetrical consolidation, and prominent air bronchograms. These resolve over several days. Meconium aspiration syndrome is the commonest cause of respiratory distress in full-term neonates. Hyperinflation, pneumothorax and pleural effusions are seen, as are diffuse patchy opacities due to atelectasis and consolidation. No air bronchograms are seen. Changes usually resolve in 48 hours.

Dähnert (2007), 513, 527–8.

78) d. ***

Subependymal haemorrhage (grade 1) usually has no long-term consequence. Mortality rates for intraventricular haemorrhage, intraventricular haemorrhage with ventricular dilatation and intraparenchymal haemorrhage are 10%, 20% and more than 50%, respectively. These represent grades 2, 3 and 4 haemorrhage. Normal choroid plexus pulsates while haematoma at the same location is not pulsatile.

Weissleder et al (2007), 890.

79) c. ***

Infantile polycystic kidney disease is autosomal recessive. Both parents and half the children will be carriers. The sonographic hallmark is enlarged echogenic kidneys. The individual cysts are small, measuring 1–2 mm, and can be defined only with a high-resolution probe. Autosomal kidney disease affects the liver also. The less severe the renal disease, the more severe the hepatic periportal fibrosis.

Weissleder et al (2007), 861–2.

80) a. ***

Congenital biliary atresia is a destructive inflammatory process resulting in atresia of the bile ducts, which presents in neonates with persistent jaundice. Diagnosis is usually made with a combination of liver biopsy and hepatobiliary scintigraphy with a ^{99m}Tc-labelled iminodiacetic acid (IDA) analogue. Phenobarbital is given for 5 days prior to imaging to stimulate biliary secretion. Normal findings are of activity within the small bowel due to biliary excretion by 60 minutes, but in biliary atresia no biliary clearance is seen by 24 hours. Patients with non-obstructive causes of neonatal jaundice usually demonstrate biliary clearance into the bowel during the first 24 hours. Choledochal cyst usually presents in children, and cholescintigraphy may be used to confirm that the cystic structure is connected to the biliary system. The ^{99m}Tc-labelled IDA analogue will fill the cyst, and may show prolonged retention depending on the degree of obstruction. Cystic fibrosis may be associated with steatosis and biliary cirrhosis. Physiological jaundice resolves spontaneously within 2 weeks.

Zeissman et al (2006), 180–2.

81) e. *

Avulsion fractures occur in both adults and children due to a tensile force being applied through a tendon or ligament where the skeleton is the weakest link. The mechanism can be either a powerful normal contraction (as seen in sportspersons) or an abnormal force, as in anterior teardrop fractures of the cervical spine seen in road traffic collisions. They may be acute or chronic from repetitive minor trauma. In the paediatric skeleton, the spectrum of avulsion injuries is larger, as many of the growing apophyses are weaker than the soft-tissue structures that attach to them. For example, avulsion of the tibial spine in the knee is the paediatric equivalent of a ruptured anterior cruciate ligament, and it follows therefore that the ligament rupture is rarely seen in children. Fractures of the radial head in both adults and children are usually due to compressive forces, although one can see avulsion of the radial tuberosity by the biceps brachii tendon.

Tehranzadeh (1987).

82) d. ****

Juvenile angiofibromas are the commonest benign tumour of the nasopharynx and can grow to enormous sizes. They tend to present in teenagers with recurrent and severe epistaxis, as well as nasal obstruction. They are highly vascular and biopsy is contraindicated. In most cases, they are supplied primarily by the internal maxillary artery.

Dähnert (2007), 387.

83) b. ****

Neonatal hypoxic ischaemic encephalopathy occurs in 1–2/1000 live births. Clinically, it manifests as disturbed neurological function such as difficulty with respiration, abnormal tone, depressed reflexes, altered level of consciousness, feeding difficulties or seizures. Initial MRI findings, particularly in the first week of life, can be T1 shortening (bright) rather than a high T2 signal. This is because the unmyelinated white matter is brighter on T2W images and can disguise pathological lesions. T1 shortening is thought to be due to lipid breakdown products of damaged myelin or to mineralization.

Khong et al (2003).

84) c. ***

Osteogenesis imperfecta is one of the more common heritable connective tissue disorders and is characterized by micromelic dwarfism. In all four major types, findings include bowing of the long bones as a result of softening caused by osteomalacia and multiple fractures once the child is walking. Other findings include cortical thinning, exuberant callus formation and pseudarthroses. Rickets and Blount's disease both show abnormal metaphyses, with rickets also demonstrating a coarse trabecular pattern. Neurofibromatosis causes bowing most commonly localized to the junction of the middle and distal thirds of the tibia, with associated sclerosis and cystic changes.

Cheema et al (2003).

85) b. ***
Craniosynostosis means premature closure of a suture of the skull, and skull growth is arrested in the direction perpendicular to the affected suture. Craniosynostosis of the sagittal suture therefore results in a head shape that is abnormally long and narrow and has the appearance of an upturned boat. This is called scaphocephaly (or dolichocephaly) and accounts for 60% of all craniosynostoses. Closure of the coronal suture accounts for 20% and results in a short, wide head called brachycephaly. Trigonocephaly is caused by craniosynostosis of the metopic suture and results in a forward-pointing head. Oxycephaly is the most extreme form, and all sutures may be affected, resulting in a high head. Plagiocephaly is unilateral craniosynostosis. Early recognition of all types is important to prevent permanent deformity and allow for surgical correction. Causes may be primary or secondary to dysplasia, a number of genetic syndromes, microcephaly, and metabolic or haematological conditions.

Weissleder et al (2007), 892.

86) b. ***
Hepatoblastoma is the commonest malignant liver tumour of early childhood, typically presenting before 3 years with pain, palpable mass, jaundice and weight loss, as well as precocious puberty due to hormone production. Tumours are typically large (average 10–12 cm) and appear to be heterogeneous with areas of calcification and necrosis. Metastases to the lung are common. Hepatocellular carcinoma is the second most common malignant liver tumour of children, but usually affects children over 5 years of age. Although it also commonly appears of heterogeneous echogenicity, calcifications are rare. Haemangiomas commonly appear hyperechoic on ultrasound scan and may contain calcifications, but are usually <4 cm and are rarely seen in young children. Pyogenic abscess and choledochal cyst are typically hypoechoic lesions.

Dähnert (2007), 724.

87) b. ***
The average length of the normal neonatal kidney is 4.5 cm. Ultrasound appearances of the kidney in the neonate and infant show a number of differences from those of the older child and adult. Cortical echogenicity

is increased, as the glomeruli form 20% of the cortex in the neonate but only 9% in the adult, and may be comparable to that of the liver or the spleen. The medullary pyramids are larger and more hypoechoic than in older children and adults, and there may be little or no fat in the renal sinus. Persistent fetal lobulation may give the kidneys a lobulated contour. In addition, echogenic septa may be normally seen at the anterosuperior or posteroinferior margins of the kidney, representing the sites of fusion of metanephric elements. Most kidneys attain an adult pattern by 6 months of age.

Butler et al (1999), 425.

88) d. **
Renal artery stenosis and aneurysms plus abdominal coarctation are associated with neurofibromatosis type 1 (NF1). Renal cysts are found in von Hippel–Lindau syndrome (VHL) and tuberous sclerosis, while renal cell carcinoma is found in VHL. NF1 and VHL are associated with phaeochromocytoma. Angiomyolipomas, usually multiple and bilateral, are found in 50% of cases of tuberous sclerosis.

Weissleder et al (2007), 576–80.

89) c. ***
The described features are typical of a branchial cleft cyst arising from the second branchial cleft. The mass displaces the sternocleidomastoid posteriorly, and the carotid and internal jugular vessels posteromedially. The pointing between the internal and external carotid arteries is pathognomonic. Cystic hygromas present in infancy as a cystic mass in the posterior cervical space. Abscesses present with associated symptoms and a painful red swelling, though imaging findings may be similar. Carotid body tumours are solid, highly vascular masses lying between the internal and external carotid artery origins.

Dähnert (2007), 376–7.

90) a. ****
Ewing's sarcoma is the commonest malignant bone tumour in children, and the ribs are involved in 30% of cases in children under 10. It is the commonest malignant chest wall tumour. Neuroblastoma presents in children under 5 as a well-defined, soft-tissue mass that may calcify and erodes/splays the ribs. Hodgkin's disease presents in young adults, and usually involves bones by secondary involvement with direct invasion of sternum or ribs. Osteomyelitis presents at any age with a shorter history (usually less than 2 weeks), and imaging shows rib destruction with a relatively small mass and loss of tissue planes. Hamartoma of the chest wall presents in the first year of life as an extrapleural mass, causing partial/complete destruction of adjacent ribs. Significant calcification and compression of the adjacent lung occur.

Dähnert (2007), 75–6, 449.

91) d. **

In ambulant children, spiral fractures of the tibia (toddler's fractures) are seen reasonably commonly, often with no history of significant trauma, and are not by themselves suggestive of abuse. However, a spiral fracture in a non-ambulant child is quite suggestive of non-accidental injury (NAI). The metaphyseal corner fracture is the most specific of all the findings observed in NAI and is considered virtually pathognomonic of abuse. The injury consists of a series of microfractures orientated parallel to the physis, due to a shearing injury across the bone end. This mechanism of injury is not seen in blunt trauma or falls, although similar lesions may be seen in some metabolic diseases (particularly scurvy). Older children and adults may suffer rib fractures after trauma such as falls and road traffic accidents. However, they are unusual in infants and are strongly correlated with inflicted injury caused by chest wall compression.

Lonergan et al (2003).

92) d. ****

Tethering of the cord results in the conus lying lower than normal and is associated with scoliosis, thickening of the filum terminale (>2 mm at the L5–S1 level on axial T1 image) and spinal lipoma. Less frequent associations are Chiari malformations, syrinx, myelomeningocele, diastematomyelia and dermal sinus. Diastematomyelia is a midline sagittal cleft in the cord, often with a bony/fibrous septum. Syringomyelia is dissection of cerebrospinal fluid through the cord, producing high T2 signal within the cord. This is associated with several neurological abnormalities. Developmental scoliosis occurs in adolescent girls, is convex to the right and has no associated neurological symptoms.

Redla et al (2001).

93) a. ****

Infantile haemangioendothelioma is the commonest benign hepatic tumour occurring in the first 6 months of life, consisting of multiple sinusoidal vascular channels with surrounding connective tissue stroma. Patients typically present with an abdominal mass, or high-output cardiac failure secondary to arteriovenous shunting. Kasabach–Merritt syndrome (consumptive coagulopathy) is seen in 11% of patients. Typical CT features are of early peripheral enhancement and variable delayed central enhancement. Hepatoblastomas tend to occur in slightly older infants (peak 18–24 months) and congestive cardiac failure is not usually a feature. Mesenchymal hamartoma is a rare developmental liver tumour, which appears typically as a multiloculated cystic mass, but may appear solid and echogenic in infants due to innumerable microcysts. However, these are generally hypovascular lesions. Hepatocellular carcinoma is more commonly seen in older children and adolescents. Cavernous haemangiomas are rarely seen in young children.

Sutton (2002), 879.

94) d. ***

Dermoid and epidermoid cysts are ectoderm-lined congenital inclusion cysts. They may not present until early adulthood due to slow growth (particularly epidermoids). Epidermoids contain only squamous epithelium whereas dermoids contain hair, sebaceous and sweat glands, and squamous epithelium. Unlike teratomas, neither is a true neoplasm. Clinical presentation is often with chemical meningitis from rupture of fatty contents. Epidermoids usually have imaging characteristics similar to water and can be differentiated from arachnoid cysts by restricted diffusion on DWI. Attenuation varies according to the keratin:cholesterol ratio and therefore can be similar to fat but is usually homogeneous. The cyst wall is very thin and is often not visible in epidermoids, and areas of calcification can infrequently be seen. Dermoids may appear more complex but are still unilocular. The wall may be thicker and calcification is more frequent. The sebaceous lipid material in a dermoid has attenuation and signal intensity characteristics of fat on CT (low attenuation) and MR (high signal on T1). 'White epidermoids' with high signal on T1 may be seen rarely; they are due to haemorrhage or a high fat content. However, the latter usually produces a homogeneous fat signal as opposed to dermoids, where the appearances are more heterogeneous due to the increased complexity of contents.

Smirniotopoulos & Chiechi (1995).

95) b. ***

Mesenteric lymphadenitis is an inflammatory process affecting the mesenteric lymph nodes; it is most frequently caused by viral infection but also by *Yersinia enterocolitica* and other pathogens. It affects children and young adults, and clinically mimics acute appendicitis. Imaging findings are of enlarged mesenteric lymph nodes, and ileal and colonic wall thickening. The normal appendix must be visualized to differentiate it from acute appendicitis. Features of acute appendicitis on ultrasound scan are of a blind-ending, non-compressible, tubular, aperistaltic, fluid-filled structure measuring over 6 mm in diameter. Mesenteric lymph nodes may also be seen anterior to the right psoas muscle, but tend to be smaller and fewer than in mesenteric lymphadenitis. Thickened bowel wall may be seen on ultrasound scan in Crohn's disease, but this would be less likely in this age group. Symptomatic Meckel's diverticulum usually presents in younger children with gastrointestinal bleeding. Small bowel duplication cyst usually presents under 2 years of age, and lymphadenopathy is not a feature.

Dähnert (2007), 857.

96) b. ***

Haematometrocolpos is described, which at this age can be due to a transverse vaginal septum or imperforate hymen. There is an association with imperforate anus, hydronephrosis, renal agenesis and dysplasia, polycystic kidneys, duplication of the vagina and uterus, sacral hypoplasia and oesophageal atresia. Cervical dysgenesis and obstructed uterine horn would produce haematometra.

Dähnert (2007), 1046–7.

97) a. *
Elevation of the anterior humeral fat pad into a triangular shape (the sail sign) occurs secondary to elbow effusion. In the context of trauma, the probable cause is haemarthrosis. The posterior fat pad lies in the olecranon fossa and should not be visible on normal lateral radiographs in 90° of flexion, although it may normally be seen in extension, when it is displaced by the olecranon process. In trauma the posterior fat pad may be elevated out of the fossa by effusion, and is particularly valuable in predicting an intra-articular disease process when no bony abnormality is apparent radiographically. Rarely the fat pad sign may not be apparent, due to capsular rupture or surrounding soft-tissue swelling. In children, supracondylar fractures represent around 60% of elbow fractures; other causes include medial and lateral epicondyle injuries. The commonest adult elbow fracture is a fracture of the radial head or neck.

Goswami (2002).

98) b. ****
Total anomalous pulmonary venous return presents in the first year of life with cyanosis. It is due to failure of the pulmonary veins to drain into the left atrium, with drainage instead into another vascular structure. There are four types – the commonest, type I (supracardiac), has the four pulmonary veins draining into one common vein, the vertical vein, which drains into the left brachiocephalic vein. This dilated vein, along with the dilated left brachiocephalic vein and superior vena cava, causes widening of the superior mediastinum, which is the 'head' of the 'snowman'. The body is formed by enlargement of the right atrium, producing a rounded appearance of the lower mediastinum. There may be increased pulmonary vascularity. Partial anomalous pulmonary venous return presents later in life with symptoms similar to atrial septal defect. Transposition of the great vessels presents in the first 2 weeks of life with cyanosis. Chest radiograph shows an 'egg-on-string' appearance of the mediastinum with increased pulmonary vascularity. Infantile-type coarctation presents with symptoms and signs of congestive heart failure in infancy. The classic figure-3 sign seen in coarctation is often hidden by the thymus in infants.

Ferguson et al (2007).

99) b. ***
Typhlitis is acute inflammation of the caecum, appendix and occasionally terminal ileum, initially described in neutropenic children with leukaemia, but also seen with lymphoma, following immunosuppressive therapy and with clinical AIDS. Patients present with abdominal pain and

diarrhoea, and may have a palpable, right lower quadrant mass. Characteristic findings are of circumferential caecal wall thickening, with oedematous bowel wall and inflammatory changes. Pericolonic fluid and intramural pneumatosis may be seen. Leukaemic deposits would be expected to cause more eccentric bowel wall thickening. Appendicitis may result in apical caecal wall thickening but would be accompanied by abnormal appendix. Crohn's disease may produce a similar picture, but, in this clinical setting, typhlitis is the most likely diagnosis. Diverticulitis would be very unlikely in this age group.

Dähnert (2007), 872–3.

100) a. ***

Necrotizing enterocolitis is an acute inflammatory bowel condition seen predominantly in preterm infants. It usually presents 2–3 days after birth, with abdominal distension, vomiting and blood-stained stools. Plain film signs include distended small and large bowel, and bowel wall thickening, but the hallmark of the condition is pneumatosis intestinalis, seen in 80% of cases. This may be curvilinear (subserosal) or bubbly (submucosal) and may also be associated with portal venous gas. Hirschsprung's disease is characterized by an aganglionic segment of distal colon, resulting in abnormal peristalsis and impaired evacuation of the colon. In this age group, it presents with failure to pass meconium, but is extremely rare in preterm infants. Meconium ileus and imperforate anus also present with failure to pass meconium. Pneumatosis intestinalis may be seen in association with mechanical obstruction resulting from these three conditions, but it is rare. It is not a feature of viral gastroenteritis.

Dähnert (2007), 861.

MODULE 6
CENTRAL NERVOUS SYSTEM AND
HEAD & NECK

Module 6: Central Nervous System and Head & Neck: Questions

1) A 70-year-old woman presents with a sudden onset of right-sided hemiplegia and expressive dysphasia. She is otherwise well and has normal blood pressure on examination. Emergency CT shows a small subcortical acute haemorrhage in the inferior posterior left frontal lobe. Elsewhere, throughout the brain, there are smaller acute and subacute haemorrhages in the subcortex and a background of lacunar infarction. There is also marked brain atrophy in excess of that expected for the patient's age. Changes consistent with diffuse leukoencephalopathy are also seen. What is the most likely underlying pathological condition?

   a. malignant hypertension
   b. acute disseminated encephalomyelitis
   c. neurosarcoidosis
   d. neuroamyloidosis
   e. haemorrhagic metastases

2) A child who undergoes MR of the brain for clinically apparent facial abnormalities is shown to have a defect of midline cleavage of the brain. What structure is abnormal or absent in all forms of holoprosencephaly, and therefore is the most sensitive indicator of a midline cleavage abnormality?

   a. falx cerebri
   b. third ventricle
   c. fourth ventricle
   d. corpus callosum
   e. septum pellucidum

3) A 37-year-old man with AIDS presents with confusion, lethargy and memory loss. CT of the brain demonstrates multiple supratentorial enhancing masses. Which imaging feature favours a diagnosis of toxoplasmosis rather than primary CNS lymphoma?

   a. subependymal distribution
   b. lesions hyperdense on unenhanced CT
   c. lesion size >3 cm
   d. hypovascularity on MR perfusion study
   e. increased uptake of thallium-201 on SPECT

4) An 80-year-old man presents acutely with a dense hemiplegia. CT perfusion is performed soon after admission, which suggests that the entire involved arterial territory is beyond recovery. Which of the following options represents the most likely combination of cerebral blood flow, mean transit time and cerebral blood volume, respectively, seen within the affected brain parenchyma, compared with unaffected parenchyma?

a. increased, increased, increased
b. increased, increased, decreased
c. increased, decreased, decreased
d. decreased, decreased, decreased
e. decreased, increased, decreased

5) A 14-year-old boy with a recent history of viral upper respiratory tract infection presents with a 2-day history of rapid onset of fever and lethargy progressing to reduced consciousness and seizures. MRI shows several large lesions in the cerebral white matter, and a diagnosis of acute disseminated encephalomyelitis is made. Which additional finding is associated with the most fulminant course of this disease, with a median survival of only 6 days?

a. grey matter involvement
b. high signal in the CSF on FLAIR images
c. generalized brain oedema
d. areas of petechial haemorrhage
e. enhancement with intravenous gadolinium

6) Which of the following conditions will typically demonstrate unrestricted diffusion on MR DWI and ADC map?

a. epidermoid cyst
b. acute infarction
c. cerebral abscess
d. glioblastoma multiforme
e. viral encephalitis

7) A 77-year-old patient presents with amaurosis fugax. A carotid Doppler ultrasound scan is performed. Which of the following findings would be suggestive of an internal carotid artery stenosis of >70% (using Consensus Conference of Society of Radiologists in Ultrasound 2002 criteria)?

a. internal carotid artery peak systolic velocity of 120 cm/s
b. internal carotid artery end-diastolic velocity of 80 cm/s
c. ratio of peak systolic velocities in internal and common carotid arteries of >4.0
d. loss of flow in common carotid artery during diastole
e. no spectral broadening

8) A 62-year-old man with a history of falls and confusion undergoes MR of the brain. This demonstrates a subdural haematoma of high signal intensity on T1W images and of high signal intensity with a hypointense rim on T2W images. What is the most likely age of the haematoma?

   a. <6 hours
   b. 8–72 hours
   c. 3 days to 1 week
   d. 1 week to several months
   e. several months to several years

9) A 75-year-old man undergoes an aortic valve replacement. His GCS remains low as the general anaesthetic effect wears off, and a new left-sided weakness is observed. Unenhanced CT of the brain is performed. The CT reveals a hypodensity (of attenuation value −30 HU) within the first segment of the right middle cerebral artery. Which of the following options is most likely to explain the patient's abnormal neurology?

   a. right middle cerebral artery thromboembolic occlusion
   b. cerebral embolism as part of the fat embolism syndrome
   c. right middle cerebral artery fat embolism
   d. right middle cerebral artery air embolism
   e. right middle cerebral artery dissection

10) A 46-year-old patient presents with an enlarged level IV lymph node in the neck. Histology from FNA demonstrates metastatic squamous cell carcinoma. Which of the following is the most likely site of the primary malignancy?

   a. oral cavity
   b. nasopharynx
   c. tongue
   d. salivary gland
   e. larynx

11) Degenerative spinal vertebral body endplate changes, as seen on MRI, may have which of the following appearances?

   a. type I – high T1W and low T2W signal
   b. type I – low T1W and low T2W signal
   c. type II – high T1W and high T2W signal
   d. type II – low T1W and high T2W signal
   e. type II – high T1W and low T2W signal

12) A 14-year-old boy presents with a grossly abnormal gait, kyphoscoliosis and upper limb tremors. MRI shows mild atrophy of the cerebellum and much more marked cervicomedullary junction thinning with decreased anteroposterior diameter of the upper cervical spinal cord, which returns normal signal. What is the most likely diagnosis?

   a. Friedreich's ataxia
   b. Creutzfeldt–Jakob disease
   c. olivopontocerebellar atrophy
   d. Huntington's disease
   e. tuberous sclerosis

13) What are the typical appearances of a pituitary microadenoma on early, contrast-enhanced T1W MR images?

   a. focus of hypointensity within normal enhancing gland
   b. focus of enhancement within normal, non-enhancing gland
   c. lesion and normal gland enhance similarly
   d. hyperenhancing focus within normal, mildly enhancing gland
   e. not usually visualized on this sequence

14) A 20-year-old man presents with gradual onset of neck pain and a painful lump in the upper neck posteriorly. Plain films show an apparent destructive lesion of the C2 vertebra. MRI shows a large lesion arising from the posterior elements of C2 and comprising multiple cysts with fluid–fluid levels, with preservation of the vertebral body. What is the most likely diagnosis?

   a. aneurysmal bone cyst
   b. giant cell tumour
   c. chordoma
   d. fibrous dysplasia
   e. telangiectatic osteosarcoma

15) A 32-year-old man of African descent presents to the neurologist with a several-month history of headache followed by rapid onset of bilateral facial weakness and blurring of vision. An MRI shows thickening of the basal leptomeninges, which enhance with intravenous gadolinium. Abnormal areas are identified in the pituitary gland, and optic and facial nerves, which all return low signal on T1W images and high signal on FLAIR images. What is the most likely diagnosis?

   a. multiple sclerosis
   b. tuberculous meningitis
   c. neuroamyloidosis
   d. neurosarcoidosis
   e. lymphoma

16) A 46-year-old female presents with back pain and increasing weakness of the lower limbs. An MR scan shows a lesion in the cord at the level of T11. Which of the following features would suggest an ependymoma rather than demyelination?

a. multiple lesions
b. expansion of the cord
c. high signal on T2W images
d. enhancement with gadolinium
e. peripheral low signal on all sequences

17) A mass is seen peripherally in the middle cranial fossa on MR of the brain. Which of the following imaging features favours an intra-axial rather than an extra-axial location?

a. buckling of the grey–white matter interface
b. expansion of the cortex of the brain
c. expansion of the subarachnoid space
d. medial displacement of pial blood vessels by the mass
e. the mass has a dural base

18) A 35-year-old woman presents with progressive deafness and tinnitus in the left ear. She undergoes MRI, which demonstrates a 2 cm mass at the left cerebellopontine angle. Which of the following features would favour a diagnosis of meningioma rather than vestibular schwannoma?

a. acute angle with the petrous bone
b. hyperintensity on T2W images
c. expansion of the internal auditory canal
d. presence of a dural tail
e. internal cystic degeneration and haemorrhage

19) A 64-year-old woman presents with progressive headache and confusion. On CT, she is found to have multiple, well-defined, rounded, low-attenuation masses of varying sizes in both hemispheres at the grey–white matter junction. The masses demonstrate intense enhancement following intravenous contrast, and there is considerable surrounding oedema. Which of the following is the most appropriate next imaging investigation?

a. mammography
b. thyroid ultrasound scan
c. barium enema
d. renal ultrasound scan
e. chest radiograph

20) A 78-year-old male patient presents with signs of acute lumbar myelopathy. Lumbar spine radiographs show collapse of the L3 vertebral body, which is encroaching upon the spinal canal. Additionally, throughout the remaining visualized vertebral bodies, there is diminished density of the central trabecular bone with relative preservation of the cortex and thickening of the marginal trabeculations, which appear coarse. What is the most likely underlying condition of bone?

a. Paget's disease
b. pyknodysostosis
c. osteopetrosis
d. Gaucher's disease
e. hyperparathyroidism

21) A 52-year-old female presents with increasing short-term memory problems. CT and MR scans are normal. A perfusion scintigraphy study of the brain shows reduced perfusion in the posterior parietal regions bilaterally. What is the most likely diagnosis?

a. Alzheimer's disease
b. vascular dementia
c. Lewy body dementia
d. frontotemporal dementia
e. Parkinson's disease

22) What is the most sensitive sign on non-contrast CT for detecting early hydrocephalus?

a. cortical sulcal effacement
b. uncal herniation
c. enlarged third ventricle
d. enlarged fourth ventricle
e. enlarged temporal horns of the lateral ventricles

23) A 22-year-old man presents with a 6-week history of progressive worsening confusion. Initial CT examination is normal. Following neurological review, the patient undergoes MRI, at which the only abnormality seen is high signal in the posterior portions of the thalami bilaterally on T2W and FLAIR images. What is the most likely condition?

a. acute disseminated encephalomyelitis
b. variant Creutzfeldt–Jakob disease
c. multiple sclerosis
d. metachromatic leukodystrophy
e. Rasmussen's encephalitis

24) A 60-year-old female admitted with severe, sudden-onset headache is found to have widely distributed subarachnoid haemorrhage. A saccular aneurysm is identified on CT angiography. From which of the following locations in the circle of Willis is this aneurysm most likely to arise?

a. basilar tip
b. middle cerebral artery bifurcation
c. junction of anterior cerebral and anterior communicating arteries
d. pericallosal artery
e. vertebral artery

25) A 70-year-old man is referred for CT scan of the brain due to sudden onset of left-sided hemiparesis and clinical diagnosis of stroke. Unenhanced CT shows a rounded area of low attenuation in the right posterior frontal lobe with local gyriform swelling and sulcal effacement. Upon questioning, he reveals a history of lung resection for malignancy 18 months previously. Which of the following imaging investigations would you perform next?

a. no further imaging
b. CT of the thorax
c. CT of the thorax and abdomen
d. MRI of the brain
e. contrast-enhanced CT of the brain

26) A 43-year-old man presents with cough and numerous masses in the neck bilaterally. CT confirms multiple lymph nodes that enhance peripherally and contain areas of calcification. A cavitating lesion is noted in the right lung apex. What is the most likely diagnosis?

a. tuberculosis
b. metastatic laryngeal carcinoma
c. metastatic nasopharyngeal carcinoma
d. metastatic papillary thyroid carcinoma
e. metastatic squamous cell carcinoma of the lung

27) A 22-year-old man with von Hippel–Lindau syndrome presents with headaches, vomiting and ataxia. CT of the brain demonstrates an abnormality in the posterior fossa. What are the most likely findings?

a. cystic lesion with an enhancing mural nodule
b. multiple ring-enhancing lesions with surrounding oedema
c. gyriform cortical calcifications
d. multiple calcified subependymal nodules
e. hypodense, ill-defined mass with central necrosis and marked surrounding oedema

28) With ageing, iron accumulates in tissues of the brain and is seen as low signal on both T1W and T2W sequences at MRI. Which of the following locations for iron deposition is pathological in a 60-year-old man and may indicate onset of dementia?

a. putamen
b. globus pallidus
c. red nucleus
d. dentate nucleus
e. pars reticulata

29) An 85-year-old female presents with low back pain and is tender over the sacrum. Radiographs show a generalized reduction in bone density. MRI demonstrates symmetrical, bilateral, linear areas of signal abnormality in the sacral alae, which are low signal on T1W and high signal on STIR images. There is no history of trauma, but the patient does have a history of radiotherapy for cervical carcinoma many years previously. What is the most likely diagnosis?

a. insufficiency fracture
b. metastases
c. ankylosing spondylitis
d. Reiter's syndrome
e. post-radiotherapy change

30) A patient presents with diplopia and is found to have unilateral restricted eye movements. On MRI, the extraocular muscles of the same eye are seen to be enlarged and oedematous. Which of the following additional features favours a carotid–cavernous sinus fistula as the diagnosis, over Graves' disease, lymphoma or orbital pseudotumour?

a. distal tapering of the swollen extraocular muscles
b. stranding in the orbital fat
c. extraocular muscles isointense to fat on T2W images
d. dilated superior ophthalmic vein
e. extraocular muscle swelling involving the tendons

31) A 5-year-old boy undergoes CT of the brain for investigation of headaches, vomiting and ataxia. This demonstrates a well-defined, multilobulated, isodense mass within the fourth ventricle containing areas of punctate calcification. The mass is seen to extend out of the foramina of Luschka into the cerebellopontine angles. There is associated hydrocephalus. What is the most likely diagnosis?

a. metastasis
b. haemangioblastoma
c. juvenile pilocytic astrocytoma
d. medulloblastoma
e. ependymoma

32) An 18-month-old toddler presents with progressive gait disturbance, motor developmental delay and muscle weakness. Biochemical tests show abnormally low levels of arylsulphatase A enzyme in peripheral blood leukocytes and urine. MRI demonstrates symmetrical, confluent areas of high signal on T2W images affecting the periventricular and cerebellar white matter, corpus callosum and corticospinal tracts with sparing of the subcortical U fibres. The periventricular abnormality shows a striped 'tigroid' pattern. There is no enhancement with administration of intravenous gadolinium. What is the most likely condition?

a. Alexander's disease
b. Canavan's disease
c. acute disseminated encephalomyelitis
d. mucopolysaccharidosis
e. metachromatic leukodystrophy

33) An elderly male patient presents with signs suggesting acute middle cerebral artery infarction. Around $2\frac{1}{2}$ hours after symptom onset, an unenhanced CT of the brain is performed. Among other subtle signs, the basal ganglia are obscured. Reduced perfusion through which of the following vessels best explains this sign?

a. lenticulostriate arteries
b. anterior choroidal artery
c. callosomarginal artery
d. recurrent artery of Heubner
e. angular artery

34) An unenhanced CT scan of the brain is performed 3 hours after the onset of signs suggestive of ischaemic stroke. Which of the following image window parameters is most likely to reveal the early CT changes?

a. width 400 HU, centre 40 HU
b. width 80 HU, centre 20 HU
c. width 8 HU, centre 32 HU
d. width 0 HU, centre 0 HU
e. width 1500, centre −500 HU

35) A 9-month-old boy presents to the paediatric neurologist with general developmental delay, left-sided weakness from birth and tonic–clonic seizures. MRI performed under anaesthetic reveals a thin cleft containing CSF extending from the right lateral ventricle to the cortical surface of the right frontal lobe. The margins of the cleft are opposed and lined with heterotopic grey matter that shows polymicrogyria. Which disorder of cortical formation is described?

a. porencephaly
b. schizencephaly
c. holoprosencephaly
d. lissencephaly
e. hemimegalencephaly

36) A patient is investigated by catheter angiogram for a giant anterior communicating artery aneurysm. Soon after the procedure, the patient experiences excessive nausea. Unenhanced CT of the brain offers no explanation, but a small bright focus is seen in the cerebellum on T2W MR images. Which of the following is the most likely explanation?

a. iodinated contrast media reaction
b. rupture of the aneurysm
c. embolism of vertebral arterial plaque
d. dissection of internal carotid artery
e. vasospasm of common carotid artery

37) A 39-year-old man known to have HIV and with clinically deteriorating dementia undergoes MRI of the brain with a provisional diagnosis of HIV encephalopathy. Images show abnormal high signal on T2W and FLAIR images affecting the white matter, caudate nucleus and basal ganglia on a background of brain atrophy. Which additional MR characteristic of these lesions is likely to suggest progressive multifocal leukoencephalopathy over HIV encephalopathy?

a. frontal white matter preponderance
b. clustering around the basal ganglia
c. involvement of subcortical U fibres
d. areas of haemorrhagic necrosis
e. enhancement with intravenous gadolinium

38) Which of the following MR sequences is most sensitive for detecting subcortical and periventricular lesions in multiple sclerosis?

a. axial T1W
b. axial T2W
c. axial FLAIR
d. axial proton density
e. axial T1W post-gadolinium contrast

39) A 65-year-old, previously well man with a short history of headaches and behavioural change undergoes CT of the brain. This demonstrates an irregular, ill-defined mass in the left frontal lobe extending across the corpus callosum to involve the right frontal lobe. The mass is of low attenuation and contains cystic areas, demonstrates ring enhancement following intravenous contrast, and has considerable surrounding oedema. What is the most likely diagnosis?

a. progressive multifocal leukoencephalopathy
b. glioblastoma multiforme
c. lymphoma
d. abscess
e. metastasis

40) A 35-year-old man is involved in a low-velocity road traffic accident. Within minutes, he experiences an occipital headache and neck pain. On arrival in hospital, he complains of nausea, vertigo and diplopia. An unenhanced CT scan of the brain is performed. Which of the following abnormal findings is most likely?

a. high density seen in CSF of the sylvian fissure
b. low density and loss of grey–white matter differentiation in the insular region
c. expansion of a vertebral artery with a peripheral, high-density crescent
d. lenticular high attenuation between the temporal lobe and temporal bone
e. crescent-shaped high attenuation between the temporal lobe and temporal bone

41) A 70-year-old man has severe rhinorrhoea and then develops a cough with haemoptysis. A chest radiograph shows a large nodule in the right lung, and a subsequent CT thorax demonstrates a cavitary, left-lung nodule. A cerebral catheter angiogram, undertaken to investigate a focal motor deficit, is most likely to reveal which of the following?

a. a giant berry aneurysm
b. multiple aneurysms with stenoses and occlusions
c. dural arteriovenous malformation
d. contrast extravasation
e. numerous collaterals supplying the anterior circle of Willis

42) An elderly man undergoes CT for gradual onset of confusion and memory loss. A pattern of generalized global brain atrophy showing marked temporal lobe predominance with an increase in size of the hippocampal–choroidal fissure is seen. Coronal T2W images show atrophy of the hippocampus bilaterally. Which condition is most likely to result in such a pattern of volume loss?

a. Pick's disease
b. Alzheimer's disease
c. Parkinson's disease
d. Lewy body dementia
e. multi-infarct dementia

43) A patient with multiple previous ischaemic strokes has an MRI including T2W and DWI sequences. In the left frontal lobe, there is a region of increased T2 signal. The same area is dark on the DWI and bright on the ADC map. Which of the following is the most likely age of this region of ischaemia?

a. 10 minutes
b. 30 minutes
c. 3 days
d. 2 weeks
e. 4 months

44) A 62-year-old male patient presents with a mass in the right side of his neck. CT shows an enlarged, right-sided lymph node anterior to sternocleidomastoid, below the level of the hyoid bone and above the cricoid ring. At which level does the node lie?

a. level I
b. level II
c. level III
d. level IV
e. level V

45) A 21 year old presents with back pain, increasing over time. There are no neurological symptoms. A radiograph of the lumbar spine shows a grade II spondylolisthesis at L5–S1. Which of the following features would suggest the presence of bilateral spondylolysis as the cause?

a. narrowing of AP diameter of spinal canal at L5–S1
b. widening of AP diameter of spinal canal at L5–S1
c. lucencies through the laminae of L5
d. sclerosis of the pedicles of L5
e. reduced height of the L5–S1 disc

46) A 17-year-old boy presents with headache and is found to have paralysis of upward gaze (Parinaud's syndrome) on examination. MR scan of the brain identifies an abnormality. What is the most likely site of the lesion?

a. thalamus
b. occipital lobe
c. optic chiasm
d. pineal gland
e. cerebellar vermis

47) A 28-year-old woman presents with a history of headaches and refractory temporal lobe epilepsy. CT of the brain demonstrates a mixed solid–cystic, intraparenchymal mass located peripherally in the right temporal lobe, which contains calcification and demonstrates faint enhancement following intravenous contrast. There is minimal surrounding oedema. What is the most likely diagnosis?

a. arachnoid cyst
b. ganglioglioma
c. epidermoid
d. meningioma
e. dysembryoplastic neuroepithelial tumour

48) Which of the following represents an appropriate window width and level for viewing the bony structures on a CT scan of the brain?

a. width 80, level 35
b. width 400, level 40
c. width 250, level 70
d. width 2000, level 500
e. width 1500, level −500

49) A 24-year-old male patient presents following a head injury with GCS of 13. There is bruising over the right temporal region. A CT scan shows no intracranial haemorrhage but does identify a longitudinal fracture through the petrous temporal bone. What complication should be considered?

a. sensorineural hearing loss
b. conductive hearing loss
c. vertigo
d. carotid artery injury
e. sigmoid sinus injury

50) A 44-year-old man presents with a long history of headaches and more recent onset of seizures. CT of the brain demonstrates an oval, well-defined, heterogeneous, hypodense mass containing large nodular clumps of calcification located peripherally in the right frontal lobe. The mass extends to the cortical margin, and there is erosion of the inner table of the skull. There is minimal surrounding vasogenic oedema. What is the most likely diagnosis?

a. meningioma
b. oligodendroglioma
c. astrocytoma
d. glioblastoma multiforme
e. ganglioglioma

51) A patient presents with colicky, right-sided, abdominal pain and is found to have multiple renal calculi. Blood tests reveal hypercalcaemia and hyperparathyroidism. Ultrasound scan shows a hypoechoic nodule posterior to the left lobe of the thyroid suggestive of parathyroid adenoma. Which features on parathyroid scintigraphy, using pertechnetate and sestamibi (with delayed washout images), would suggest a functioning parathyroid adenoma at this site?

a. increased uptake on pertechnetate and sestamibi studies with delayed washout
b. no uptake on pertechnetate; increased uptake on sestamibi with normal washout
c. no uptake on pertechnetate; increased uptake on sestamibi with delayed washout
d. no uptake on pertechnetate or sestamibi studies including delayed image
e. increased uptake on pertechnetate and no uptake on sestamibi study including delayed image

52) A 19-year-old man with axillary freckling has a cerebral angiogram for recurrent hemiparetic episodes. There is bilateral occlusion of the distal internal carotid arteries extending into the proximal anterior and middle cerebral arteries. This is associated with an extensive network of upper brain-stem collaterals. Which of the following is the most likely cause of the angiographic findings in this patient?

a. sickle cell disease
b. atherosclerosis
c. radiation vasculopathy
d. Moyamoya syndrome
e. amyloid angiopathy

53) A 50-year-old female presents with a 'thunder-clap' headache and fluctuating level of consciousness. Unenhanced CT of the brain shows high-density material layered in the occipital horns of the lateral ventricles. Which of the following is the most appropriate next imaging investigation?

a. CT angiography
b. CT venography
c. MR angiography
d. catheter angiography
e. radionuclide regional cerebral blood flow imaging

54) A 20-year-old male is involved in an accident in which one femur is fractured. No other significant injury is revealed by CT of the brain, cervical spine, chest, abdomen and pelvis. Several hours after the injury, petechial skin haemorrhages appear, associated with respiratory distress and hypoxia. The patient complains of headache shortly before a seizure is witnessed. Repeat CT of the brain is unchanged and looks normal. Which of the following brain MRI findings best accounts for the patient's condition?

a. diffuse low T2 signal in subarachnoid space
b. crescent-shaped, space-occupying, extra-axial, low-T2-signal abnormality
c. lenticular, space-occupying, extra-axial, low-T2-signal abnormality
d. multiple, small, non-confluent, hyperintense lesions on T2W images and DWI within the cerebral deep white and deep grey matter
e. multiple, small, non-confluent, hypointense lesions on T2W and DWI within the cerebral deep white and deep grey matter

55) One week following a subarachnoid haemorrhage, a 50-year-old female, who had thus far been making a good recovery, develops intractable vomiting, vertigo and ataxia. An unenhanced CT of the brain demonstrates unchanged ventricular size but a new hypodense region in a cerebellar hemisphere. Which of the following complications of subarachnoid haemorrhage is most likely to have occurred?

a. acute obstructive hydrocephalus
b. delayed communicating hydrocephalus
c. vasospasm and infarction
d. transtentorial herniation
e. rebleed from a berry aneurysm

56) A 30-year-old female presents with left-sided hearing loss and facial nerve palsy. CT shows a solid mass in the left middle ear behind an intact tympanic membrane, occupying an enlarged attic and eroding the scutum and middle-ear ossicles. What is the most likely diagnosis?

a. Bell's palsy
b. cholesteatoma
c. malignant otitis externa
d. acoustic neuroma
e. squamous cell carcinoma

57) A 46-year-old man presents with headaches and visual disturbance and is found to have bitemporal hemianopia on visual field testing. CT of the brain demonstrates a multilobulated, heterogeneous, suprasellar mass containing cystic areas and rim-like calcification. Enhancement of the solid component is observed following intravenous contrast. What is the most likely diagnosis?

a. epidermoid
b. craniopharyngioma
c. pituitary macroadenoma
d. meningioma
e. Rathke's cleft cyst

58) A 27-year-old, previously well man gives a history of positional headaches. He undergoes unenhanced CT of the brain, which demonstrates a well-defined, hyperdense, spherical lesion in the anterosuperior portion of the third ventricle, with asymmetrical enlargement of the lateral ventricles. What is the most likely diagnosis?

a. meningioma
b. colloid cyst
c. ependymoma
d. subependymal giant cell astrocytoma
e. choroid plexus papilloma

59) A 47-year-old female presents with gradual onset back pain over 4 weeks, with associated pyrexia and tenderness at the thoracolumbar junction. Radiographs show destruction of the endplates at the T12–L1 disc level. Which of the following features on further imaging would suggest tuberculous over pyogenic discitis as a cause?

a. single-level involvement
b. paravertebral, soft-tissue mass
c. epidural abscess
d. disc-space loss
e. calcification

60) Which of the following is the most common radiation-induced CNS tumour?

a. ependymoma
b. oligodendroglioma
c. lymphoma
d. glioblastoma multiforme
e. meningioma

61) On an axial section of the brain at the level of the third ventricle, which structure lies immediately lateral to the putamen?

a. internal capsule
b. globus pallidus
c. external capsule
d. thalamus
e. insular cortex

62) Ultrasound examination of the face and neck is performed to investigate a buccal, soft-tissue mass that became noticeable during pregnancy. The lesion is heterogeneous and hypoechoic, and has sinusoidal spaces demonstrating slow flow and circular calcifications. Which of the following is the most likely diagnosis?

a. benign lymph node
b. malignant lymph node
c. pleomorphic parotid adenoma
d. arteriovenous malformation
e. venous vascular malformation

63) A 20-year-old male patient has an MR scan of his spine for investigation of back pain. He has low IQ and multiple skin patches. The MR scan shows bilateral branching tubular paraspinal masses, with widening of the intervertebral foramina and posterior scalloping of the vertebral bodies. A sharply angulated kyphosis is present at the thoracolumbar junction. What is the most likely diagnosis?

a. neurofibromatosis type 1
b. neurofibromatosis type 2
c. tuberous sclerosis
d. Marfan's syndrome
e. Ehlers–Danlos syndrome

64) A 56-year-old male presents with a mass in the anterior triangle of the neck and is referred for ultrasound scan and biopsy. Ultrasound scan shows a vascular mass splaying the internal and external carotid arteries at their origin. How should cell sampling of the mass be undertaken?

a. perform FNA rather than core biopsy
b. use multiple passes
c. use a single pass
d. ensure that needle midway between internal and external carotid arteries
e. both FNA and core biopsy contraindicated

65) A severely hypoplastic cerebellar vermis in an enlarged bony posterior fossa, with associated hydrocephalus and communication of the fourth ventricle with a posterior midline CSF cyst, are features of which of the following posterior fossa malformations?

a. mega cisterna magna
b. Dandy–Walker malformation
c. Dandy–Walker variant
d. Arnold–Chiari malformation
e. Joubert's syndrome

66) Following a large postpartum haemorrhage, a 25-year-old woman develops a severe headache and sudden visual field defect. What is the most likely diagnosis?

a. intracerebral haemorrhage
b. reversible posterior leukoencephalopathy
c. subarachnoid haemorrhage
d. Sheehan's syndrome
e. vertebral artery dissection

67) Which paired vein forms in the sylvian fissure and travels in the ambient cistern around the midbrain to enter the vein of Galen along with the internal cerebral vein?

a. superficial middle cerebral or sylvian vein
b. basal vein of Rosenthal
c. vein of Labbe
d. vein of Trolard
e. thalamostriate vein

68) Carotid Doppler examination is performed on a patient following a transient ischaemic attack. All other factors are in favour of surgical treatment for carotid stenosis. At what peak internal carotid artery velocity would ultrasound scan also support this management?

a. >50 cm/s
b. >75 cm/s
c. >100 cm/s
d. >200 cm/s
e. >250 cm/s

69) In the presence of raised intracranial pressure, the anterior cerebral artery is at risk of compression during which of the following types of brain herniation?

a. transforaminal herniation
b. sphenoid herniation
c. ascending transtentorial herniation
d. descending transtentorial herniation
e. subfalcine herniation

70) A 30-year-old man with a history of metastatic malignant melanoma presents with sudden onset of visual loss of the upper right quadrant in both eyes (right superior homonymous quadrantanopia). Emergency CT of the brain demonstrates a haemorrhagic cerebral metastasis with surrounding oedema. Which of the following is the most likely location of the lesion?

a. optic chiasm
b. right temporal lobe
c. left temporal lobe
d. left thalamus
e. right thalamus

71) Sequelae and complications of meningitis that may be identified on contrast-enhanced CT of the brain in the acute phase of the disease include all but which of the following?

a. venous sinus thrombosis
b. leptomeningeal enhancement
c. encephalomalacia
d. ring-enhancing mass lesion
e. infarction

72) A 23-year-old man presents with acute headache. Unenhanced CT of the brain demonstrates a heterogeneous mass at the inferior cerebellar vermis. It is predominantly of fat attenuation with areas of calcification and does not enhance following administration of intravenous contrast. Multiple droplets of fat attenuation are noted throughout the subarachnoid space. What is the most likely diagnosis?

a. lipoma
b. arachnoid cyst
c. dermoid
d. epidermoid
e. teratoma

73) Between which structures do the dural venous sinuses lie?

a. skull and dura mater
b. dura mater and dura mater
c. dura mater and arachnoid mater
d. arachnoid mater and pia mater
e. pia mater and brain

74) A 65-year-old man presents with back stiffness and painful hips. Radiographs of the thoracolumbar spine and pelvis show ossification of the iliolumbar and sacroiliac ligaments with whiskering of the ischial tuberosities. Which of the following additional features is most likely to be seen on the spine radiographs?

a. flowing osteophytes over several vertebral levels
b. squaring of vertebral bodies
c. reduced disc spaces
d. sclerosis of vertebral bodies
e. posterior longitudinal ligament calcification

75) Which of the following imaging features of an intraparenchymal haemorrhage is most likely to suggest that the haemorrhage originates from an underlying tumour?

a. homogeneous CT appearance
b. complete haemosiderin ring
c. complete resolution on follow-up imaging
d. solitary haemorrhage
e. post-contrast enhancement of non-haemorrhagic areas

76) Bilateral globus pallidus injury manifest radiologically as high signal on T2W MR sequences is indicative of poisoning by which of the following substances?

a. lead
b. methanol
c. carbon monoxide
d. carbon dioxide
e. mercury

77) A 31-year-old woman presents with a painless mass involving the right side of the mandible. Radiographs show a well-defined, lucent lesion. Which of the following additional findings favour a diagnosis of ameloblastoma over a radicular cyst?

a. absence of matrix mineralization
b. location at the symphysis menti
c. location at the root of a tooth
d. soap-bubble appearance
e. rim of cortical bone

78) The fourth branch of the external carotid artery crosses the inferior border of the mandible before traversing the cheek, and forms an important connection between the external and internal carotid arteries by anastomosing with branches of the ophthalmic artery. Which artery is described?

a. ascending pharyngeal
b. lingual
c. facial
d. maxillary
e. superficial temporal

79) A hypertensive, 75-year-old female admitted with an acute stroke is found, on unenhanced CT of the brain, to have an acute basal ganglia haemorrhage. If an MRI were performed 2 weeks later, what signal characteristics would the region of haemorrhage return?

a. isointense on T1W images and hyperintense on T2W images
b. hyperintense on T1W images and hyperintense on T2W images
c. isointense on T1W images and hypointense on T2W images
d. hyperintense on T1W images and hypointense on T2W images
e. hypointense on T1W images and a rim of hypointensity on T2W images

80) A 24-year-old man is an unrestrained passenger in a car involved in a high-speed collision. He is found unconscious at the scene. CT of the brain is normal. MR scan of the brain demonstrates multiple small foci of high signal on T2W images in the white matter of the parasagittal regions of the frontal lobes and the periventricular regions of the temporal lobes. What is the most likely diagnosis?

a. acute subdural haematoma
b. diffuse axonal injury
c. cortical contusions
d. intracerebral haematoma
e. subcortical grey matter injury

81) A 31-year-old woman presents to the neurologist with a transient episode of facial numbness. On close questioning, she reveals a transient episode of blurred vision which occurred several months previously. MRI, including MR angiography, shows several small areas of low signal on T1W and high signal on T2W images in the optic nerves and cerebellar peduncles. The FLAIR sequence demonstrates further multiple, ovoid, high-signal areas in the corpus callosum and periventricular white matter. The angiogram demonstrates normal head and neck vessels. These imaging findings support which of the following diagnoses?

a. internal carotid artery dissection
b. multiple sclerosis
c. progressive multifocal leukoencephalopathy
d. acute disseminated encephalomyelitis
e. wallerian degeneration

82) In normal anatomy of the nasal cavity, which structure opens into the inferior meatus below the inferior nasal turbinate?

a. anterior ethmoidal ostium
b. posterior ethmoidal ostium
c. frontal sinus ostium
d. maxillary sinus ostium
e. nasolacrimal duct

83) Regional cerebral blood flow imaging is required to localize an epileptic focus. Of the following radiopharmaceuticals, which is the most appropriate for this purpose?

a. ^{99m}Tc-labelled MAA
b. ^{99m}Tc-labelled DTPA
c. ^{99m}Tc-labelled pertechnetate
d. ^{99m}Tc-labelled glucoheptonate
e. ^{99m}Tc-labelled ECD

84) A 30-year-old woman presents acutely with seizures, fever and headache, followed by rapid deterioration to coma. Emergency MRI shows asymmetrical swelling of the anterior temporal lobes on T1W images. T2W images reveal concordant asymmetrical but bilateral areas of high signal in the anterior temporal lobes, insular cortices and hippocampi. There is no enhancement following administration of intravenous gadolinium. What is the most likely condition?

a. lymphoma
b. HIV encephalitis
c. cytomegalovirus encephalitis
d. herpes simplex encephalitis
e. toxoplasmosis

85) A young patient presents with double vision and is found on examination to have a ptosis and dilated left pupil. The gaze in the same eye is fixed inferiorly and laterally and, when the ipsilateral light reflex is tested, there is constriction of the contralateral pupil only. CT shows a small spontaneous brain-stem haemorrhage thought to be due to an arteriovenous malformation. Which of the following locations of the haemorrhage best explains the presenting symptoms?

a. superior pons
b. inferior pons
c. superior midbrain
d. inferior midbrain
e. superior medulla

86) A 27-year-old female presents with emotional lability and headaches. MRI of the brain demonstrates a well-defined mass in the pericallosal region. The mass is hyperintense on T1W images and demonstrates no enhancement with intravenous gadolinium. There is associated agenesis of the corpus callosum. What is the most likely diagnosis?

a. dermoid
b. lipoma
c. interhemispheric arachnoid cyst
d. epidermoid
e. lymphoma

87) A 38-year-old male presents with a history of recent head injury and unilateral, painful, pulsatile exophthalmos with reduced visual acuity. CT shows swelling of the extraocular muscles with dilatation of the superior ophthalmic vein and cavernous sinus on the ipsilateral side, both of which enhance avidly. What is the most likely diagnosis?

a. ophthalmic varix
b. arteriovenous malformation
c. lymphangioma
d. carotid–cavernous fistula
e. pseudotumour of orbit

88) A 30-year-old female with a past medical history of spontaneous pulmonary embolus presents 2 weeks after giving birth with severe headache, vomiting and drowsiness. Unenhanced CT of the brain shows areas of low attenuation with sulcal effacement and small areas of parenchymal haemorrhage. These changes do not conform to an arterial distribution. What is the most likely finding on the post-contrast CT brain?

   a. ring enhancement of the low-attenuation regions
   b. demonstration of a basilar tip aneurysm
   c. 'empty delta' sign
   d. anterior pituitary enlargement
   e. vertebral artery dissection flap

89) Which of the following structures lies in the parapharyngeal space?

   a. internal carotid artery
   b. hypoglossal nerve
   c. maxillary artery
   d. lingual tonsil
   e. vagus nerve

90) A 43-year-old female presents on an ultrasound list for a thyroid FNA. She has an enlarging thyroid gland, right lobe more so than the left, and is biochemically euthyroid. Ultrasound scan shows multiple solid nodules with some cystic areas and foci of calcification throughout both lobes and the isthmus, with no obvious dominant nodule. Regarding FNA, how should the radiologist proceed?

   a. target solid lesion
   b. target calcification
   c. use multiple passes in both lobes
   d. use single pass at multiple sites
   e. do not perform FNA

91) A 31-year-old woman attends neurology clinic with a history of orthostatic headache, worst on standing, which sometimes induces vomiting, and relieved by lying down. MRI of the brain and cervical spine shows crowding of the foramen magnum due to low-lying cerebellar tonsils, elongation of the fourth ventricle, effacement of the prepontine cistern and a prominent pituitary gland. In the spine, an extradural fluid-signal collection is identified ventral to the cord. Administration of intravenous gadolinium reveals smooth areas of intracranial pachymeningeal enhancement. Which of the following diagnoses is best supported by these findings?

   a. intracranial hypotension
   b. intracranial hypertension
   c. migraine
   d. Chiari I malformation
   e. Dandy–Walker malformation

92) A 40-year-old male presents with pain in the jaw associated with dental caries. An orthopantomogram demonstrates a lytic lesion of 1 cm in diameter, associated with the apex of a carious tooth. The lesion has a thin rim of cortical bone and there is some resorption of the root. What is the likely diagnosis?

a. ameloblastoma
b. odontogenic keratocyst
c. dentigerous cyst
d. radicular cyst
e. odontoma

93) A 14-year-old boy is hit by a vehicle while riding his bike and sustains a left-sided head injury. Paramedics report a transient loss of consciousness at the scene. On examination, he is confused with a GCS of 13/15. Unenhanced CT of the brain is performed, which shows a biconvex extra-axial collection in the left temporoparietal region with attenuation value of 65 HU. On bone windows, there is an undisplaced, linear, left temporoparietal skull fracture. What is the most likely diagnosis?

a. acute subdural haematoma
b. acute extradural haematoma
c. acute subarachnoid haemorrhage
d. acute intracerebral haematoma
e. cerebral cortical contusion

94) The Wada test is performed before surgical treatment for medically refractory epilepsy. It involves intra-arterial injections of sodium amobarbital with ^{99m}Tc-labelled HMPAO followed by SPECT imaging to map the distribution of the barbiturate. What is the main indication for this test?

a. chemical ablation of epileptic foci
b. localization of speech and memory centres
c. mapping symmetry of brain vascular distribution
d. identification of interhemispheric collateral circulation
e. evaluation of cerebrovascular reserve

95) A 64-year-old man with squamous cell carcinoma of the lung presents with difficulty in speaking. On examination, he is noted to have dysarthric speech and deviation of the tongue to the left. CT of the brain is unremarkable, but review on bone windows reveals a destructive lesion of the left side of the skull base consistent with a bony metastasis. Which of the following skull base structures is most likely to be involved?

a. foramen ovale
b. foramen rotundum
c. foramen lacerum
d. jugular foramen
e. hypoglossal canal

96) A 65-year-old man has an unenhanced CT of the brain for recent-onset, unilateral hand weakness. The CT shows multiple, bilateral, small supratentorial regions of low attenuation. Which of the following is the most likely associated finding?

a. unilateral carotid atherosclerosis
b. cardiac valve disease
c. coarctation of proximal descending thoracic aorta
d. subclavian stenosis
e. sinus tachycardia

97) In brain imaging performed to characterize a chronic subdural collection, which feature is more likely to favour a diagnosis of subdural empyema over a sterile effusion?

a. isointense MR signal on T1W images
b. hyperintense MR signal on T2W images
c. subfalcine herniation
d. restricted diffusion on MR DWI
e. low attenuation on CT

98) A 50-year-old female presents with increasing weakness of the lower limbs and sensory disturbance. MRI shows an extramedullary, intradural ovoid mass in the mid-thoracic region. The lesion has signal isointense to the cord on T1W and T2W images, and enhances avidly with intravenous gadolinium. What is the most likely diagnosis?

a. meningioma
b. nerve sheath tumour
c. ependymoma
d. dermoid
e. arachnoid cyst

99) A 21-year-old man presents with acute headache. He undergoes CT of the brain, which demonstrates a well-circumscribed, lobulated, partially cystic, calcified mass in the frontal horn of the left lateral ventricle, attached to the septum pellucidum. There is acute blood seen layering in the left lateral ventricle and mild hydrocephalus. What is the most likely diagnosis?

a. choroid plexus papilloma
b. colloid cyst
c. intraventricular oligodendroglioma
d. central neurocytoma
e. subependymoma

100) A 2-year-old boy presents with involuntary saccadic eye movements (opsoclonus) and myoclonus of the trunk and limbs. What are the most likely findings on MRI of the brain?

a. normal appearances
b. cystic lesion in the posterior fossa with enhancing mural nodule
c. cerebellar atrophy
d. central symmetrical lesions in the pons of high signal intensity on T2W images
e. caudally displaced brain stem and fourth ventricle with tonsillar herniation

1) d. ***
Cerebral amyloid angiopathy is characterized by deposition of β-amyloid protein in cortical, subcortical and leptomeningeal vessels. It usually occurs in sporadic form and increases in frequency and severity with increasing age. The condition produces a wide variety of clinical symptoms and varied imaging appearances. Many cases are asymptomatic but progressive neurological symptomatology and cognitive decline may be a feature. Chronic haemorrhage in a distinctive distribution, or catastrophic acute intracerebral/subarachnoid haemorrhage, may also occur. Amyloid angiopathy should be strongly considered in elderly normotensive patients with spontaneous intracranial haemorrhage, particularly when associated with leukoencephalopathy and atrophy related to small-vessel cerebrovascular disease. Definitive diagnosis is usually only made *postmortem*, with a presumptive diagnosis made on clinical presentation and imaging findings.

Chao et al (2006).

2) e. ***
Holoprosencephaly is failure of the primitive brain to cleave into two hemispheres, and is commonly associated with midline facial abnormalities (ranging from cyclopia to hypertelorism) and absence of many intracranial midline structures. There are three types, the most severe being the alobar form, which shows no cleavage at all, with absence of the falx cerebri and third ventricle, fusion of the cerebral hemispheres and thalami, and a single large lateral ventricle. The semilobar form has variable cleavage with a partially formed falx, rudimentary third ventricle, and variable cleavage of the thalami, lateral ventricles and cerebral hemispheres. In the lobar type of holoprosencephaly, brain formation may be nearly normal, but the septum pellucidum is always absent, as in all forms. The falx, corpus callosum and ventricular system may be normal in the lobar type.

Weissleder et al (2007), 573–4.

3) d. ****
Toxoplasmosis is the most common cause of a cerebral mass lesion in patients with AIDS. Typical appearances are of multiple, hypoattenuating, <2 cm lesions with a predilection for the basal ganglia. Lymphoma is the second commonest mass lesion, with characteristic features including hyperdense lesions (though less frequently than in non-AIDS lymphoma) in a periventricular location with subependymal spread. Lesions in both conditions may show solid or ring enhancement. Haemorrhage is unusual in lymphoma but may be seen in toxoplasmosis,

323

particularly following treatment. Thallium scanning may be useful to distinguish the two if there is diagnostic uncertainty. CNS lymphoma is thallium avid whereas toxoplasmosis does not show uptake. MR perfusion studies may also help to differentiate the two conditions. Lymphomas demonstrate increased perfusion relative to surrounding tissue, while toxoplasmosis is hypovascular. Differentiation is important, as early radiation therapy confers a significant survival advantage in CNS lymphoma.

Grossman & Yousem (2003), 153–6; Brant & Helms (2007), 133.

4) e. ****
Cerebral perfusion CT can distinguish viable but ischaemic tissue (the penumbra) from tissue that is beyond recovery. Other uses include evaluation of vasospasm after subarachnoid haemorrhage, assessment of cerebrovascular reserve with acetazolamide (cerebral arteriole vasodilator) in cases of vascular stenosis, evaluation of collateral flow and cerebrovascular reserve in patients having temporary balloon occlusion and assessment of microvascular permeability of intracranial neoplasms. Cerebral perfusion CT utilizes the central volume principle. This states that CBF=CBV/MTT, where CBF is cerebral blood flow, CBV is cerebral blood volume and MTT is mean transit time. In practice, two CT perfusion techniques can be used. One is perfused-blood-volume mapping, in which a quantity is assigned to cerebral blood volume by subtracting unenhanced CT data from CT angiographic data. It has the advantage of imaging the whole brain. The second technique is a dynamic, contrast-enhanced technique that acquires data from a limited number of axial slices, and monitors the first pass of an iodinated contrast agent bolus through the cerebral circulation. This requires an unenhanced CT brain, followed by a dynamic CT performed during injection of 50 ml of iodinated contrast (300 mg I/ml) at 4 ml/s. The first pass of contrast is observed in the brain. Cerebral perfusion is related to the concentration of iodinated contrast, which is directly related to the attenuation measured. Several maps are produced, including the CBV, CBF and MTT. MTT is derived from arterial and venous enhancement curves, measured by using regions of interest placed on an artery (one that is not occluded as part of an acute event) and a venous sinus. CBV is the area under the enhancement curves, and CBF is obtained from the central volume equation. Differentiation of infarcted brain from penumbra is important because, while penumbra can be saved by timely thrombolysis, infarcted tissue has an increased risk of bleeding from thrombolysis with no chance of recovery. CBF is decreased in both ischaemia and infarction, MTT is longer (>6 s) in both, while CBV is decreased in infarct but increased (or normal) in the penumbra due to cerebral autoregulatory mechanisms. MTT is the most sensitive for stroke. So this or CBF can be used to detect stroke while CBV is used to determine whether there is infarct or reversible ischaemia.

Hoeffner et al (2004).

5) d. ****

Acute disseminated encephalomyelitis is an acute autoimmune demyelinating disease of the central nervous system that affects children more commonly than adults. It is usually triggered by an inflammatory response to viral infections or vaccinations. The main symptoms are decreased level of consciousness, varying from lethargy to coma, convulsions, and multifocal neurological symptoms. MR imaging findings are of multifocal, large, confluent or punctate, high-signal, white matter lesions on T2W/FLAIR images. Lesions are responsive to treatment with steroids and in 80% of cases completely resolve. A haemorrhagic, hyperacute variant (acute haemorrhagic leukoencephalitis) has also been described and is known as Hurst's disease. In addition to the usual findings, there are multiple, white matter haemorrhages and rapid development of profound generalized mass effect. Hurst's disease is usually fatal within a few days.

Honkaniemi et al (2001).

6) d. **

Diffusion-weighted MRI provides image contrast which is different from that provided by conventional MR techniques. The sequence enables the measurement of net macroscopic water movement, which is anisotropic (varies in different directions) particularly in white matter. Restricted diffusion is seen as high signal on DWI (which is a T2W image with signal degraded by diffusion) and low signal on the ADC map. Restricted diffusion occurs in tissue that does not allow free movement of water molecules, such as areas of infection due to the high viscosity and cellularity of pus. Similarly, epidermoid cysts are very cellular and so also show restricted diffusion, a feature that helps distinguish them from arachnoid cysts, which are fluid structures. In stroke, restriction in water diffusion occurs within minutes after the onset of ischaemia. The basis of this change is not completely clear but is thought to be related to the cytotoxic oedema seen in ischaemic cells due to the impairment of the Na^+/K^+ ATPase pumps (which are very energy dependent), leading to loss of ionic gradients and a net translocation of water from the extracellular to the intracellular compartment, where water mobility is relatively more restricted.

Schaefer et al (2000).

7) c. ***

A peak systolic velocity of >230 cm/s (250 cm/s in some texts) in the internal carotid artery, an end-diastolic velocity of >100 cm/s and a ratio of peak systolic velocities between the internal and common carotid arteries of >4.0 are all features that suggest a stenosis of $>70\%$. Loss of flow, or even reversal of flow, in the common carotid artery suggests an occlusion or very-high-grade stenosis. The grade of stenosis that is suitable for surgical rather than medical treatment has been shown to be 70%.

Dähnert (2007), 379.

8) d. ****

In the first 3–6 hours (hyperacute stage) following haemorrhage, the intact red cells contain mostly oxyhaemoglobin, which appears hyperintense on T2W images. Desaturation occurs peripherally, forming deoxyhaemoglobin, which is seen as hypointensity on T2W images. In the acute stage (8–72 hours), there is rapid deoxygenation of the oxyhaemoglobin to deoxyhaemoglobin, which, together with the high protein content of the clot and susceptibility effects, results in iso- to hypointensity on T1W images and hypointensity on T2W images. In the early subacute stage (3–7 days), oxidation of deoxyhaemoglobin to methaemoglobin occurs inside the red cell, resulting in characteristic hyperintensity on T1W images due to paramagnetic effects, and marked hypointensity on T2W images. In the late subacute stage (1 week to months), extracellular methaemoglobin results in persistent hyperintensity on T1W images, but increasing signal intensity on T2W images, with peripheral susceptibility effects causing a low intensity rim. In the chronic stage (months to years), iron atoms are deposited as haemosiderin and ferritin, which cause susceptibility effects resulting in low signal intensity on both T1W and T2W images.

Grossman & Yousem (2003), 208–15.

9) c. ***

The hypodense artery sign is described, representing a single, large, macroscopic fat embolus within the middle cerebral artery, giving rise to a stroke syndrome. It may occur during cardiac surgery, resulting in dislodgement of fat from the surrounding tissue. This is distinct from the shower of microscopic fat emboli that occurs in the fat embolism syndrome.

Lee et al (2005).

10) e. ***

The lymph node chains in the neck are complex and consist of a superficial circular nodal group and a deep cervical chain. Supraglottic laryngeal squamous cell carcinoma tends to spread to the high internal jugular vein chain of nodes, which are in level II, with tumours of the epiglottis, aryepiglottic folds and pyriform sinuses most likely to present with adenopathy. This can be ipsilateral (most common), contralateral or bilateral. Subglottic tumours tend to spread to bilateral middle- or lower-level nodes of the internal jugular vein chain in level III or IV. The level IV lymph nodes also drain the hypopharynx, thyroid and upper oesophagus. The oral cavity, including the tongue and nasopharynx, drains to the level II nodes. The salivary glands drain to level I or II nodes. Tumours confined to the vocal folds do not normally metastasize to lymph nodes.

Werner et al (2003).

11) c. ***
The endplates in degenerative disc disease have three described appearances during their evolution, which are also known as Modic changes. Type I (marrow oedema) changes show low signal on T1W and high signal on T2W sequences. Type II (fatty marrow) changes show high signal on both T1W and T2W sequences. Type III (sclerosis) changes are low signal on both T1W and T2W sequences.

Tehranzadeh et al (2000).

12) a. ****
Loss of myelinated fibres and gliosis in the posterior and lateral columns of the spinal cord are the histopathological hallmarks of Friedreich's ataxia. On MRI, the predominant radiological finding is thinning of the cervical spinal cord and medulla, and there may be associated mild cerebellar atrophy. Conversely, in the majority of other forms of ataxia such as early onset cerebellar ataxia and olivopontocerebellar atrophy, atrophy of the cerebellum and pons predominates with relative sparing of the cord. Although cerebellar atrophy may be seen in Friedreich's ataxia, it is less pronounced than in these other diseases.

Mascalchi et al (1994).

13) a. ***
Pituitary microadenomas are typically hypointense compared with the normal gland on unenhanced T1W images, and the diagnosis can usually be made without contrast. Following contrast, the microadenoma does not initially enhance, and maximal contrast between enhancing normal gland and pituitary tumour is seen on dynamic images obtained within the first minute. Contrast enhancement may therefore be useful in identifying lesions that are not obviously hypointense on the unenhanced images. However, contrast enhancement of the tumour relative to the normal gland may be seen on delayed (>20 min) images.

Grossman & Yousem (2003), 532–3.

14) a. ****
Aneurysmal bone cysts are seen mainly in patients under 20 years of age (75%) and affect the posterior elements when involving the spine. They may arise de novo, or secondary to another lesion such as a giant cell tumour (GCT) or fibrous dysplasia. Both GCTs and telangiectatic osteosarcomas may cause cysts with fluid–fluid levels on MRI, but GCTs arise from vertebral bodies and usually occur in the sacrum. Telangiectatic osteosarcomas usually affect long bones. Chordomas are

malignant tumours that usually affect the vertebral body, with destruction and invasion of the discs and adjacent structures.

Laredo et al (2001).

15) d. ***
Neurosarcoidosis is seen in up to 8% of cases of sarcoidosis and has a tendency to involve the base of the brain. Cranial nerve involvement occurs frequently and nerve palsies are a common presenting feature. Bilateral facial nerve palsies, particularly in young adults, are most commonly due to neurosarcoidosis. The most common imaging manifestation is diffuse basomeningeal thickening, which typically shows enhancement with intravenous gadolinium. Also frequently seen are meningeal nodules and deep white matter lesions with high T2 signal. Multiple or solitary parenchymal masses may also occur, which can have a ring-like appearance and may therefore mimic primary or metastatic neoplasia.

Koyama et al (2004).

16) b. **
Ependymomas are the commonest tumour of the spinal cord in adults, accounting for 40–60% of cord tumours. They present with a long history of pain, and sensory or motor disturbance. Less commonly, bladder and bowel dysfunction may occur. Expansion of the cord is more often seen with ependymomas than with demyelination. Both lesions may enhance and have high signal on T2W images, but multiplicity is more often seen with demyelination. Peripheral low signal, usually indicating haemosiderin, is not a feature of either of these lesions.

Sutton (2002), 1666–8; Dähnert (2007), 213–14.

17) b. ***
Once the presence of a mass has been established, the radiologist must determine whether the mass is intra-axial (arising within the brain parenchyma) or extra-axial (arising outside the brain substance) in order to formulate an appropriate differential diagnosis. An extra-axial mass characteristically causes buckling of the grey–white matter interface, expansion of the subarachnoid space at its borders, and medial displacement of the vessels in the subarachnoid space. A dural base is also a feature of an extra-axial mass. Intra-axial masses characteristically cause expansion of the cortex of the brain but no expansion of the subarachnoid space, and pial vessels may be seen peripheral to the mass.

Grossman & Yousem (2003), 97–8.

18) d. ***

The most common causes of a cerebellopontine angle mass are vestibular schwannoma (also called acoustic neuroma) (75%), meningioma (10%) and epidermoid cyst (5%). Features suggestive of a meningioma include a dural tail (thickening of enhancing adjacent dura resembling a tail extending from the mass), adjacent hyperostosis and an obtuse angle with the petrous bone (vestibular schwannomas make an acute angle). Distinguishing features of schwannomas include extension into the internal auditory canal, causing expansion of the canal and flaring of the porus acousticus (bony opening of the internal auditory canal). Meningiomas may show a small tongue of extension into the canal but usually no expansion. Schwannomas undergo cystic degeneration and haemorrhage more commonly than meningiomas (particularly larger lesions), and may show very high signal on T2W images, which is unusual for a meningioma.

Grossman & Yousem (2003), 105–8.

19) e. ***

Brain metastases are the most common intracranial tumours. Six primary tumours account for 95% of all brain metastases. Primary bronchial carcinoma is the most common (47% of cases), though squamous cell carcinoma rarely metastasizes to the brain. Other common primary tumours are breast carcinoma (17%), gastrointestinal malignancy (15%), renal cell carcinoma, melanoma and choriocarcinoma. Metastases characteristically occur at the grey–white matter junction, are multiple in 66% of cases, and typically appear as hypodense masses that demonstrate solid or ring enhancement.

Dähnert (2007), 309.

20) a. ***

The described appearance is of 'picture-frame' vertebral bodies and is seen in Paget's disease. The central osteoporosis can lead to insufficiency fractures and complications thereof. 'Rugger jersey spine' has a similar appearance due to sclerosis of the endplates (but the anterior and posterior cortices are spared) and is seen with both hyperparathyroidism (usually secondary and associated with renal failure) and osteopetrosis. Pyknodysostosis is a congenital disorder with sclerosis of long bones, causing obliteration of the medullary canal. Gaucher's disease causes osteosclerosis secondary to bone infarcts, often causing H-shaped vertebra due to central endplate collapse.

Resnick & Kransdorf (2005), 578–81.

21) a. ****

Alzheimer's disease typically presents with atrophy and reduced perfusion to the mesiotemporal regions bilaterally, but, in younger patients, it often presents with posterior parietal perfusion abnormalities. Vascular dementia shows patchy cortical and subcortical perfusion defects, with involvement of the cerebellum. Lewy body dementia is similar to Alzheimer's disease but with less occipital sparing; Parkinson's dementia is also similar but with less mesiotemporal change and more involvement of the visual cortex.

Ell & Gambhir (2004), 1437.

22) e. ***

In many cases of hydrocephalus due to subarachnoid haemorrhage, the temporal horns of the lateral ventricles become dilated sooner than the frontal horns. Dilatation of the temporal horn is often particularly conspicuous, as it is frequently not visualized at all on CT of normal brains. Uncal herniation is herniation of the medial temporal lobe into a subtentorial location, where it may exert pressure on the brain stem and is a late sign of raised intracranial pressure, often presenting with oculomotor nerve palsy resulting in a fixed dilated pupil.

Hosoya et al (1992).

23) b. ***

Variant Creutzfeldt–Jakob disease is a rare but important, transmissible, rapidly progressive spongiform encephalopathy and a cause of dementia and death in young patients. The transmissible agent is thought to be a prion protein (proteins devoid of nucleic acid), and the condition is causally linked to bovine spongiform encephalopathy. CT is typically normal, but symmetrical hyperintensity in the pulvinar nuclei of the posterior thalami (pulvinar sign) on T2W or FLAIR MR images has been described as a specific sign for the variant form. The classic form affects an older age group and is often genetically linked, whereas the variant form is sporadic. The pulvinar sign is seen only in the variant form, with the classic type typically showing similar hyperintense abnormalities located in the caudate nucleus and putamen.

Collie et al (2003).

24) c. **

It is at this location that 35% of berry aneurysms are found. This is the same proportion that occurs at the junction of the internal carotid and posterior communicating arteries. Five per cent occur at the basilar tip and 20% at the middle cerebral artery bifurcation. Two per cent of the population have cerebral aneurysms. They are multiple in 20% of cases and giant in 25% (over 25 mm in diameter). They are caused by degenerative vascular changes, trauma, infection, tumour and vasculopathy. The incidence is increased in adult polycystic renal disease, aortic coarctation, fibromuscular dysplasia, and Marfan's and Ehlers–Danlos syndromes.

Weissleder et al (2007), 513.

25) e. **

In this scenario, the low attenuation and surrounding changes most likely represent brain oedema. This may be due to an evolving infarction or oedema around a metastatic deposit from the previous lung cancer. Differentiation between the two will immediately affect patient treatment, as anti-platelet therapy for ischaemic stroke will increase the risk of haemorrhage from a metastasis and therefore should be withheld if a metastatic deposit is suspected or diagnosed. The primary factor in determining whether a lesion will enhance on CT after administration of intravenous iodinated contrast is the integrity of the blood–brain barrier in that region of the brain substance. A large molecule such as iodinated contrast would not be able to enter the brain unless the integrity of the barrier were compromised. The majority of aggressive tumours, including metastases, will disrupt this barrier, and so contrast enhancement will be seen in the solid component of these lesions. Acute infarction will typically not show areas of enhancement.

Grossman & Yousem (2003), 5–7; Cha (2006).

26) a. *

Tuberculous lymphadenitis is the most common form of head and neck tuberculosis, representing 15% of all extrapulmonary tuberculous infections. It is frequently bilateral and, the more inferior the involved nodes, the higher the prevalence of associated pulmonary disease. Peripherally enhancing lymph nodes are seen with tuberculosis, metastatic disease (usually squamous cell tumours), lymphoma or infection. The presence of calcification suggests tuberculosis, but it may also be seen with papillary or medullary thyroid carcinoma. The other diagnoses listed may cause cervical lymphadenopathy, but the lung lesion would be unusual in all except a cavitating squamous cell carcinoma of the lung.

Moon et al (1997).

27) a. ***

Haemangioblastomas are the most commonly recognized manifestation of von Hippel–Lindau syndrome. They usually occur in the cerebellum and may be multiple in up to 15% of cases. Patients also commonly develop renal cell carcinoma, and difficulty may occasionally arise in distinguishing metastases from multiple haemangioblastomas. Typical features are of a cystic mass in the hemisphere or vermis, with an enhancing mural nodule, though entirely solid lesions may also occur. Calcification is not a feature. Gyriform cortical calcifications are a feature of Sturge–Weber syndrome, and usually occur in the temporo-parieto-occipital region. Calcified subependymal nodules (hamartomas) are a feature of tuberous sclerosis. A hypodense, ill-defined mass with central necrosis and marked surrounding oedema is a classic appearance of a glioblastoma multiforme.

Chapman & Nakielny (2003), 450–1; Grossman & Yousem (2003), 131–2.

28) a. ******
Non-haem brain iron is normally found within oligodendroglia and astrocytes, with smaller amounts in neurons and myelinated axons. Half is found within the mitochondria and 10% in the nuclei, and 40% represents a soluble fraction. The areas of maximum iron concentration in normal adults are found in the globus pallidus, red nucleus, pars reticulata of the substantia nigra and dentate nucleus of the cerebellum. The brain concentration is independent of general body stores, and the mechanism by which it crosses the blood–brain barrier is not fully understood. By the eighth decade, the concentration of iron may increase in the caudate nucleus and putamen to levels similar to those seen in the globus pallidus. Excessive or premature accumulation in these areas has been seen in various forms of senile dementia including Alzheimer's disease. Iron deposition is identified on T1W and T2W sequences as signal hypointensity due to magnetic susceptibility.

Drayer (1988a, 1988b).

29) a. ****
Insufficiency fractures tend to occur in elderly female patients and manifest with pain. They are notoriously difficult to diagnose on plain film due to overlying soft tissues and bowel gas. MR and bone scans demonstrate them well, often in an 'H' configuration (Honda sign). Metastases tend to cause multiple focal areas of change. Ankylosing spondylitis and Reiter's syndrome are known causes of sacroiliitis, which would cause changes on MRI more localized to the iliac sides of the sacroiliac joints. Post-radiotherapy changes tend to be those of fatty marrow replacement, with high signal on both T1W and T2W, and low signal on STIR images.

Diel et al (2001).

30) d. ****
Carotid–cavernous sinus fistula can be caused by penetrating injury, base of skull fracture or rupture of an intracavernous internal carotid artery aneurysm. Drainage from the affected cavernous sinus is via the superior ophthalmic vein, contralateral cavernous sinus, petrosal sinus and, rarely, cortical veins. Pulsatile exophthalmos and orbital bruit are evident, as are chemosis, conjunctival oedema and increased intraocular pressure. On imaging, the cavernous sinus may be enlarged, and can cause erosion of the sella and enlargement of the superior orbital fissure. Regarding the differentials for extraocular muscle swelling, Graves' disease typically spares the muscle attachments whereas

inflammatory orbital pseudotumour affects the tendons while also causing orbital fat stranding.

Dähnert (2007), 344.

31) e. ****
Ependymomas most commonly arise in the floor of the fourth ventricle and are usually isodense. They have a greater incidence of calcification than other posterior fossa paediatric tumours; it is typically punctate and seen in 40–50% of cases. A characteristic feature of ependymomas is their propensity to extend through and widen the foramina of Luschka and Magendie. Juvenile pilocytic astrocytomas are the commonest paediatric infratentorial neoplasms and typically occur in the cerebellar hemispheres. They appear cystic with an enhancing mural nodule. Medulloblastomas tend to be homogeneous hyperdense lesions located in the vermis, and the presence of calcification is uncommon. Metastases are the commonest infratentorial tumour to occur in adults, but are uncommon in children. Haemangioblastomas usually occur in young adults and are classically cystic masses with a solid mural nodule.

Grossman & Yousem (2003), 119–28.

32) e. ****
Dysmyelinating diseases (leukodystrophies) are a wide spectrum of inherited neurodegenerative disorders affecting myelin in the brain and peripheral nerves. Most fall into one of three categories: lysosomal storage diseases, peroxisomal disorders and diseases caused by mitochondrial dysfunction. The most common, metachromatic leukodystrophy, is an autosomal recessive disorder caused by a deficiency of the lysosomal enzyme arylsulphatase A, which leads to accumulation of sulphatides in tissues. It usually manifests as a late infantile subtype in children at 12–18 months of age, and is characterized by motor signs of peripheral neuropathy followed by deterioration in intellect, speech and coordination, leading to death within a few years. On T2W MRI, symmetrical confluent areas of high signal intensity are seen in the periventricular white matter with sparing of the subcortical U fibres. Sparing of the perivascular white matter gives a striped or tigroid appearance to the periventricular area of abnormality, particularly well seen in the centrum semiovale. Other sites often affected are the corpus callosum, internal capsule and corticospinal tracts.

Cheon et al (2002).

33) a. ***
The lenticulostriate arteries are vessels arising from the M1 segment of the middle cerebral artery; there are medial and lateral groups. Collectively, they supply the thalamus, caudate and lentiform nuclei. The callosomarginal artery and the recurrent artery of Heubner are anterior cerebral artery branches. The latter provides some supply to the

anterior limb of the internal capsule, and parts of the caudate nucleus and globus pallidus. The angular artery is a cortical branch of the middle cerebral artery. The anterior choroidal artery also supplies parts of the internal capsule and basal ganglia but is a branch of the internal carotid artery. The nuclei of the basal ganglia are the amygdala, claustrum, lentiform and caudate nuclei, with the internal, external and extreme capsules being associated white matter tracts.

Butler et al (1999), 50–5.

34) c. ***
Loss of grey–white matter differentiation, obscuration of the lentiform nucleus and the insular ribbon sign are manifestations of cytotoxic oedema that can be seen on CT as early as 2 hours after middle cerebral artery infarction. With normal window settings (width 80 HU, centre 20 HU), the sensitivity and specificity for acute ischaemic stroke detection on unenhanced CT are 57% and 100% respectively. The sensitivity is improved to 71% with window settings of width 8 HU and centre 32 HU. This setting accentuates the difference between normal and oedematous brain tissue.

Srinivasan et al (2006).

35) b. **
The development of the cerebral cortex takes place in three stages: cell proliferation, cell migration and cortical organization. Schizencephaly is a disorder of the final stage where there is a CSF-containing cleft lined with grey matter (which is often polymicrogyric) connecting the subarachnoid CSF space with the ventricular system. Differentiation can be made from the cyst or cavity of porencephaly, by the presence in schizencephaly of a lining of heterotopic grey matter, whereas a porencephalic cyst is lined by white matter. To result in schizencephaly, the insult must involve the entire thickness of the cerebral hemisphere during cortical organization, as in injuries due to prenatal infection, ischaemia or chromosomal abnormalities. Clinical presentation varies but often includes developmental delay, motor impairment and seizures.

Abdel Razek et al (2009).

36) c. ***
Cerebral catheter angiograms are indicated: to investigate an intracranial haemorrhage where aneurysm or arteriovenous malformation is sought; to investigate aneurysms identified on other imaging techniques; to investigate cavernous sinus syndromes, caroticocavernous fistula and venous sinus thrombosis; for preoperative assessment of tumours; and to investigate cerebral ischaemia. Idiosyncratic and dose-related renal iodinated contrast reactions are among the complications of cerebral angiography. Groin puncture site complications are also possible, as with any angiogram. Complications specific to cerebral angiography include embolism of plaque, thrombus

or other particulate matter. Catheter-induced spasm or dissection can also occur.

Chapman & Nakielny (2001), 302–5.

37) c. ****
HIV encephalopathy is a progressive subcortical dementia caused by direct infection of the central nervous system by HIV. It is therefore not an opportunistic infection and is seen in up to 60% of AIDS cases. The most striking feature is cerebral atrophy and diffuse myelin pallor, manifested as ill-defined, confluent areas of high signal in the white matter on T2W sequences or low attenuation on CT. Changes are usually bilateral but asymmetrical, with characteristic sparing of the grey matter. Progressive multifocal leukoencephalopathy occurs in only 2–4% of AIDS cases and is a reactivation of the JC (John Cunningham) virus, resulting in destruction of oligodendrocytes. The most common location is posterior whereas HIV encephalopathy is more commonly frontal; however, this is an unreliable discriminator. Progressive multifocal leukoencephalopathy characteristically involves the subcortical U fibres and also affects grey matter. It has a very poor prognosis, death occurring within 2–5 months.

Balakrishnan et al (1990).

38) c. **
The FLAIR MR sequence is a heavily T2-weighted inversion recovery sequence designed to nullify the signal from CSF. This highlights any T2 high-signal lesions that may be masked on standard T2W images by adjacent high signal of CSF. This is of particular benefit in the periventricular region and corpus callosum, and studies have shown that FLAIR has higher accuracy than intermediate and T2W sequences in the detection of supratentorial cortical, subcortical and periventricular multiple sclerosis lesions. Depending on location, some lesions can be best seen on standard T2W images; these areas include the posterior fossa, brain stem and spinal cord.

Pikus et al (2006).

39) b. ***
Glioblastoma multiforme is the most malignant form of astrocytoma. It occurs in older patients, and most commonly affects the deep white matter of the frontal lobes. Classic appearances are of an irregular, ill-defined hypodense mass with necrosis, haemorrhage and extensive surrounding white matter oedema. Ninety per cent of cases show enhancement, which may be diffuse, heterogeneous or ring like. Tumour spread is directly along white matter tracts, and commonly occurs across the corpus callosum to involve both frontal lobes (butterfly glioma). Lymphomas also have a propensity to involve the corpus callosum but usually are slightly hyperdense due to a high nuclear-to-cytoplasmic ratio. Metastases may also involve the corpus callosum

but tend to be better defined and would be less likely in the absence of a known primary tumour. Progressive multifocal leukoencephalopathy may involve the corpus callosum but occurs in immunocompromised patients. Involvement of the corpus callosum is not usually a feature of abscesses.

Brant & Helms (2007), 129–131; Dähnert (2007), 247, 288–9.

40) c. ***

Minor trauma stretching the vertebral artery over the lateral mass of C2 can cause vertebral artery dissection. Symptoms include headache and neck pain, and as many as 95% of patients develop a stroke after hours to weeks. Imaging will show an axially enlarged vessel with a narrow lumen and a periarterial rim sign. Angiography may demonstrate tapering or occlusion of the artery or the dissection flap. Predisposing factors to spontaneous arterial dissection include fibromuscular dysplasia, Marfan's syndrome, collagen vascular disease and homocysteinuria.

Dähnert (2007), 384.

41) b. ***

Nasal and paranasal involvement and migratory lung nodules, which can be cavitary, are typical features of Wegener's granulomatosis. Cerebral vasculitis can also be a feature. MRI findings are non-specific and include hyperintensities on T2W images, infarcts and haemorrhage. Angiography may demonstrate occlusion, stenoses and aneurysms.

Weissleder et al (2007), 525–6.

42) b. ***

Alzheimer's disease is a progressive neurodegenerative disorder and the most common cause of dementia in elderly people. Current thinking is that imaging can help in the early diagnosis by documenting or quantifying atrophy in certain regions of the brain such as the hippocampus and entorhinal cortex. However, conventional structural imaging has a relatively low sensitivity in Alzheimer's disease and may be normal. Therefore, use is limited to identification of patterns of atrophy and the exclusion of other potential causes of dementia such as normal pressure hydrocephalus, vascular dementia or space-occupying lesion. Patterns of atrophy, when seen, may be relatively specific for different causes of dementia, with hippocampal atrophy a cardinal radiological sign of Alzheimer's disease. Pick's disease has a frontal and temporal preponderance and is part of the rarer group of diseases under the umbrella term 'frontotemporal lobar degeneration'. Lewy body dementia typically affects the parietal and occipital lobes and the cerebellum, which are usually spared in Alzheimer's disease. Multi-infarct dementia is vascular in origin and will show a patchy distribution of change. The different patterns of atrophy have also been recently demonstrated with [18]FDG PET.

Petrella et al (2003).

43) e. ***
The imaging findings are in keeping with a chronic infarct, in which the unrestricted extra water within gliosis gives a high T2 signal, dark DWI and bright ADC. Cytotoxic oedema occurs because of early ischaemic damage to the cell membrane Na^+/K^+ ATPase pump. This can be seen as early as 30 minutes after symptom onset as a bright DWI region. T2W images will be normal this early and the corresponding ADC map dark. DWI signal increases during the first week due to restricted diffusion but may remain bright for a prolonged period due to T2 'shine-through'. ADC will return to normal at 1–4 weeks (pseudonormalization) when restricted diffusion is matched by increasing amounts of vasogenic oedema that is not restricted. Long-term gliosis has extra water that is not restricted. DWI can be usefully thought of as a T2 signal diminished by net water movement. Since the DWI can be bright because of T2 'shine-through' rather than restricted diffusion, comparison of DWI findings with the ADC map is mandatory.

Srinivasan et al (2006).

44) c. **
Levels II, III and IV lie anterior to the sternocleidomastoid. Level II is from base of skull to hyoid, level III from hyoid to cricoid, and level IV from cricoid to clavicle. Level I is the submandibular space. Level V is posterior to sternocleidomastoid.

Weissleder et al (2007), 627–8.

45) b. ***
Spondylolysis (pars defect) is seen in 3–7% of the population, with 50% being symptomatic. L5 is the most commonly affected level. There are fractures through the pars interarticularis, which may be unilateral or bilateral. Spondylolisthesis can occur only when pars defects are bilateral. The AP diameter of the canal is widened, as the vertebral body and pedicles are detached from the posterior elements and migrate anteriorly. Narrowing of the canal is seen with other causes of spondylolisthesis, particularly degenerative causes. Sclerosis of one pedicle is seen with unilateral pars defects, as the contralateral pedicle undergoes reactive sclerosis due to excessive stress.

Dähnert (2007), 224–5.

46) d. ****
Parinaud's syndrome (also known as dorsal midbrain syndrome) is characterized by supranuclear paralysis of upward gaze. It results from

injury or compression of the dorsal midbrain, in particular the superior colliculi, and is most commonly seen in young patients with tumours of the pineal gland or midbrain, with pineal germinoma being the most common lesion producing the syndrome. Young women with multiple sclerosis and elderly patients with brain-stem stroke may also present with Parinaud's syndrome.

Grossman & Yousem (2003), 156–7.

47) b. ****
Gangliogliomas are low-grade tumours with a good prognosis, generally occurring in patients under the age of 30. Typical presentation is with focal seizures, and ganglioglioma is the most common tumour seen in patients with chronic temporal lobe epilepsy. They are usually well-circumscribed, hypo- or isodense lesions in the temporal lobes. Calcification (30%) and cyst formation (>50%) are common features. There is usually minimal mass effect and surrounding oedema. Meningiomas commonly calcify and have minimal surrounding oedema, but are extra-axial, and usually demonstrate intense uniform enhancement following intravenous contrast. Dysembryoplastic neuroepithelial tumours are commonly associated with partial complex seizures, but usually occur before the age of 20, and characteristically appear as a soap-bubble, multicystic lesion, which may remodel the calvarium. Epidermoids and arachnoid cysts are of CSF density, do not enhance with contrast and are extra-axial lesions.

Grossman & Yousem (2003), 136–7, 139.

48) d. *
CT images are displayed with different window levels and widths to highlight differences in CT attenuation between the structures of interest. Narrow window widths (80–400 HU) and lower levels (20–80 HU) are used to emphasize differences between soft tissues, whereas wide widths (2000–3000 HU) and higher levels (300–600 HU) are used for optimal visualization of bony structures. Images are usually also reconstructed using specific bone algorithms to accentuate the bone–soft tissue interface.

Grossman & Yousem (2003), 6–7.

49) b. ****
Longitudinal fractures of the temporal bone represent 75% of temporal bone fractures and run parallel to the axis of the petrous pyramid. They may cause dislocation of the auditory ossicles, usually the incus, causing a conductive deafness. Sensorineural hearing loss is associated with transverse fractures of the temporal bone, as is vertigo. Facial nerve palsy is seen in both fracture types, but is less common in longitudinal fractures, where it frequently recovers spontaneously. Carotid artery

and major sinus injuries are not directly associated with petrous temporal fractures.

Dähnert (2007), 208–9.

50) b. **
Oligodendrogliomas are slow-growing tumours, usually presenting in adults aged 30–50 years. They occur most commonly in the frontal lobe, and often extend to the cortex, where they may erode the inner table of the skull. Calcification is seen in 70% of cases, typically appearing as large nodular clumps. There is usually a relative absence of surrounding oedema. Astrocytomas also usually appear as hypodense calcified lesions with little surrounding oedema, but calvarial erosion is not usually a feature. Glioblastoma multiforme usually has considerable surrounding oedema and rarely calcifies. Gangliogliomas show calcification in a third of cases but tend to occur in children and young adults, and have a predilection for the temporal lobes.

Brant & Helms (2007), 132–3.

51) c. **
Parathyroid adenomas do not take up pertechnetate, which is accumulated by thyroid tissue, whereas sestamibi is taken up by both thyroid and parathyroid tissue. Subtraction of these two images can then be used to show any difference that can be attributed to a parathyroid adenoma. The delayed image typically shows retention of sestamibi in parathyroid adenomas (delayed washout) compared with normal parathyroid and thyroid. Small parathyroid adenomas are often missed by scintigraphy.

Smith & Oates (2004).

52) d. *
Moyamoya disease is progressive arteritis typically affecting both supraclinoid internal carotid arteries and the anterior two vessels of the circle of Willis – the anterior and middle cerebral arteries. It is termed 'Moyamoya syndrome' when associated with neurofibromatosis, bacterial meningitis, head trauma, tuberculosis, oral contraceptives, atherosclerosis or sickle cell anaemia. Sickle cell anaemia and atherosclerosis are not associated with axillary freckling, unlike neurofibromatosis type I. Amyloid angiopathy should be suspected in elderly normotensive patients with multiple areas of intra-axial haemorrhage sparing the basal ganglia.

Dähnert (2007), 310.

**53) a. **
Some 80–90% of subarachnoid haemorrhage is due to aneurysmal rupture. Therefore, when the diagnosis is proven or strongly suspected,

the cerebral arterial circulation requires assessment. Sixteen-slice CT angiography (CTA) is as accurate for aneurysm detection as 2D catheter digital subtraction angiography (DSA). CTA can be used as primary imaging and DSA reserved for difficult cases. It has the advantages of being safe, immediate, swift and less likely to need sedation or general anaesthetic. CTA also offers anatomical information beyond just the cerebral vasculature, in contrast to DSA. With 16-slice CTA, the spatial resolution is similar to DSA: 0.40 mm for CTA and 0.32 mm in DSA (2D DSA 33 cm FOV, 1024 × 1024 matrix, resolution 0.32 × 0.32 mm). When DSA is performed with AP and lateral projections, aneurysms may be masked, but 3D rotational DSA avoids this problem. The CTA parameters are as follows: 0.5 rotation/s with a 10 mm table advance per rotation and a 5-s scan, 16 rows of 0.75 mm reconstructed to 0.4 mm, kVp 120, mA 130.

Tipper et al (2005).

54) d. *****
The syndrome described is the fat embolism syndrome. This consists of the triad of acute respiratory distress with hypoxia, petechial skin haemorrhage and varying degrees of neurological dysfunction. The last includes headache, diminished GCS, seizures and irritability. Other features are tachycardia, fever, thrombocytopenia and anaemia. It occurs in 0.5–3.5% of long-bone fractures. The cause is likely to be the release of bone marrow elements into the circulation as a result of trauma. These act as emboli and they initiate a systemic inflammatory response when free fatty acids are released by the action of pulmonary lipases. The brain lesions seen on MRI are believed to be a combination of these two insults. Microinfarcts result from cerebral fat embolism, and oedema results from blood–brain barrier disruption which occurs because of the toxic effect of free fatty acids on brain tissue. Acute extra-axial haemorrhage might explain the neurological features of this case but would not account for the rash or hypoxia.

Butteriss et al (2006).

55) c. **
Infarction in this case is cerebellar. Vasospasm is the leading cause of death and morbidity following subarachnoid haemorrhage. It occurs after 72 hours with a peak at 5–17 days. Acute obstructive hydrocephalus results from intraventricular blood or the resultant ependymitis obstructing the aqueduct of Sylvius or the outlet of the fourth ventricle. Communicating hydrocephalus usually occurs after 1 week when the haemorrhage causes impaired CSF absorption.

Dähnert (2007), 327.

56) b. **
Cholesteatoma is an abnormal collection of keratinized debris arising from an ingrowth of stratified squamous epithelium and occurs in

primary (2%) or acquired (98%) types. The acquired type can be further subdivided, with the most common being a primary, acquired, epidermoid-type lesion of the pars flaccida, located in the attic of the middle ear. Cholesteatomas are benign lesions but cause bone erosion, including the auditory ossicles, resulting in conductive hearing loss. Local extension may compress the geniculate ganglion in the facial canal.

Fatterpekar et al (2006).

57) b. ***

Craniopharyngiomas are the most common suprasellar mass, predominantly occurring in the first and second decades, but with a second peak in the fifth decade. Presenting symptoms include headache secondary to hydrocephalus, bitemporal hemianopia (compression of the optic chiasm) and diabetes insipidus (compression of the pituitary gland). Typical imaging features are calcification, cyst formation and enhancement that may be solid or nodular. Meningiomas may arise in the suprasellar region and commonly demonstrate calcification but are generally not cystic. Epidermoids may occasionally demonstrate rim calcification but rarely enhance following intravenous contrast. Pituitary macroadenomas may undergo haemorrhage, resulting in heterogeneity that can cause confusion with craniopharyngioma, but this typically occurs in adolescence. Calcification in macroadenomas is infrequent. Rathke's cleft cysts are thin-walled, benign cysts arising in the anterior sellar or suprasellar region. They show no contrast enhancement and rarely calcify.

Grossman & Yousem (2003), 541–8.

58) b. **

Colloid cysts arise from the inferior aspect of the septum pellucidum and protrude into the anterior aspect of the third ventricle, where they may cause positional headaches and hydrocephalus due to transient obstruction at the foramen of Monro. They usually contain mucinous fluid, desquamated cells and proteinaceous debris, making them hyperdense on CT. On MR scan, the high protein content, as well as the paramagnetic effect of magnesium, copper and iron in the cyst, results in high signal intensity on T1W and T2W sequences in 60% of cases. Meningiomas and ependymomas may also appear hyperdense, but location within the third ventricle is uncommon for both. Subependymal giant cell astrocytoma is a benign tumour occurring in the region of the foramen of Monro, which may cause obstruction, but it is usually hypodense and is nearly always seen in association with tuberous sclerosis. Choroid plexus papilloma predominantly occurs in children under 5 years of age, and location in the third ventricle is unusual.

Dähnert (2007), 277–8.

59) e. **

Tuberculous discitis tends to occur in children and adults around the age of 50 years. It most commonly affects T12–L1, compared with pyogenic discitis, which tends to occur more distally. Tuberculous discitis often affects more than one level contiguously. Paravertebral masses and epidural abscesses are seen as complications in all types of discitis, but calcification within an abscess is virtually diagnostic for tuberculosis. Disc-space loss is also seen in all types of discitis, although it tends to be better preserved with tuberculous infection.

Burrill et al (2007).

60) e. ****

Meningioma is the most common radiation-induced CNS tumour, and has been particularly associated with low-dose radiation treatment for tinea capitis. For the diagnosis of radiation-induced meningioma to be made, the meningioma must arise in the radiation field, appear after a latency period of years and should not have been the primary tumour irradiated. Radiation-induced meningiomas are more frequently multiple and have higher recurrence rates than non-radiation-induced tumours.

Grossman & Yousem (2003), 104–5.

61) c. ***

The lentiform nucleus is composed of a larger lateral component (the putamen) and a smaller medial component (the globus pallidus), separated by a sheet of white matter. The lentiform nucleus is bounded medially by the internal capsule. Lateral to the lentiform nucleus lies the white matter of the external capsule, and then the claustrum, a thin sheet of grey matter. The extreme capsule lies lateral to the claustrum, and separates it from the insular cortex.

Butler et al (1999), 41.

62) e. ***

Phleboliths if present are unique to vascular malformations. Arterial malformations are high flow, while venous, capillary or combined malformations are low flow. MRI is required to assess the full extent, particularly intraosseous and intracranial, of head and neck vascular malformations. Benign lymph nodes are smooth, elliptical and hypoechoic with hilar architecture and vascularity. Malignant lymph nodes are typically round, are hypoechoic, have no hilum and show peripheral vascularity. Malignant lymph nodes with necrosis are seen with squamous cell and papillary cell carcinoma of the thyroid. Internal punctate calcification is seen in metastases from papillary or medullary carcinoma of the thyroid.

Connor et al (2005).

63) a. ******

Neurofibromatosis type 1 (peripheral neurofibromatosis or von Recklinghausen's disease) is a multisystem disorder affecting the majority of organ systems. The presence of plexiform neurofibroma is pathognomonic. In the spine, there is abnormal development of the vertebral bodies with hypoplasia of pedicles and posterior elements. Dural ectasia is seen secondary to weakness of the meninges. Neurofibromatosis type 2 (central neurofibromatosis) is characterized by bilateral acoustic neuromas, meningiomas and ependymomas. Tuberous sclerosis produces multiple hamartomas and malformations of several organ systems. Marfan's and Ehlers–Danlos syndromes may also cause posterior scalloping of vertebral bodies.

Dähnert (2007), 315–19.

64) e. *******

The imaging appearances are highly suggestive of a carotid body tumour (paraganglioma), and biopsy should not be performed, as haemorrhage would be certain due to the high vascularity of the lesion (in addition to the proximity of the carotid system). They present as painless, pulsatile masses in the neck of adults, below the angle of the jaw, and are laterally mobile but vertically fixed. There is splaying of the carotid bifurcation but preservation of calibre of the two arteries. Contrast imaging shows avid enhancement.

Dähnert (2007), 394.

65) b. ******

Classically, the Dandy–Walker malformation consists of partial or total absence of the cerebellar vermis, dilatation of the fourth ventricle into a large cystic mass, an enlarged posterior fossa, hydrocephalus (in 75% of cases) and torcular–lambdoid inversion (elevation of the torcular herophili above the lambdoid suture). The proposed aetiology is obstruction of CSF outflow at the foramina of Magendie and Luschka. The vermis abnormality is the key component in all forms of the Dandy–Walker complex. The variant is less severe with a better prognosis. Chiari malformations have the fundamental abnormality of an underdeveloped, small posterior fossa, in contrast to the Dandy–Walker complex where it is normal or enlarged.

Grossman & Yousem (2003), 432.

66) d. *******

Many of the acute neurological conditions of pregnancy occur with rising blood pressure. Sheehan's syndrome results from haemorrhage-induced hypotension causing pituitary infarction. Early on, this appears as an enlarged homogeneous pituitary with low T1 signal, high T2 signal and post-contrast ring enhancement. Later, there is an empty sella. Clinical manifestations include visual field loss, headache, ophthalmoplegia and pituitary dysfunction (diabetes insipidus). Reversible posterior leukoencephalopathy produces cortical blindness, headaches, confusion and seizures. Those affected are often taking immunosuppressant treatment. Imaging features can be identical to eclampsia, peripartum cerebral angiopathy and hypertensive encephalopathy, but with a posterior predominance. On CT, there is low attenuation change. On MRI, there is high signal on T2W/FLAIR images. ADC maps can differentiate between likely reversible vasogenic oedema (high signal on ADC map showing unrestricted diffusion) and cytotoxic oedema (low signal due to restricted diffusion), which is more likely to progress to infarct. Microangiopathic haemolytic anaemias, such as thrombotic thrombocytopenic purpura and haemolytic uraemic syndrome, give widespread ischaemia/infarction and haemorrhagic transformation. There is no increased risk in pregnancy of vasculitis such as systemic lupus erythematosus, Takayasu's syndrome or Moyamoya syndrome. Arteriovenous malformation is no more likely to bleed in pregnancy, but there is an increased risk with arterial aneurysms. Haemorrhage, sepsis and pulmonary embolism cause hypotension that can cause watershed infarction as well as Sheehan's syndrome.

Dineen et al (2005).

67) b. **

These veins are all part of the supratentorial venous system. The superficial middle cerebral vein forms an arc along the surface of the sylvian fissure and is continuous with the sphenoparietal sinus. The veins of Trolard and Labbe are anastomotic veins that connect the superficial middle cerebral vein to the superior sagittal and transverse sinuses respectively. The thalamostriate vein is a subependymal vein that passes across the floor of the lateral ventricle, over the thalamus and into the internal cerebral vein behind the foramen of Monro. The paired internal cerebral veins run along the roof of the third ventricle and enter the vein of Galen with the paired basal veins of Rosenthal. The vein of Galen joins the inferior sagittal sinus and the straight sinus at the 'venous confluence' within the quadrigeminal plate cistern. The straight sinus lies along the junction of the falx and tentorium. The straight sinus, transverse sinus and superior sagittal sinus meet as the torcular herophili.

Butler et al (1999), 57–8.

68) e. **

Carotid ultrasound scan can be used to assess the common, external and internal carotid arteries and the carotid bulb, including the vessel walls and the presence of plaques and stenoses. Doppler scan can display velocity profiles and allow waveform analysis and peak velocity measurement. Flow velocity increases proportionally with the degree of stenosis, except when the affected vessel is almost completely or totally occluded. Here flow velocity drops off. Stenosis above 70% is considered for surgery. This corresponds to a flow rate of greater than 250 cm/s.

Weissleder et al (2007), 508–9.

69) e. ****
Transtentorial herniation may be descending (towards the posterior fossa) or ascending (upward displacement of the cerebellum through the tentorial incisura). Descending transtentorial herniation causes shift of the temporal lobe over the tentorium, which may compress the third cranial nerve, the posterior cerebral and anterior choroidal arteries, and the midbrain. Contralateral hemiparesis may occur due to compression of the ipsilateral cerebral peduncle. Ipsilateral hemiparesis may also occur due to compression of the contralateral cerebral peduncle against the tentorial edge (Kernohan's notch phenomenon, a false localizing sign). Subfalcine herniation occurs when the cingulate gyrus shifts beneath the falx, due to medially directed supratentorial mass effect. This may cause compression of the anterior cerebral artery (resulting in ipsilateral distal anterior cerebral infarction) and internal cerebral veins. Sphenoid herniation involves herniation of the frontal lobe posteriorly across the edge of the sphenoid ridge, and rarely produces significant clinical symptoms. Transforaminal herniation results in herniation of the inferior cerebellum downward through the foramen magnum, which can result in obtundation and death.

Dähnert (2007), 234.

70) c. ****
The optic radiation runs from the optic chiasm posteriorly to the occipital visual cortex. Each radiation carries with it optical fibres carrying information from the contralateral half of the visual field of each eye. This means a lesion in the left optic radiation will result in loss of vision of the right half of the visual field in both eyes (right homonymous hemianopia). However, as the radiation passes posteriorly from the lateral geniculate nucleus of the thalamus, it divides into two, with one division taking a relatively direct course posteriorly and the other a longer course through the temporal lobe. This is known as Meyer's loop, and the lengthier course means that these fibres are more prone to disruption. The fibres in Meyer's loop carry information from the upper visual field only, so a left temporal lobe lesion that affected Meyer's loop would result in loss of vision only of the upper right quadrants of each eye (right superior homonymous quadrantanopia). A lesion at the optic chasm, such as a pituitary macroadenoma, will affect only the fibres that decussate at the chiasm, causing bitemporal loss of vision (bitemporal hemianopia).

Kier et al (2004).

71) c. *
Diagnosis of meningitis is made by clinical examination and examination of CSF. Imaging is reserved for complications and to identify

contraindications to lumbar puncture. The mechanism of spread is usually haematogenous, common organisms being *Neisseria meningitidis* (meningococcus) in young adults, *Escherichia coli* and *Haemophilus influenzae*. Complications that can be identified on CT include subdural empyema (sterile effusion can be seen with *H. influenzae*), venous sinus thrombosis, infarction, cerebritis and abscess formation. Leptomeningeal thickening and enhancement may be seen, but its absence does not exclude a diagnosis of uncomplicated meningitis. CT may also identify a potential source of infection such as otitis media, mastoiditis, sinusitis or orbital cellulitis.

Castillo (2006), 152–4.

72) c. ****
Epidermoids and dermoids are congenital lesions resulting from inclusion of ectodermal elements during closure of the neural tube. Both have a squamous epithelial lining and produce keratin, but dermoids contain both ectodermal and mesodermal elements (hair follicles, sweat and sebaceous glands), while epidermoids contain only ectodermal elements. Epidermoids are lobulated masses, usually located off the midline, which compress adjacent structures such as cranial nerves, and tend to have appearances on CT and MR scan following that of CSF. Dermoids are usually midline in location and cause symptoms by obstruction of CSF pathways or by rupture and leakage of fat contents, causing chemical meningitis. They have appearances on CT and MR scan following that of fat, and are often heterogeneous with areas of calcification and other soft-tissue components. This heterogeneity helps to distinguish a dermoid from a lipoma. Arachnoid cysts are of CSF density, but may be distinguished from epidermoids on DWI, where they do not show evidence of water restriction. Teratomas are composed of ectodermal, mesodermal and endodermal elements, and also appear heterogeneous with areas of fat, calcification and cystic components, but these lesions occur most commonly in the pineal and suprasellar regions.

Brant & Helms (2007), 151–4.

73) b. *
Dural venous sinuses are large venous channels located between the two layers of dura. They also contain arachnoid granulations that are responsible for CSF resorption.

Weissleder et al (2007), 507.

74) a. ****
The pelvic features are suggestive of diffuse idiopathic skeletal hyperostosis (DISH). Flowing anterior vertebral osteophytes, especially in the lower thoracic region, are very suggestive of this condition, and

disc spaces are usually well preserved. Vertebral body squaring is seen in a number of conditions, including ankylosing spondylitis, but not DISH.

Haller et al (1989).

75) e. **
Haemorrhage occurs in 5–10% of tumours. Features suggesting tumour rather than benign haemorrhage include complex CT pattern, incomplete haemosiderin ring, persisting oedema or mass on follow-up studies, and multiple lesions.

Weissleder et al (2007), 512.

76) c. ****
Carbon monoxide poisoning results in irreversible formation of carboxyhaemoglobin in the blood, causing anoxic ischaemic encephalopathy. These changes are usually bilateral and affect the basal ganglia, most commonly the globus pallidus. Injury is demonstrated as high signal on T2W and FLAIR images, and shows restricted diffusion on DWI. Areas less commonly affected acutely are the putamen (which is characteristically involved in methanol poisoning) and caudate nucleus. Involvement elsewhere can occur but is less common than basal ganglia changes. Delayed post-anoxic encephalopathy may develop several weeks after carbon monoxide poisoning, and MRI then shows further high T2 signal changes in the corpus callosum, subcortical U fibres, and internal and external capsules, with low T2 signal changes in the thalamus and putamen.

O'Donnell et al (2000).

77) d. ***
Both ameloblastoma and radicular cysts most commonly present in the third to fifth decades of life as a painless lump, often as an incidental finding. Neither typically shows matrix mineralization. Ameloblastoma represents 10% of all odontogenic (developing during or after the formation of teeth) tumours, with the majority located in the posterior body or ramus. They are frequently associated with the crown of an impacted or unerupted tooth. They can vary in radiographic appearance, an expansile, multiloculated lesion being typical. They are often resected due to locally aggressive infiltration. Radicular cysts are unilocular with a rim of cortical bone and usually develop at the root apex of a carious tooth as the end stage of the inflammatory process.

Scholl et al (1999).

78) c. **
The external carotid artery is usually described as having 8 branches but may have 4–12. The terminal branches are the superficial temporal and maxillary arteries. The usual branches in the order in which they arise

are superior thyroid, ascending pharyngeal, lingual, facial, occipital and posterior auricular. There is a plethora of anastomotic connections between branches of the external carotid artery, between external and internal carotid artery branches, and between external and vertebral artery branches.

Butler et al (1999), 116–17.

79) b. ***

The MRI signal of blood depends first on whether it is moving or static, since on most sequences movement produces a signal void. When it is static, the signal returned by blood reflects the magnetic properties of the blood products and their location. Hyperacute haemorrhage is intracellular oxyhaemoglobin that is diamagnetic, returning an isointense T1 and bright T2 signal. At 1–2 days, deoxygenation has occurred, making the iron paramagnetic. It remains intracellular and returns an isointense T1 signal and is dark on T2W images. At 2–7 days, haemorrhage contains paramagnetic intracellular methaemoglobin. This is bright on T1W images and dark on T2W images. The methaemoglobin becomes extracellular from 1 week to 4 weeks, and the MRI signal is bright on both T1W and T2W sequences. Chronic haemorrhage contains haemosiderin/ferritin, which is ferromagnetic, is dark on T1W images and has a dark rim on T2W sequences.

Weissleder et al (2007), 511.

80) b. ***

Diffuse axonal injury is characterized by widespread axonal disruption occurring in response to acceleration or deceleration forces – direct impact is not necessary. Typically, patients are immediately unconscious after the injury. CT is commonly negative, though 20% of lesions contain sufficient haemorrhage to be visible. On MR scan, typical findings are of multiple small foci of decreased signal intensity on T1W images and increased signal intensity on T2W images. Characteristic locations are the frontal and temporal white matter near the grey–white matter junction. More severe injuries may involve the lobar white matter and corpus callosum, with the brain stem involved in the most severe cases. Cortical contusions usually involve the superficial grey matter, and patients are less likely to present with immediate loss of consciousness. They characteristically occur near bony protuberances and are more commonly haemorrhagic. Subcortical grey matter injury is an uncommon type of injury seen after severe head trauma, with petechial haemorrhages in the basal ganglia and thalamus.

Brant & Helms (2007), 62–7.

81) b. *

MRI is an important paraclinical tool to support the clinical diagnosis of multiple sclerosis. Multiple sclerosis is an inflammatory autoimmune disease of the brain and spine characterized by demyelination and damage to axons. It typically presents in a relapsing and remitting way with symptoms dependent on the location of lesions. MR enables identification of areas of tissue injury and disease progression, and location of active lesions. The lesions are high signal on T2W sequences (including FLAIR) and can be found throughout the brain, but have a predilection for periventricular white matter, appearing perpendicular to the ventricles with an ovoid conformation (Dawson's fingers). The corpus callosum and cranial nerves are also common sites, and the FLAIR sequence helps to reveal lesions that would otherwise be masked by the high T2 signal of CSF. The corpus callosum is best examined on sagittal sequences. On T1W sequences, lesions are often isointense, but low signal can indicate areas of severe inflammation (so-called black holes) resulting in disease progression and disability. Enhancement with intravenous gadolinium is sometimes seen in lesions during the acute inflammatory phase and is thought to be the earliest detectable sign on MRI.

Ge (2006).

82) e. **

The lateral nasal wall is separated into superior, middle and inferior meatuses by three curled bony shelves called turbinates (or conchae). The nasolacrimal duct opens into the anterior aspect of the inferior meatus and is usually the only opening seen there. The other ostia all open into the middle meatus, with the exceptions of the posterior ethmoidal ostia (superior meatus) and sphenoidal ostia (posterior to the superior turbinate in the sphenoethmoidal recess). The sphenopalatine foramen lies inferior to the sphenoethmoidal recess posterior to the middle turbinate.

Dähnert (2007), 367.

83) e. *****

Conventional radionuclide brain scans are not indicated when CT or MRI can be used. Brain accumulation of radiotracer occurs at sites of blood–brain barrier disruption and increased vascularity such as cerebral metastases, meningioma and high-grade glioma. Reagents used are ^{99m}Tc-labelled pertechnetate, ^{99m}Tc-labelled DTPA, and, when it was available, ^{99m}Tc-labelled glucoheptonate. Radionuclide imaging is also able to provide regional blood flow mapping, which is used to localize epileptic foci, map cerebrovascular disease, investigate dementia, assess treatments and confirm brain death. ^{99m}Tc-labelled HMPAO is the most used radiopharmaceutical overall. It is lipophilic and therefore crosses the blood–brain barrier, and in doing so is distributed in proportion to cerebral blood flow. ^{99m}Tc-labelled ECD is another regional blood flow imaging tracer and can therefore also be used in the localization of epileptic foci. ^{18}FDG PET tracers are distributed through the brain according to metabolic activity.

Chapman & Nakielny (2001), 295–300.

84) d. **

Herpes simplex virus is the most common cause of fatal endemic encephalitis, often leaving survivors with severe memory and personality problems. Both oral (type I) and genital (type 2) strains may produce encephalitis with a multimodal distribution, affecting neonates (due to cross-infection with type 2 from the mother during birth), children and adults. Childhood and adult infection is caused by the type I virus and results in fulminant necrotizing encephalitis presenting with acute confusion and deteriorating rapidly to coma. Focal neurological deficits are seen in only 30% of cases. The virus asymmetrically affects the temporal lobes, insula, orbitofrontal region and cingulate gyrus, causing oedema. This is seen as high signal on T2W/FLAIR images, with DWI appearances variable depending on the presence of infarction. The putamen is characteristically spared, and the areas of encephalitis typically do not show enhancement on CT or MRI.

Grossman & Yousem (2003), 288–92.

85) c. ***

The signs describe oculomotor nerve palsy. This will result in a characteristic down-and-out position of the affected eye due to the unantagonized action of the superior oblique and lateral rectus muscles, which are supplied by the trochlear and abducent nerves respectively. The palsy will also cause ptosis and pupillary dilatation due to loss of the motor component of the light reflex. The nuclei of the oculomotor nerves are found in the superior midbrain within the tegmentum, at the level of the superior colliculi. Those of the trochlear nerve are situated at the level of the inferior colliculi. The oculomotor nerve arises from the anterior surface of the midbrain on the medial side of the cerebral peduncle, passing between the posterior cerebral and superior cerebellar arteries to enter the cavernous sinus and pass into the orbit via the superior orbital fissure.

Butler et al (1999), 37.

86) b. ***

Intracranial lipomas appear as well-circumscribed masses of fat density on CT with occasional rim calcification. On MR scan, characteristic appearances are of hyperintensity on T1W images, with chemical shift artefact or signal suppression on fat-saturated sequences.
Approximately 30% of intracranial lipomas occur in the pericallosal region, and there is a high incidence of associated congenital anomalies, most commonly agenesis of the corpus callosum, but also encephalocele and cutaneous frontal lipomas. Interhemispheric arachnoid cysts may occur in association with agenesis of the corpus callosum, but they are of CSF density and, like epidermoids, appear hypointense on T1W images. Dermoids have signal characteristics following those of fat, but are usually more heterogeneous and not associated with callosal

anomalies. Lymphoma may involve the corpus callosum but appears iso- or hypointense on T1W images.

Grossman & Yousem (2003), 117–118, 424–5.

87) d. ***
Carotid–cavernous sinus fistula may occur spontaneously (secondary to aneurysm rupture, dural sinus thrombosis or atherosclerosis) or after trauma/surgery. It presents with a classic triad of pulsatile exophthalmos, conjunctival chemosis and auscultatory bruit. However, reduction in visual acuity may be the only sign. Secondary findings such as proptosis, congestive extraocular muscle enlargement, and distension with enhancement of the superior ophthalmic vein and cavernous sinus are usually identified on routine CT or MRI. However, catheter angiography is usually required for lesion classification and treatment planning prior to embolization. Drainage may also occur into the contralateral cavernous sinus, resulting in dilatation and enhancement. Ophthalmic varices present with intermittent exophthalmos related to straining, with dilatation of superior and/or inferior ophthalmic veins, which may thrombose. Orbital pseudotumour is an idiopathic inflammatory condition affecting all orbital contents, but vascular dilatation is not a feature.

Smoker et al (2008).

88) c. **
The patient has a venous sinus thrombosis causing congestion and venous infarction. Veno-occlusive disease is commoner in the first 3 weeks postpartum, especially if there is underlying hypercoagulability, including factor V Leiden abnormality, antiphospholipid antibody syndrome, and protein C, protein S or antithrombin III deficiency. On unenhanced CT, there may be hyperdense veins, grey–white matter junction haemorrhage and brain oedema. On CT venography, an 'empty delta' can be seen because thrombus rather than iodinated contrast occupies the affected dural venous sinus.

Dineen et al (2005).

89) c. ***
The parapharyngeal space is triangular shaped and extends from the skull base to the hyoid. It contains fat, branches of the mandibular division of the trigeminal nerve, maxillary artery, ascending pharyngeal artery and pharyngeal venous plexus. The internal carotid artery, vagus nerve and hypoglossal nerve lie in the carotid space. The lingual tonsils lie in the pharyngeal mucosal space.

Butler et al (1999), 111.

90) e. ***

The appearances are characteristic of a multinodular goitre, and FNA can be misleading in these cases. Imaging diagnosis alone is usually sufficient. If there is a dominant nodule that is clearly larger than the others or a solitary enlarging nodule found on follow-up, then FNA should be performed to exclude malignancy.

Kim et al (2008).

91) a. ***

Spontaneous intracranial hypotension is a syndrome of low CSF pressure characterized by postural headaches in patients without any history of dural puncture or penetrating trauma. It is thought to arise from an occult CSF leak due to dural defects reducing CSF volume and subsequently pressure. Intracranial findings include downward displacement of the brain, subdural effusions, engorgement of other venous structures (including the hyperaemic pituitary) and low-lying cerebellar tonsils. There may be flattening of the pons as the brain sags against the skull base. Diffuse pachymeningeal enhancement is due to increased venous supply in an attempt to maintain intracranial volume and therefore pressure, according to the Monro–Kellie doctrine. In the spine, extradural fluid collection is indicative of an occult leak. Treatment is with an epidural blood patch where autologous blood is introduced into the extradural (epidural) space in an attempt to seal the microscopic dural defects.

Schievink et al (2008).

92) d. ***

A radicular cyst is the commonest type of cyst in the jaw and is associated with the apex of a tooth. It may displace teeth and cause mild root resorption. Ameloblastoma (adamantinoma of the jaw), odontogenic keratocyst and dentigerous cyst are all associated with the crown of a tooth, usually unerupted, and can be difficult to distinguish from each other on imaging alone. They are all odontogenic with no mineralization, and may be large and expand the mandible. Odontomas are the commonest odontogenic mass (67%) and show mineralization. They are seen in 10–20 year olds presenting with single or multiple, tooth-like masses.

Dähnert (2007), 180–2.

93) b. **

Acute extradural haematomas are traumatic in origin and tend to be commoner in younger patients. Two-thirds of cases involve the temporoparietal region, and 75–95% of patients have an associated skull fracture. Bleeding is usually from the underlying middle meningeal artery, though it may also be due to disruption of the middle meningeal vein, dural venous sinuses or diploic veins. Typical appearances are of a high-density lentiform or biconvex collection, which forms between the inner table of the skull and the dura mater. The dura is firmly bound to the skull at sutural margins, so extradural haematomas tend not to cross suture lines. Acute subdural haematomas usually follow severe trauma, and have a poorer prognosis than acute extradural haematomas due to a high incidence of associated contusions and other brain injuries. They tend to be crescentic in shape and may freely extend across suture lines, being limited only by the interhemispheric fissure and tentorium. They are commonly bilateral, particularly in infants, and have no particular association with skull fractures.

Dähnert (2007), 286–7.

94) b. ****
SPECT of the central nervous system allows assessment of the collateral circulation during balloon occlusion, mapping the extent and distribution of vasospasm associated with subarachnoid haemorrhage, evaluation of cerebrovascular reserve prior to carotid endarterectomy, identification of seizure foci and guiding of stereotactic brain biopsy in tumour recurrence. The Wada test is used to predict the probability of memory and speech complications in patients before they undergo anterior temporal lobectomy with amygdalohippocampectomy, a surgical treatment for medically refractory epilepsy. The test involves injection of radiopharmaceutical and short-acting barbiturate (usually sodium amobarbital) into each of the carotid arteries in turn. Loss of memory or speech following one of the injections indicates that these centres lie in the ipsilateral temporal lobe. The results of the Wada test can be negated by vessels crossing the midline, and the presence of such collateral circulation may not be readily apparent without SPECT.

Berger et al (1996).

95) e. **
Hypoglossal nerve (cranial nerve XII) palsy is uncommon, characteristically producing unilateral atrophy of the tongue musculature, and resulting in deviation of the tongue towards the weak side and dysarthric speech. Supranuclear lesions cause contralateral paralysis (tongue deviation away from the side of the lesion) whereas nuclear and infranuclear lesions cause ipsilateral paralysis (tongue deviation towards the side of the lesion). The hypoglossal nerve exits the skull base via the hypoglossal canal, and this segment of the nerve may be affected by benign or malignant tumours and trauma of the skull base. Metastatic tumours most commonly arise from the lung, breast or prostate primaries. Direct extension from nasopharyngeal squamous cell carcinoma may also produce skull base erosion involving the hypoglossal canal. Other pathological conditions that can affect the nerve at this site include skull base infections, Paget's disease and fibrous dysplasia.

Thompson & Smoker (1994).

96) b. ***

Thromboembolic cerebral infarction occurs in atrial fibrillation, cardiac valve disease, fibromuscular dysplasia, intracranial aneurysms, sickle cell disease, atherosclerosis and thrombotic thrombocytopenic purpura. Multiple infarcts are more likely with extracranial disease and can take the form of a shower of emboli. In these cases, the distribution is typically bilateral and more commonly supratentorial.

Dähnert (2007), 233.

97) d. ***

Abscess cavities and empyemas are homogeneously hyperintense on MR DWI and low on ADC map due to the increased viscosity of the purulent material that they contain, resulting in restricted diffusion of water. Sterile effusions are hypointense on DWI and have an ADC appearance similar to that of CSF due to their lower viscosity and free macro-diffusion of water. Diffusion images can therefore be important when deciding whether to intervene surgically or conservatively manage subdural collections, as empyema requires timely surgical drainage. Contrast enhancement of the wall of the collection may be seen on CT and MRI, but its absence does not exclude the diagnosis of a purulent collection. Likewise, one may expect to see additional mass effect with an infected collection, but this too is not sensitive enough to exclude infection by its absence.

Schaefer et al (2000).

98) a. ***

Meningiomas in the spine are seen mainly in females (80%) and in those over 40 years of age. They have similar signal characteristics to the cord on MRI and enhance avidly. They can cause symptoms related to cord compression. Bone erosion is seen in <10%. Nerve sheath tumours produce fusiform masses arising from the nerve roots, often extending through the intervertebral foramen, causing them to be dumb-bell shaped. They are isointense to muscle on T1W and hyperintense to fat on T2W images. Ependymomas are usually located in the filum terminale and show low/intermediate signal on T1W images, with foci of high signal on T2W images, and they often enhance. Dermoids usually occur in the conus or cauda equina and are associated with spinal dysraphism in one-third of cases. They are variable in signal on T1W but are high signal on T2W images.

Dähnert (2007), 216–17.

99) d. *****

Central neurocytomas (also known as intraventricular neurocytomas) are benign tumours of the lateral and third ventricles usually presenting in adults aged 20–40 years. They frequently calcify (69%) and contain cystic spaces. Attachment to the septum pellucidum is a characteristic feature. Lesions appear isointense to grey matter on all MR sequences and show mild-to-moderate contrast enhancement. Central neurocytomas were previously frequently mistaken for intraventricular oligodendrogliomas, which have very similar imaging features but are actually quite rare. In addition, neurocytomas undergo haemorrhage into the tumour or ventricle more frequently, helping to distinguish the two. Colloid cysts arise within the third ventricle, and rarely calcify. Subependymomas may arise in the lateral ventricles with an attachment to the septum pellucidum, and cyst formation and calcification may be seen in large tumours. However, most occur in patients over 40 years of age. Choroid plexus papillomas generally occur in children under 5 years of age.

Brant & Helms (2007), 143–5.

100) a. ****

Opsoclonus–myoclonus syndrome is characterized by opsoclonus in combination with myoclonus of the trunk, limbs or head. It may be idiopathic or occur as a paraneoplastic syndrome, when it may follow a relapsing–remitting course. In adults, it is most commonly associated with breast and squamous cell lung carcinoma, while in children it is associated with neuroblastoma. The syndrome usually precedes diagnosis of the underlying malignancy, and in children should prompt investigation to identify an underlying neuroblastoma. MIBG whole-body scintigraphy may be helpful in identifying occult disease if conventional imaging is negative. MR scan of the brain is usually normal.

Rutherford et al (2007).

References

Abdel Razek AAK, Kandell AY, Elsorogy LG, Bassett AA. Disorders of cortical formation: MR imaging features. *AJNR Am J Neuroradiol* 2009; **30**: 4–11.

Adam A, Dixon AK, Grainger RG, Allison DJ, eds. *Grainger and Allison's Diagnostic Radiology: A textbook of medical imaging*, 5th edn. London: Churchill Livingstone, 2007.

Afshani E, Kuhn JP. Common causes of low back pain in children. *Radiographics* 1991; **11**: 269–91.

Akisik MF, Sandrasegaran K, Aisen AA, et al. Dynamic secretin-enhanced MR cholangiopancreatography. *Radiographics* 2006; **26**: 665–77.

Akman C, Kantarci F, Cetinkaya S. Imaging in mediastinitis: a systematic review based on aetiology. *Clin Radiol* 2004; **59**: 573–85.

Akpinar E, Turkbey B, Karcaaltincaba M, et al. MDCT of inferior mesenteric vein: normal anatomy and pathology. *Clin Radiol* 2008; **63**: 819–23.

Alford BA, McIlhenny J. An approach to the asymmetric neonatal chest radiograph. *Radiol Clin North Am* 1999; **37**: 1079–92.

Altman NR, Purser RK, Post MJD. Tuberous sclerosis: characteristics at CT and MR imaging. *Radiology* 1988; **167**: 527–32.

Anthony S, Milburn S, Uberoi R. Multi-detector CT: review of its use in acute GI haemorrhage. *Clin Radiol* 2007; **62**: 938–49.

Apfelberg DB, Maser MR, Lash H, et al. Rheumatoid hand deformities: pathophysiology and treatment. *West J Med* 1978; **129**: 267–72.

Applegate KE, Anderson JM, Klatte EC. Intestinal malrotation in children: a problem-solving approach to the upper gastrointestinal series. *Radiographics* 2006; **26**: 1485–1500.

Araujo CR Jr, Montandon S, Montandon C, et al. Best cases from the AFIP: dysplasia epiphysealis hemimelica of the patella. *Radiographics* 2006; **26**: 581–6.

Aspelin P, Aubry P, Fransson SG, et al. Nephrotoxic effects in high-risk patients undergoing angiography. *N Engl J Med* 2003; **348**: 491–9.

Baker PN, ed. *Obstetrics by Ten Teachers*, 18th edn. London: Hodder Arnold, 2006.

Balakrishnan J, Becker PS, Kumar AJ, et al. Acquired immunodeficiency syndrome: correlation of radiologic and pathologic findings in the brain. *Radiographics* 1990; **10**: 201–15.

Ballesteros MC, Hansen PE, Soila K. MR imaging of the developing human brain. Part 2. Postnatal development. *Radiographics* 1993; **13**: 611–22.

Barwick TD, Rockall AG, Barton DP, Sohaib SA. Imaging of endometrial adenocarcinoma. *Clin Radiol* 2006; **61**: 545–55.

Berger JD, Witte RJ, Holdeman KP, et al. Neuroradiologic applications of central nervous system SPECT. *Radiographics* 1996; **16**: 777–85.

Berrocal T, López-Pereira P, Arjonilla A, Gutiérrez J. Anomalies of the distal ureter, bladder, and urethra in children: embryologic, radiologic, and pathologic features. *Radiographics* 2002; **22**: 1139–64.

Blum AG, Zabel JP, Kohlmann R, et al. Pathologic conditions of the hypothenar eminence: evaluation with multidetector CT and MR imaging. *Radiographics* 2006; **26**: 1021–44.

Boles CA, El-Khoury GY. Slipped capital femoral epiphysis. *Radiographics* 1997; **17**: 809–23.

Boström A, Weinzierl M, Spangenberg P, et al. Radiographic and clinical features in Morquio's syndrome. *Clin Neuroradiol* 2006; **16**: 249–53.

Boudiaf M, Soyer P, Pelage JP, et al. CT of radiation-induced injury of the gastrointestinal tract: spectrum of findings with barium studies correlation. *Eur Radiol* 2000; **10**: 920–5.

Brant WE, Helms CA, eds. *Fundamentals of Diagnostic Radiology*, 3rd edn. Philadelphia: Lippincott Williams & Wilkins, 2007.

Burrill J, Williams CJ, Bain G, et al. Tuberculosis: a radiological review. *Radiographics* 2007; **27**: 1255–73.

Butler P, Mitchell A, Ellis H, eds. *Applied Radiological Anatomy*. Cambridge: Cambridge University Press, 1999.

Butteriss DJA, Mahad D, Soh C, et al. Reversible cytotoxic cerebral edema in cerebral fat embolism. *AJNR Am J Neuroradiol* 2006; **27**: 620–3.

Caoili EM, Korobkin M, Francis IR, et al. Adrenal masses: characterization with combined unenhanced and delayed enhanced CT. *Radiology* 2002; **222**: 629–33.

Carty H. Non-accidental injury: a review of the radiology. *Eur Radiol* 1997; **7**: 1365–76.

Castillo M. *Neuroradiology Companion: Methods, guidelines and imaging fundamentals*, 3rd edn. Philadelphia: Lippincott Williams & Wilkins, 2006.

Catterall A. The natural history of Perthes' disease. *J Bone Joint Surg Br* 1971; **53**: 37–53.

Cerezal L, del Piñal F, Abascal F, et al. Imaging findings in ulnar-sided wrist impaction syndromes. *Radiographics* 2002; **22**: 105–21.

Cha S. Update on brain tumor imaging: from anatomy to physiology. *AJNR Am J Neuroradiol* 2006; **27**: 475–87.

Chao CP, Kotsenas AL, Broderick DF. Cerebral amyloid angiopathy: CT and MR imaging findings. *Radiographics* 2006; **26**: 1517–31.

Chapman S, Nakielny R, eds. *A Guide to Radiological Procedures*, 4th edn. London: WB Saunders, 2001.

Chapman S, Nakielny R, eds. *Aids to Radiological Differential Diagnosis*, 4th edn. London: WB Saunders, 2003.

Cheema JI, Grissom LE, Harcke HT. Radiographic characteristics of lower-extremity bowing in children. *Radiographics* 2003; **23**: 871–80.

Chen L, Chantra PK, Larsen LH, et al. Imaging characteristics of malignant lesions of the male breast. *Radiographics* 2006; **26**: 993–1006.

Cheon JE, Kim IO, Hwang YS, et al. Leukodystrophy in children: a pictorial review of MR imaging features. *Radiographics* 2002; **22**: 461–76.

Choi YJ, Kim JK, Kim N, et al. Functional MR imaging of prostate cancer. *Radiographics* 2007; **27**: 63–75.

Chu WCW, Lee V, Howard RG, et al. Imaging findings of paediatric oncology patients presenting with acute neurological symptoms. *Clin Radiol* 2003; **58**: 589–603.

Chun KA, Ha KH, Yu ES, et al. Xanthogranulomatous cholecystitis: CT features with emphasis on differentiation from gallbladder carcinoma. *Radiology* 1997; **203**: 93–7.

Collie DA, Summers DM, Sellar RJ, et al. Diagnosing variant Creutzfeldt–Jakob disease with the pulvinar sign: MR imaging findings in 86 neuropathologically confirmed cases. *AJNR Am J Neuroradiol* 2003; **24**: 1560–9.

Connor SEJ, Flis C, Langdon JD. Vascular masses of the head and neck. *Clin Radiol* 2005; **60**: 856–68.

Creasy JD, Chiles C, Routh WD, et al. Overview of traumatic injury of the thoracic aorta. *Radiographics* 1997; **17**: 27–45.

Cuénod CA, Laredo JD, Chevret S, et al. Acute vertebral collapse due to osteoporosis or malignancy: appearance on unenhanced and gadolinium-enhanced MR images. *Radiology* 1996; **199**: 541–9.

Dähnert W. *Radiology Review Manual*, 6th edn. Philadelphia: Lippincott Williams & Wilkins, 2007.

Davies H, Unwin A, Aichroth P. The posterolateral corner of the knee. Anatomy, biomechanics and management of injuries. *Injury* 2004; **35**: 68–75.

De Lacey G, Morley S, Berman L. *The Chest X-Ray. A survival guide*. Philadelphia: Saunders, 2007.

De Smet AA, Ilahi OA, Graf BK. Reassessment of the MR criteria for stability of osteochondritis dissecans in the knee and ankle. *Skeletal Radiol* 1996; **25**: 159–63.

DeGroot III H. Bizarre parosteal osteochondromatous proliferation (Nora's lesion), 2001. www.bonetumor.org/tumors/pages/page178.

Denis F. The three column spine and its significance in the classification of acute thoracolumbar spinal injuries. *Spine* 1983; **8**: 817–31.

Desai SR. Acute respiratory distress syndrome: imaging of the injured lung. *Clin Radiol* 2002; **57**: 8–17.

Dhillon R, Depree P, Metcalf C, et al. Screen-detected mucinous breast carcinoma: potential for delayed diagnosis. *Clin Radiol* 2006; **61**: 423–30.

Diel J, Ortiz O, Losada RA, et al. The sacrum: pathologic spectrum, multimodality imaging, and subspecialty approach. *Radiographics* 2001; **21**: 83–104.

Dineen R, Banks A, Lenthall R. Imaging of acute neurological conditions in pregnancy and the puerperium. *Clin Radiol* 2005; **60**: 1156–70.

Doyle DJ, Hanbidge AE, O'Malley ME. Imaging of hepatic infections. *Clin Radiol* 2006; **61**: 737–48.

Drayer BP. Imaging of the aging brain. Part I. Normal findings. *Radiology* 1988a; **166**: 785–96.

Drayer BP. Imaging of the aging brain. Part II. Pathologic conditions. *Radiology* 1988b; **166**: 797–806.

Duncan KA. Antenatal renal pelvic dilatation; the long-term outlook. *Clin Radiol* 2007; **62**: 134–9.

Dyde R, Chapman AH, Gale R, et al. Precautions to be taken by radiologists and radiographers when prescribing hyoscine-N-butylbromide. *Clin Radiol* 2008; **63**: 739–43.

Eich GF, Babyn P, Giedion A. Pediatric pelvis: radiographic appearance in various congenital disorders. *Radiographics* 1992; **12**: 467–84.

Eisenberg RL. *Clinical Imaging: An atlas of differential diagnosis*, 4th edn. Philadelphia: Lippincott Williams & Wilkins, 2003.

Ejindu VC, Hine AL, Mashayekhi M, et al. Musculoskeletal manifestations of sickle cell disease. *Radiographics* 2007; **27**: 1005–21.

Ell PJ, Gambhir SS. *Nuclear Medicine in Clinical Diagnosis and Treatment*, 3rd edn. Oxford: Churchill Livingstone, 2004.

Euathrongchit J, Thoongsuwan N, Stern EJ. Nonvascular mediastinal trauma. *Radiol Clin North Am* 2006; **44**: 251–8.

Fabian TC. Unravelling the fat embolism syndrome. *N Engl J Med* 1993; **329**: 961–3.

Failinger MS, McGanity PL. Unstable fractures of the pelvic ring. *J Bone Joint Surg Am* 1992; **74**: 781–91.

Fatterpekar GM, Doshi AH, Dugar M, et al. Role of 3D CT in the evaluation of the temporal bone. *Radiographics* 2006; **26**: S117–32.

Ferguson EC, Krishnamurthy R, Oldham SAA. Classic imaging signs of congenital cardiovascular abnormalities. *Radiographics* 2007; **27**: 1323–34.

Ganeshan A, Anderson EM, Upponi S, et al. Imaging of obstructed defecation. *Clin Radiol* 2008; **63**: 18–26.

Gandhi SN, Brown MA, Wong JG, et al. MR contrast agents for liver imaging: what, when, how? *Radiographics* 2006; **26**: 1621–36.

Ge Y. Multiple sclerosis: the role of MR imaging. *AJNR Am J Neuroradiol* 2006; **27**: 1165–76.

Gentry LR. Imaging of closed head injury. *Radiology* 1994; **191**: 1–17.

Glass RBJ, Norton KI, Mitre SA, Kang E. Pediatric ribs: a spectrum of abnormalities. *Radiographics* 2002; **22**: 87–104.

Glass RBJ, Fernbach SK, Norton KI, et al. The infant skull: a vault of information. *Radiographics* 2004; **24**: 507–22.

Goldfarb CA, Yin Y, Gilula LA, et al. Wrist fractures: what the clinician wants to know. *Radiology* 2001; **219**: 11–28

Goswami GK. Signs in imaging. The fat pad sign. *Radiology* 2002; **222**: 419–20.

Greenfield GB, Warren DL, Clark RA. MR imaging of periosteal and cortical changes of bone. *Radiographics* 1991; **11**: 611–23.

Grossman RI, Yousem DM. *Neuroradiology: The requisites*, 2nd edn. Philadelphia: Mosby, 2003.

Haller J, Resnick D, Miller CW, et al. Diffuse idiopathic skeletal hyperostosis: diagnostic significance of radiographic abnormalities of the pelvis. *Radiology* 1989; **172**: 835–9.

Halpert RD. *Gastrointestinal Imaging: The requisites*, 3rd edn. Philadelphia: Mosby, 2006.

Hamer OW, Aguirre DA, Casola G, et al. Fatty liver: imaging patterns and pitfalls. *Radiographics* 2006; **26**: 1637–53.

Hansen MW, Merchant N. MRI of hypertrophic cardiomyopathy: part I, MRI appearances. *AJR Am J Roentgenol* 2007; **189**: 1335–43.

Harms SE, Wilk RM. Magnetic resonance imaging of the temporomandibular joint. *Radiographics* 1987; **7**: 521–42.

Hartman TE. Radiologic evaluation of the solitary pulmonary nodule. *Radiol Clin North Am* 2005; **43**: 459–65.

Hayes CW, Conway WF, Daniel WW. MR imaging of bone marrow edema pattern: transient osteoporosis, transient bone marrow edema syndrome, or osteonecrosis. *Radiographics* 1993; **13**: 1001–11.

Helms CA. *Fundamentals of Skeletal Radiology*, 3rd edn. Philadelphia: Saunders, 2005.

Hemker M. Radiographic Skull Series, 1999. www.bethesda.med.navy. mil/careers/postgraduate_dental_school/comprehensive_dentistry/ Pearls/pearlsc3.htm.

Herlinger H, Maglinte DDT, Birnbaum BA. *Clinical Imaging of the Small Intestine*, 2nd edn. New York: Springer-Verlag, 1999.

Hermann KA, Althoff CE, Schneider U, et al. Spinal changes in patients with spondyloarthritis: comparison of MR imaging and radiographic appearances. *Radiographics* 2005; **25**: 559–69.

Hoeffner EG, Case I, Jain R, et al. Cerebral perfusion CT: technique and clinical applications. *Radiology* 2004; **231**: 632–44.

Hogan MJ. Neonatal vascular catheters and their complications. *Radiol Clin North Am* 1999; **37**: 1109–25.

Honkaniemi J, Dastidar P, Kähärä V, Haapasalo H. Delayed MR imaging changes in acute disseminated encephalomyelitis. *AJNR Am J Neuroradiol* 2001; **22**: 1117–24.

Hopper KD, Sherman JL, Boal DK, et al. CT and MR imaging of the pediatric orbit. *Radiographics* 1992; **12**: 485–503.

Hopper RA, Salemy S, Sze RW. Diagnosis of midface fractures with CT: what the surgeon needs to know. *Radiographics* 2006; **26**: 783–93.

Hosoya T, Yamaguchi K, Adachi M, et al. Dilatation of the temporal horn in subarachnoid haemorrhage. *Neuroradiology* 1992; **34**: 207–9.

Hricak H, Husband J, Panicek DM, eds. *Oncologic Imaging: Essentials of reporting common cancers*. Philadelphia: Saunders, 2007.

Hueftle MG, Modic MT, Ross JS, et al. Lumbar spine: postoperative MR imaging with Gd-DTPA. *Radiology* 1988; **167**: 817–24.

Hulse PA, Carrington BM. *MRI Manual of Pelvic Cancer*. London: Martin Dunitz, 2004.

Hunter TB, Peltier LF, Lund PJ. Radiologic history exhibit. Musculoskeletal eponyms: who are those guys? *Radiographics* 2000; **20**: 819–36.

Hwang S, Panicek DM. Magnetic resonance imaging of bone marrow in oncology, Part 1. *Skeletal Radiol* 2007; **36**: 913–20.

Jacobs P. Post-traumatic osteolysis of the outer end of the clavicle. *J Bone Joint Surg Br* 1964; **46**: 705–7.

Jeudy J, Waite S, White CS. Nontraumatic thoracic emergencies. *Radiol Clin North Am* 2006; **44**: 273–93.

Khong PL, Cheung SCW, Leong LLY, Ooi CGC. Ultrasonography of intra-abdominal cystic lesions in the newborn. *Clin Radiol* 2003; **58**: 449–54.

Khong PL, Lam BCC, Tung HKS, et al. MRI of neonatal encephalopathy. *Clin Radiol* 2003; **58**: 833–44.

Kier EL, Staib LH, Davis LM, Bronen RA. MR imaging of the temporal stem: anatomic dissection tractography of the uncinate fasciculus, inferior occipitofrontal fasciculus, and Meyer's loop of the optic radiation. *AJNR Am J Neuroradiol* 2004; **25**: 677–91.

Kier R, McCarthy S, Dietz MJ, et al. MR appearance of painful conditions of the ankle. *Radiographics* 1991; **11**: 401–14.

Kilborn TN, Teh J, Goodman TR. Paediatric manifestations of Langerhans cell histiocytosis: a review of the clinical and radiological findings. *Clin Radiol* 2003; **58**: 269–78.

Killeen KL. The fallen fragment sign. *Radiology* 1998; **207**: 261–2.

Kim MJ, Kim EK, Park SI, et al. US-guided fine-needle aspiration of thyroid nodules: indications, techniques, results. *Radiographics* 2008; **28**: 1869–86.

Kim JS, Kim HH, Yoon Y. Imaging of pericardial diseases. *Clin Radiol* 2007a; **62**: 626–31.

Kim YK, Lee KS, Chung MP, et al. Pulmonary involvement in Churg–Strauss syndrome: an analysis of CT, clinical and pathologic findings. *Eur Radiol* 2007b; **17**: 3157–65.

King J, Diefendorf D, Apthorp J, et al. Analysis of 429 fractures in 189 battered children. *J Pediatr Orthop* 1988; **8**: 585–9.

Kirsch MD, Fitzgerald SW, Friedman H. Transient lateral patellar dislocation: diagnosis with MR imaging. *AJR Am J Roentgenol* 1993; **161**: 109–13.

Kluetz PG, White CS. Acute pulmonary embolism: imaging in the emergency department. *Radiol Clin North Am* 2006; **44**: 259–71.

Kock MC, Dijkshoorn ML, Pattynama PM, et al. Multi-detector row computed tomography angiography of peripheral arterial disease. *Eur Radiol* 2007; **17**: 3208–22.

Koyama T, Ueda H, Togashi K, et al. Radiologic manifestations of sarcoidosis in various organs. *Radiographics* 2004; **24**: 87–104.

Kraft JK, Hughes T. Polypoid endometriosis and other benign gynaecological complications associated with tamoxifen therapy – a case to illustrate features on magnetic resonance imaging. *Clin Radiol* 2006; **61**: 198–201.

Kransdorf MJ, Murphey MD. Diagnosis please. Case 12: Mazabraud syndrome. *Radiology* 1999; **212**: 129–32.

Kransdorf MJ, Stull MA, Gilkey FW, et al. From the archives of the AFIP. Osteoid osteoma. *Radiographics* 1991; **11**: 671–96.

Kulkarni K, Abraham S, McNeish I. Understanding tumour markers. *Student BMJ* 2008; **1**: 35–7.

Lan XL, Zhang YX, Wu ZJ, et al. The value of dual time point (18)F-FDG PET imaging for the differentiation between malignant and benign lesions. *Clin Radiol* 2008; **63**: 756–64.

Laredo JD, El Quessar A, Bossard P, Vuillemin-Bodaghi V. Vertebral tumors and pseudotumors. *Radiol Clin North Am* 2001; **39**: 137–63.

Lee DH, Gao FQ, Rogers JM, et al. MR in temporal lobe epilepsy: analysis with pathologic confirmation. *AJNR Am J Neuroradiol* 1998; **19**: 19–27.

Lee TC, Bartlett ES, Fox AJ, Symons SP. The hypodense artery sign. *AJNR Am J Neuroradiol* 2005; **26**: 2027–9.

Lektrakul N, Chung CB, Lai Y, et al. Tarsal sinus: arthrographic, MR imaging, MR arthrographic, and pathologic findings in cadavers and retrospective study data in patients with sinus tarsi syndrome. *Radiology* 2001; **219**: 802–10.

Lenton J, Kessel D, Watkinson AF. Embolization of renal angiomyolipoma: immediate complications and long-term outcomes. *Clin Radiol* 2008; **63**: 864–70.

Levy AD, Remotti HE, Thompson WM, et al. From the archives of the AFIP. Gastrointestinal stromal tumors: radiologic features with pathologic correlation. *Radiographics* 2003; **23**: 283–304.

Lewis S, Patel U. Major complications after percutaneous nephrostomy – lessons from a departmental audit. *Clin Radiol* 2004; **59**: 171–9.

Lim JH, Lee G, Oh YL. Radiologic spectrum of intraductal papillary mucinous tumor of the pancreas. *Radiographics* 2001; **21**: 323–40.

Lindell RM, Hartman TE. Chest imaging in iatrogenic respiratory disease. *Clin Chest Med* 2004; **25**: 15–24.

Llauger J, Palmer J, Monill JM, et al. MR imaging of benign soft-tissue masses of the foot and ankle. *Radiographics* 1998; **18**: 1481–98.

Lockhat F, Corr P, Ramphal S, Moodley J. The value of magnetic resonance imaging in the diagnosis and management of extra-uterine abdominal pregnancy. *Clin Radiol* 2006; **61**: 264–9.

Lonergan GJ, Baker AM, Morey MK, Boos SC. From the archives of the AFIP. Child abuse: radiologic-pathologic correlation. *Radiographics* 2003; **23**: 811–45.

Love C, Din AS, Tomas MB, et al. Radionuclide bone imaging: an illustrative review. *Radiographics* 2003; **23**: 341–58.

Lubner M, Menias C, Rucker C, et al. Blood in the belly: CT findings of hemoperitoneum. *Radiographics* 2007; **27**: 109–25.

Lui KW, Gervais DA, Arellano RA, et al. Radiofrequency ablation of renal cell carcinoma. *Clin Radiol* 2003; **58**: 905–13.

Lustrin ES, Karakas SP, Ortiz AO, et al. Pediatric cervical spine: normal anatomy, variants and trauma. *Radiographics* 2003; **23**: 539–60.

Mackintosh M, Tucker S. The mechanisms of spinal injury. *Curr Anaesth Crit Care* 2002; **13**: 97–102.

Madani G, Katz RD, Haddock JA, et al. The role of radiology in the management of systemic sclerosis. *Clin Radiol* 2008; **63**: 959–67.

Manaster BJ. From the RSNA refresher courses. Total hip arthroplasty: radiographic evaluation. *Radiographics* 1996; **16**: 645–60.

Manaster BJ. From the RSNA refresher courses. Adult chronic hip pain: radiographic evaluation. *Radiographics* 2000; **20**: S3–25.

Manaster BJ, Disler DG, May DA. *Musculoskeletal Imaging: The requisites*, 3rd edn. Philadelphia: Mosby, 2006.

Maravilla KR, Cohen WA. *Magnetic Resonance Imaging Atlas of the Spine*. London: Informa Healthcare, 1991.

Marchiori E, Souza AS Jr, Franquet T, Müller NL. Diffuse high-attenuation pulmonary abnormalities: a pattern-oriented diagnostic approach on high-resolution CT. *AJR Am J Roentgenol* 2005; **184**: 273–82.

Martinez CR, Di Pasquale TG, Helfet DL, et al. Evaluation of acetabular fractures with two- and three-dimensional CT. *Radiographics* 1992; **12**: 227–42.

Mascalchi M, Salvi F, Piacentini S, Bartolozzi C. Friedreich's ataxia: MR findings involving the cervical portion of the spinal cord. *AJR Am J Roentgenol* 1994; **163**: 187–91.

Mayo-Smith WW, Boland GW, Noto RB, et al. State-of-the-art adrenal imaging. *Radiographics* 2001; **21**: 995–1012.

McAuley G, Delaney H, Colville J, et al. Multimodality preoperative imaging of pancreatic insulinomas. *Clin Radiol* 2005; **60**: 1039–50.

McCarty DJ. Milwaukee shoulder syndrome. *Trans Am Clin Climatol Assoc* 1991; **102**: 271–83.

Mengiardi B, Pfirrmann CWA, Gerber C, et al. Frozen shoulder: MR arthrographic findings. *Radiology* 2004; **233**: 486–92.

Mesgarzadeh M, Moyer R, Leder DS, et al. MR imaging of the knee: expanded classification and pitfalls to interpretation of meniscal tears. *Radiographics* 1993; **13**: 489–500.

Middleton WD, Kurtz AB, Hertzberg BS. *Ultrasound: The requisites*, 2nd edn. St. Louis, MO: Mosby, 2004.

Miller LA. Chest wall, lung and pleural space trauma. *Radiol Clin North Am* 2006; **44**: 213–24.

Mito K, Maruyama R, Uenishi Y, et al. Hypertrophic pulmonary osteoarthropathy associated with non-small cell lung cancer demonstrated growth hormone-releasing hormone by immunohistochemical analysis. *Intern Med* 2001; **40**: 532–5.

Modic MT, Ross JS. Lumbar degenerative disk disease. *Radiology* 2007; **245**: 43–61.

Moon WK, Han MH, Chang KH, et al. CT and MR imaging of head and neck tuberculosis. *Radiographics* 1997; **17**: 391–402.

Moulopoulos LA, Dimopoulos MA, Alexanian R, et al. Multiple myeloma: MR patterns of response to treatment. *Radiology* 1994; **193**: 441–6.

Murphey MD, Choi JJ, Kransdorf MJ, et al. From the archives of the AFIP. Imaging of osteochondroma: variants and complications with radiologic-pathologic correlation. *Radiographics* 2000; **20**: 1407–34.

Murphey MD, Flemming DJ, Boyea SR, et al. From the archives of the AFIP. Enchondroma versus chondrosarcoma in the appendicular skeleton: differentiating features. *Radiographics* 1998; **18**: 1213–37.

NICE. *Percutaneous Vertebroplasty (Interventional Procedure Guidance 12)*. London: National Institute for Health and Clinical Excellence, 2003.

Nosher JL, Chung J, Brenetti LS, et al. Visceral and renal artery aneurysms: a pictorial essay on endovascular therapy. *Radiographics* 2006; **26**: 1687–704.

Numaguchi Y, Rigamonti D, Rothman MI, et al. Spinal epidural abscess: evaluation with gadolinium-enhanced MR imaging. *Radiographics* 1993; **13**: 545–59.

O'Donnell P, Buxton PJ, Pitkin A, Jarvis LJ. The magnetic resonance imaging appearances of the brain in acute carbon monoxide poisoning. *Clin Radiol* 2000; **55**: 273–80.

O'Donoghue DH. The unhappy triad: etiology, diagnosis and treatment. *Am J Orthop* 1964; **6**: 242–7.

Osborn GD, Beer H, Wade R, et al. Two-view mammography at the incident round has improved the rate of screen-detected breast cancer in Wales. *Clin Radiol* 2006; **61**: 478–82.

Outwater EK, Siegelman ES, Hunt JL. Ovarian teratomas: tumor types and imaging characteristics. *Radiographics* 2001; **21**: 475–90.

Pannier S, Legeai-Mallet L. Hereditary multiple exostoses and enchondromatosis. *Best Pract Res Clin Rheumatol* 2008; **22**: 45–54.

Pantongrag-Brown L, Nelson AM, Brown AE, et al. Gastrointestinal manifestations of acquired immunodeficiency syndrome: radiologic-pathologic correlation. *Radiographics* 1995; **15**: 1155–78.

Park Y, Kim TS, Yi CA, et al. Pulmonary cavitary mass containing a mural nodule: differential diagnosis between intracavitary aspergilloma and cavitating lung cancer on contrast-enhanced computed tomography. *Clin Radiol* 2007; **62**: 227–32.

Petrella JR, Coleman RE, Doraiswamy PM. Neuroimaging and early diagnosis of Alzheimer disease: a look to the future. *Radiology* 2003; **226**: 315–36.

Pfirrmann CW, Mengiardi B, Dora C, et al. Cam and pincer femoroacetabular impingement: characteristic MR arthrographic findings in 50 patients. *Radiology* 2006; **240**: 778–85.

Pikus L, Woo JH, Wolf RL, et al. Artificial multiple sclerosis lesions on simulated FLAIR brain MR images: echo time and observer performance in detection. *Radiology* 2006; **239**: 238–45.

Pipavath S, Godwin JD. Imaging of interstitial disease. *Radiol Clin North Am* 2005; **43**: 589–99.

Planner AC, Anderson EM, Slater A, et al. An evidence-based review for the management of cystic pancreatic lesions. *Clin Radiol* 2007; **62**: 930–7.

Plas E, Daha K, Riedl CR, et al. Long-term followup after laparoscopic nephropexy for symptomatic nephroptosis. *J Urol* 2001; **166**: 449–52.

Porter GJ, Evans AJ, Lee AH, et al. Unusual benign breast lesions. *Clin Radiol* 2006; **61**: 562–9.

Quiroga S, Sebastià MC, Margarit C, et al. Complications of orthotopic liver transplantation: spectrum of findings with helical CT. *Radiographics* 2001; **21**: 1085–1102.

Raby N, Bergman L, de Lacey G. *Accident and Emergency Radiology: A survival guide*, 2nd edn. Philadelphia: Saunders, 2005.

Ramachandran I, Sinha R, Rodgers P. Pseudomembranous colitis revisited: spectrum of imaging findings. *Clin Radiol* 2006; **61**: 535–44.

Ramos-Remus C, Gomez-Vargas A, LeClercq S, Russell AS. Radiologic features of DISH may mimic ankylosing spondylitis. *Clin Exp Rheumatol* 1993; **11**: 603–8.

Reddy D, Salomon C, Demos TC, Cosar E. Mesenteric lymph node cavitation in celiac disease. *AJR Am J Roentgenol* 2002; **178**: 247.

Redla S, Sikdar T, Saifuddin A. Magnetic resonance imaging of scoliosis. *Clin Radiol* 2001; **56**: 360–71.

Remer EM, Fitzgerald SW, Friedman H, et al. Anterior cruciate ligament injury: MR imaging diagnosis and patterns of injury. *Radiographics* 1992; **12**: 901–15.

Resnick DL, Kransdorf MJ. *Bone and Joint Imaging*, 3rd edn. Philadelphia: Saunders, 2005.

Restrepo CS, Martinez S, Lemos JA, et al. Manifestations of Kaposi sarcoma. *Radiographics* 2006; **26**: 1169–85.

Richardson JD, McElvein RB, Trinkle JK. First rib fracture: a hallmark of severe trauma. *Ann Surg* 1975; **181**: 251–4.

Rimon U, Duvdevani M, Garniek A, et al. Large renal angiomyolipomas: digital subtraction angiographic grading and presentation with bleeding. *Clin Radiol* 2006; **61**: 520–6.

Rodallec MH, Feydy A, Larousserie F, et al. Diagnostic imaging of solitary tumors of the spine: what to do and say. *Radiographics* 2008; **28**: 1019–41.

Rodríguez-Merchán CE. Pediatric skeletal trauma: a review and historical perspective. *Clin Orthop Relat Res* 2005; **432**: 8–13.

Royal College of Obstetricians and Gynaecologists. *Ovarian Cysts in Postmenopausal Women*. RCOG Green Top Guideline no. 34. London: RCOG, 2003.

Royal College of Radiologists. *Recommendations for Cross-Sectional Imaging in Cancer Management*, Issue 2. London: Royal College of Radiologists, 2006.

Royal College of Radiologists. *Making the Best Use of Clinical Radiology Services: Referral Guidelines (MBUR6)*, 6th edn. London: Royal College of Radiologists, 2007.

Roy-Choudhury SH, Nelson WM, El Cast J, et al. Technical aspects and complications of laparoscopic banding for morbid obesity – a radiological perspective. *Clin Radiol* 2004; **59**: 227–36.

Russell RCG, Williams NS, Bulstrode CJK, eds. *Bailey and Love's Short Practice of Surgery*, 24th edn. London: Arnold, 2004.

Rutherford GC, Dineen RA, O'Connor A. Imaging in the investigation of paraneoplastic syndromes. *Clin Radiol* 2007; **62**: 1021–35.

Rutten MJCM, Jager GJ, Blickman JG. From the RSNA refresher courses. US of the rotator cuff: pitfalls, limitations, and artifacts. *Radiographics* 2006; **26**: 589–604.

Sakamoto I, Sueyoshi E, Uetani M. MR imaging of the aorta. *Radiol Clin North Am* 2007; **45**: 485–97.

Salter RB, Harris WR. Injuries involving the epiphyseal plate. *J Bone Joint Surg Am* 1963; **45**: 587–622.

Scarsbrook AF, Moore NR. MRI appearances of Müllerian duct abnormalities. *Clin Radiol* 2003; **58**: 747–54.

Schaefer PW, Grant PE, Gonzalez RG. Diffusion-weighted MR imaging of the brain. *Radiology* 2000; **217**: 331–45.

Schievink WI, Maya MM, Louy C, et al. Diagnostic criteria for spontaneous spinal CSF leaks and intracranial hypotension. *AJNR Am J Neuroradiol* 2008; **29**: 853–6.

Scholl RJ, Kellett HM, Neumann DP, Lurie AG. Cysts and cystic lesions of the mandible: clinical and radiologic-histopathologic review. *Radiographics* 1999; **19**: 1107–24.

Schwartz DS, Reyes-Mugica M, Keller MS. Imaging of surgical diseases of the newborn chest. Intrapleural mass lesions. *Radiol Clin North Am* 1999; **37**: 1067–78.

Semelka RC, Helmberger TKG. Contrast agents for MR imaging of the liver. *Radiology* 2001; **218**: 27–38.

Sheldon PJ, Forrester DM, Learch TJ. Imaging of intraarticular masses. *Radiographics* 2005; **25**: 105–19.

Siegel MJ. *MRI of Bone Marrow*. Leesburg, VA: American Roentgen Ray Society, 2008.

Singh AK, Gervais DA, Hahn PF, et al. Acute epiploic appendagitis and its mimics. *Radiographics* 2005a; **25**: 1521–34.

Singh AK, Saokar A, Hahn PF, et al. Imaging of penile neoplasms. *Radiographics* 2005b; **25**: 1629–38.

Sinha R, Verma R. Multidetector row computed tomography in bowel obstruction. Part 1: small bowel obstruction. *Clin Radiol* 2005; **60**: 1058–67.

Sivit CJ, Taylor GA, Bulas DI, et al. Posttraumatic shock in children: CT findings associated with hemodynamic instability. *Radiology* 1992; **182**: 723–6.

Slone RM, MacMillan M, Montgomery WJ. Spinal fixation. Part 1. Principles, basic hardware, and fixation techniques for the cervical spine. *Radiographics* 1993; **13**: 341–56.

Smirniotopoulos JG, Chiechi MV. From the archives of the AFIP. Teratomas, dermoids, and epidermoids of the head and neck. *Radiographics* 1995; **15**: 1437–55.

Smith JR, Oates ME. Radionuclide imaging of the parathyroid glands: patterns, pearls, and pitfalls. *Radiographics* 2004; **24**: 1101–15.

Smith SL, Hampson F, Duxbury M, et al. Computed tomography after radical pancreaticoduodenectomy (Whipple's procedure). *Clin Radiol* 2008; **63**: 921–8.

Smoker WRK, Gentry LR, Yee NK, et al. Vascular lesions of the orbit: more than meets the eye. *Radiographics* 2008; **28**: 185–204.

Srinivasan A, Goyal M, Al Azri F, Lum C. State-of-the-art imaging of acute stroke. *Radiographics* 2006; **26**: S75–95.

Stavropoulos SW, Charagundla SR. Imaging techniques for detection and management of endoleaks after endovascular aortic aneurysm repair. *Radiology* 2007; **243**: 641–55.

Steinbach LS, Palmer WE, Schweitzer ME. Special focus session. MR arthrography. *Radiographics* 2002; **22**: 1223–46.

Strouse PJ, Close BJ, Marshall KW, Cywes R. CT of bowel and mesenteric trauma in children. *Radiographics* 1999; **19**: 1237–50.

Subhas N, Patel PV, Pannu HK, et al. Imaging of pelvic malignancies with in-line FDG PET-CT: case examples and common pitfalls of FDG PET. *Radiographics* 2005; **25**: 1031–43.

Suei Y, Taguchi A, Tanimoto K. Diagnostic points and possible origin of osteomyelitis in synovitis, acne, pustulosis, hyperostosis and osteitis (SAPHO) syndrome: a radiographic study of 77 mandibular osteomyelitis cases. *Rheumatology (Oxford)* 2003; **42**: 1398–1403.

Sutton D, ed. *Textbook of Radiology and Imaging*, 7th edn. London: Churchill Livingstone, 2002.

Suzuki S, Furui S, Okinaga K, et al. Differentiation of femoral versus inguinal hernia: CT findings. *AJR Am J Roentgenol* 2007; **189**: W78–83.

Tehranzadeh J. The spectrum of avulsion and avulsion-like injuries of the musculoskeletal system. *Radiographics* 1987; **7**: 945–74.

Tehranzadeh J, Andrews C, Wong E. Lumbar spine imaging. Normal variants, imaging pitfalls, and artifacts. *Radiol Clin North Am* 2000; **38**: 1207–53.

Tehranzadeh J, Fung Y, Donohue M, et al. Computed tomography of Paget disease of the skull versus fibrous dysplasia. *Skeletal Radiol* 1998; **27**: 664–72.

Therasse P, Arbuck S, Eisenhauer EA, et al. New guidelines to evaluate the response to treatment in solid tumors. *J Natl Cancer Inst* 2000; **92**: 205–16.

Thompson EO, Smoker WRK. Hypoglossal nerve palsy: a segmental approach. *Radiographics* 1994; **14**: 939–58.

Tipper G, U-King-Im JM, Price SJ, et al. Detection and evaluation of intracranial aneurysms with 16-row multislice CT angiography. *Clin Radiol* 2005; **60**: 565–72.

Tirman PF, Feller JF, Palmer WE, et al. The Buford complex – a variation of normal shoulder anatomy: MR arthrographic imaging features. *AJR Am J Roentgenol* 1996; **166**: 869–73.

Tomas X, Pomes J, Berenguer J, et al. MR imaging of temporomandibular joint dysfunction: a pictorial review. *Radiographics* 2006; **26**: 765–81.

Ueno T, Tanaka YO, Nagata M, et al. Spectrum of germ cell tumors: from head to toe. *Radiographics* 2004; **24**: 387–404.

Upreti L, Dev A, Kumar Puri S. Imaging in renal lymphangiectasia: report of two cases and review of literature. *Clin Radiol* 2008; **63**: 1057–62.

Vandersluis R, O'Connor HM. The seat-belt syndrome. *Can Med Assoc J* 1987; **137**: 1023–4.

Vignaux O. Cardiac sarcoidosis: spectrum of MRI features. *AJR Am J Roentgenol* 2005; **184**: 249–54.

Visser CPJ, Coene LN, Brand R, et al. The incidence of nerve injury in anterior dislocation of the shoulder and its influence on functional recovery. A prospective clinical and EMG study. *J Bone Joint Surg Br* 1999; **81**: 679–85.

Warshauer DM, Lee JKT. Imaging manifestations of abdominal sarcoidosis. *AJR Am J Roentgenol* 2004; **182**: 15–28.

Watkinson A, Nicholson A. Uterine artery embolization to treat symptomatic uterine fibroids. *BMJ* 2007; **335**: 720–2.

Weber TM, Lockhart ME, Robbin ML. Upper extremity venous Doppler ultrasound. *Radiol Clin North Am* 2007; **45**: 513–24.

Weissleder R, Wittenberg J, Harisinghani MG, Chen JW. *Primer of Diagnostic Imaging*, 4th edn. Philadelphia: Mosby, 2007.

Werner JA, Dünne AA, Myers JN. Functional anatomy of the lymphatic drainage system of the upper aerodigestive tract and its role in metastasis of squamous cell carcinoma. *Head Neck* 2003; **25**: 322–32.

Wheeless III CR. Incomplete spinal cord lesion. *Wheeless' Textbook of Orthopaedics*, 1996. www.wheelessonline.com/ortho/incomplete_spinal_cord_lesion.

Willatt JMG, Quaghebeur G. Calvarial masses of infants and children. A radiological approach. *Clin Radiol* 2004; **59**: 474–86.

Williams HJ, Davies AM, Chapman S. Bone within a bone. *Clin Radiol* 2004; **59**: 132–44.

Win T, Tasker AD, Groves AM, et al. Ventilation-perfusion scintigraphy to predict postoperative pulmonary function in lung cancer patients undergoing pneumonectomy. *AJR Am J Roentgenol* 2006; **187**: 1260–5.

Wittenberg A. The rugger jersey spine sign. *Radiology* 2004; **230**: 491–2.

Wojtowycz AR, Spirt BA, Kaplan DS, Roy AK. Endoscopic US of the gastrointestinal tract with endoscopic, radiographic and pathologic correlation. *Radiographics* 1995; **15**: 735–53.

Yim CD, Sane SS, Bjarnason H. Superior vena cava stenting. *Radiol Clin North Am* 2000; **38**: 409–24.

Zagoria RJ. *Genitourinary Radiology: The requisites*, 2nd edn. Philadelphia: Mosby, 2004.

Zeissman HA, O'Malley JP, Thrall JH. *Nuclear Medicine: The requisites*, 3rd edn. Philadelphia: Mosby, 2006.